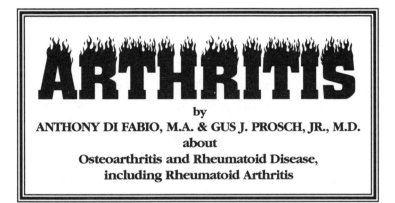

ARTHRITIS

by
ANTHONY DI FABIO, M.A. & GUS J. PROSCH, JR., M.D.
about
Osteoarthritis and Rheumatoid Disease,
including Rheumatoid Arthritis

THE EVER-POPULAR
RHEUMATOID DISEASES CURED AT LAST
DISTRIBUTED IN MORE THAN
1,500,000 COPIES!!!

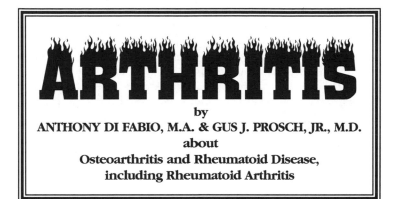

ARTHRITIS

by
ANTHONY DI FABIO, M.A. & GUS J. PROSCH, JR., M.D.
about
Osteoarthritis and Rheumatoid Disease,
including Rheumatoid Arthritis

A complete and wonderful updating of Anthony di Fabio's Rheumatoid Diseases Cured At Last with Osteoarthritis added. This book will set the standard for treatment of more than 80 forms of arthritis for years to come.

~~ Jack M. Blount, M.D.

A publication of *The Roger Wyburn-Mason and Jack M. Blount Foundation for the Eradication of Rheumatoid Disease*
a non-profit, tax-exempt foundation
a.k.a. *The Rheumatoid Disease Foundation*
a.k.a. *The Arthritis Trust of America*

Library of Congress Cataloging Card Number 97-071310

ISBN 0-9615437-3-6-$10

Copyright 1997 by Anthony di Fabio & Gus J. Prosch, Jr., M.D.

Published by
The Arthritis Trust of America
5106 Old Harding Road
Franklin, TN 37064
Printed in USA

Dedication

As a complete rewrite and update of *Rheumatoid Diseases Cured at Last*, the contents of this book are the result of hundreds of thousands of clinical studies, patient treatment hours, and other research performed by hundreds of health professionals world-wide over the span of many generations. It would be fitting to dedicate this book to all of those pioneers, many of whom risked their reputations and their licenses for the higher goal of finding truth and the power to heal dreaded, crippling diseases. And so we shall dedicate!

Special mention, however, must be made of certain pioneers who, in seeking truth and the power to heal, brought to fruition medical treatments that untangle the Gordian knots known as "arthritis." Roger Wyburn-Mason, M.D., Ph.D., Jack M. Blount, M.D., and Thomas McPherson Brown, M.D. stand at the pioneers' forefront — and so we must honor each of them, accordingly.

There is another class of pioneers who have greatly striven to bring about the freedom we need to apply newly discovered, successful treatments that have not been approved by the self-righteous, so-called, "medical establishment," which, James Carter, M.D., Dr.P.H., defines as "the American Medical Association, state medical associations, medical specialty organizations, state boards of medical examiners, medical schools and teaching hospitals, the American Hospital Association, the National Insurance Association (representing some 1,500 companies) and the entire drug, pharmaceutical, and medical equipment industry."[16]

Honest science does not drive medical advances, contrary to popular belief. And as Julian Whitaker, M.D. has said it, "What physicians do today is determined by the same forces that have always been present: cultural beliefs, current medical dogma (often irrational), financial interests, training, and peer pressure."[17]

So there's much more to getting well, than simply discovering a workable method. At least in the United States there is also the very real problem of getting legal permission to apply the necessary healing tools.

Among all those men of good will who daily fight against the suppressive nature of the medical establishment are three men who also deserve our sincere dedication. These are former Iowa Congressman Berkley Bedell, Iowa Senator Tom Harkin, both founders of the Alternative Medicine Office under the National Institute of Health, and, finally, Burton Goldberg, a grand public disseminator of workable alternative methods.

— GUS J. PROSCH, JR., M.D. & ANTHONY DI FABIO, M.A.

Table of Contents

iv

Illustrations

A complete and wonderful updating of Anthony di Fabio's Rheumatoid Diseases Cured At Last with Osteoarthritis added. This book will set the standard for treatment of more than 80 forms of arthritis for years to come.

-- Jack M. Blount, M.D.

A publication of *The Roger Wyburn-Mason and Jack M. Blount Foundation for the Eradication of Rheumatoid Disease* a non-profit, tax-exempt foundation
AKA *The Rheumatoid Disease Foundation,*
AKA *The Arthritis Trust of America*

ISBN 0-9615437-3-6-$15

Foreward
Our Purpose

We want to help <u>you</u> to get <u>you</u> well:
- by convincing you that generally it is an outright lie, that arthritis is incurable;
- by means of books and articles that expand your horizon (and your physician's) on causes of ill-health;
- with the gentle support of some self-help treatments; and
- through your committment to guided tours led by knowledgeable alternative medical health professionals of your choice, using treatments of your choice.

We can and do supply you with some of the world's best wellness advice and down-to-earth reading references and other resources. We have no vested interest or stock holdings in those whose help or products are recommended.

Considering all of the above, you're sure to run into the claim of "quackery" especially by the professional who <u>does</u> have a vested interest in holding onto your "patient" status, or suffers from his or her own hidden desire to remain ignorant. So bear with us a moment while we discuss the nature of quackery.

The Nature of Quackery

Much of the advice proferred so liberally by many health professionals while creating this book bucks traditional medicine, but represents safe, innovative, non-traditional treatments when applied properly. Given the success stories told repeatedly, it's hard to understand how anyone could or would want to continue with totally ineffective, often damaging traditional treatments for arthritis!

Those who would persuade you not to try safe, workable alternatives would call such treatments "quackery," and those who would help you toward wellness as "quacks."

John W. Campbell, Jr.[4] was a remarkable modern writer and thought-provoker, who was commemorated by naming a crater on the far side of the moon the "Campbell" crater.

A "Quack" According to John W. Campbell, Jr.

"Now let's consider for a moment what's meant by a 'quack' in the medical field.

"The usual charge is that a quack is someone who uses an improper treatment, one which does not help, or actually injures the patient, while inducing the patient to pay for his mistreatment, and keeping the patient from going to a licensed doctor and getting the treatment he needs. That a quack is in the business solely to make money at the expense of suffering humanity.

"Now any time A disapproves of B emotionally, he'll attribute B's actions to some generally demeaned motivation -- 'just for money' being the most common, with 'just for his own pleasure' being a runner-up.

"Let's be objective about this business of what a quack does. Suppose a man, calling himself Dr. Jones, treats a patient who has a lethal disease, and uses a method he knows for a positive fact will not save the man's life. He charges fees, and sees to it that the patient doesn't go to any other therapist -- just gives him some drugs that do not save him, but let him die slowly.

"That set of actions fulfills exactly what the [medical establishment] accuses those awful, nasty, wicked quacks of doing.

"It is also precisely what an [establishment medical] doctor does when he treats [an arthritis] patient; he knows that the standard treatments for [arthritis] do not work, do not save lives. [Arthritis], treated by the [medical establishment] methods, means [continuous pain, disfigurement and possibly] death.

"The [medical establishment], moreover, does everything in its power to make it impossible for the victim to get treatment from any other therapist who *might* be able to do better, and most certainly couldn't be less effective.

"The patient [may], moreover, wind up broke, and his family in debt -- a charge constantly leveled against those wicked quacks! -- by the time he dies.

"But this is not quackery, of course.

"Why not? Because the doctors know they are doing their best, with the best of intentions -- despite the [medical establishment's] convictions that he *must* be evil -- and actually does better than the [medical establishment's] best?

"Oh . . . I see. That never happens, huh . . . ?

". . . how about that unlicensed non-M.D. -- that charlatan, that fraud, who'd gotten crackpot ideas from studying silk-worms and wineries, no less! -- who started treating human beings for rabies? That chemist, with only half a brain, Louis Pasteur?

"Or how about that licensed M.D. charlatan, expelled from the hospital and the medical society -- Semmelweis? [Semmelweis solved childbed fever and demonstrated the importance of cleansing hands before touching patients.]

"Or take a few other notorious quacks like Lister -- who was most violently attacked for his temerity in opening the abdomens of living patients. (Ethical doctors of the time never opened the abdomen until after the patient died.)

"And Ehrlich, another chemist, who invented the concept of chemotherapy.

"Every time someone outside -- or even inside! -- the field of medicine brings up a break-through discovery, he'll be labeled a quack. The field is too emotional.

"He'll be charged with being a fraud, charlatan out after money, a blood-sucking leech. . . .

"Actually, it's pretty clear, the definition of 'quack' is someone I believe to be dangerous, evil, destructive and unprincipled!

"Trouble is -- the term 'quack' was -- in their own place and time -- violently hurled at many men we consider today among the greatest medical heroes. [Semmelweis], Jenner, Koch, Harvey, Ross, Lister, Pasteur, Ehrlich, Sister Kenny, even Roentgen, who didn't even try to practice medicine!

"One very certain thing about the field of medicine: it is not, and never will be a field of objective science. It's too deeply dominated by emotional factors."

Your Search for Wellness

So! You've probably been to an establishment medical physician about your present ill-health.

You've probably been told that your pain is a consequence of age or genetics, soon to lead to an incurable condition! -- Or that it is such and such a maladay, and is already incurable! That very nice man, that fine mannered, knowledgeable doctor said, "Here's a pill. Take it three times a day. Learn to live with your condition and pain!"

He may also have warned you against quackery -- people who claim to have cures, but only want your money -- also conveniently overlooking the fact that he claims not to have a cure, but is perfectly willing to take your money.

He's an Authority -- a MEDICAL DOCTOR. Possibly he's one of the very best in your region, highly educated and trained, a respectable, leading citizen, of the highest ethics, a family man, recognized by both your local hospital and your insurance company as a man to trust.

Since -- you believe -- all medical doctors are equally trained, equally knowledgeable, all have had the same education, the same training, have read the same books, and all are at the very forefront of research, you'll profer trust in this nice man (or woman), you'll go home, suffer, take the pill three or more times a day, and be emotionally stricken as your body progresses into a grotesque disease condition.

Right?

Hopefully, not any more! Not after reading this book, and others available elsewhere. Thankfully people are beginning to wake up, to realize the ineffectiveness and futility of relying on traditional medicine, as more and more folks take up alternatives -- and achieve wellness.

Not all establishment medicine is bad, of course. It simply uses a faulty standard usually designed by medical boards, insurance companies, pharmaceutical industries, trade unions such as the American Medical Association or American Dental Association, or ivory towered professors in medical schools whose research is dominated by the pocketbooks of pharmaceutical industries -- hardly an unemotional or unbiased grouping.

While the gold standard of medical scientific proof is that of controlled, double-blind studies that often cost as much as $40,000,000 to establish the fact that one kind of pain killer is slightly better than another kind of pain killer, the crux of medicine is and should be whether or not people achieve wellness, and how they do so. We have, therefore, included actual case histories (usually under pseudonyms), describing how people suffered and what they did to achieve wellness.

In the osteoarthritis chapter you'll learn that William Kaufman, M.D., Ph.D. solved one of the basic mysteries of osteoarthritis, having proved his solution under rigorous scientific studies. Others also worked on pieces of the puzzles, and these include natural-medicine-oriented Rex E. Newnham, D.O., N.D., Ph.D. and Michael T. Murray, N.D., nerve specialist Roger Wyburn-Mason, M.D., Ph.D., surgeon/acupuncturist Dr. Paul K. Pybus, reconstructive therapists William J. Faber, D.O. and James Carlson, D.O., general practitioners Jack M. Blount and one of us (Gus J. Prosch, Jr., M.D.), chiropractors like Paul Goldberg, D.C., M.P.H., and many other health professionals -- all of whom have volunteered extremely useful knowledge.

Osteoarthritis is no longer a necessary concommitant of aging, being treatable and solvable. Would it also surprise you to learn that rheumatoid arthritis has been capable of being cured for many years?

The necessary treatment factors, usually involve (1) proper nutrition, (2) detoxification [mercury, foci of infection, herbicides and pesticides] (3) strengthening of the immune system, (4) elimination of foreign organisms [parasites], (5) treatment for food allergies, and (6) treatment against candidiasis, a yeast/fungus infestation. While accounting for all of these factors, and while all are necessary ingredients to achieve wellness, in particular cases they may not be sufficient, as each of us are designed with genetic differences and reared in differing environments.

What We've Learned

Both of us have experienced nearly fifteen years of freedom from rheumatoid arthritis, and one of us has successfully treated thousands of rheumatoid arthritis patients.

We've learned two impressive fundamental truths:

(a) All health not related to genetic defects is a function of what we eat, drink, breathe, how we eliminate, the nature of our living styles, and our response to and the levels of experienced stress. "To be healthy," says the wise man, "then clean up your act."

This book describes how to start cleaning up your act!

(b) There are probably more ways known to stay or get well than there are ways to achieve illness, or to stay ill. Apparently -- from the nature of wellness principles -- we humans work very hard to stay ill!

The Many Layers to Wellness

It took one of us (Anthony di Fabio) six weeks to halt the progress of "galloping" rheumatoid arthritis, two more years to pay attention to candidiasis, nutrition and food allergies, and the next 13 years to understand what's really going on with the factors that create rheumatoid arthritis and the other 79 related rheumatoid diseases. The following are layers which, when peeled apart sheet by sheet, surely will produce wellness in virtually everyone:

1. Stress

Stress is the greatest contributor toward a sick body. As a necessary ingredient of life, stress is totally unavoidable, arriving at our doorstep because we live, and appearing as either a physical or emotional stressor.

Physical stress includes heat and cold, polluting chemicals, daylight and darkness, the pull of gravity, microorganisms, changes in humidity and air pressure, accidents and sports, and so on.

Emotional stressors include offenses against others or against ourselves, shool discipline and study, work -- particularly if detested -- marriage relationships and divorces, and certainly the loss of loved ones.

According to Derrick Lonsdale, M.D. [*Why I Left Orthodox Medicine*], "Each of us live in a dangerous world, surrounded by all kinds of invisible stressors, many of which are indeed bacteria and viruses. The defense reaction to a stressor, however, regardless of the nature of the stressor, is much the same."

Some folks can handle enormous amounts of stress, and others very little, probably as a matter of their differing nutritional intake, state of health, and genetic factors.

We can make choices to reduce stress, but, short of death, there is no way to totally eliminate stress. It is our *choices* that determine the *nature* of our stress.

Whenever undue stress is unavoidable, or even if you've conditioned yourself to believe that a stress activity is enjoyable, some folks will get well simply by choosing to remove themselves from an environment of undue stress.

Stress has many faces, and it is never solved by blaming others, although it's possible that removing yourself from others may be necessary.

There are so many faces to stress that it deserves a book by itself.

Some folks can get well from rheumatoid arthritis and related rheumatoid diseases simply by removing themselves from stressful situations.

2. **Nutrition**

As we've repeatedly written -- as has Joel Wallach, D.V.M., N.D. and Ma Lan, M.D. (*Dead Doctors Don't Lie; Rare Earths: Forbidden Cures*, etc.) -- a successful farmer knows more about nutrition than the vast majority of health professionals graduating from the standard medical school. A successful farmer knows with a certainty -- a certainty upon which his family's welfare relies -- that unless he feeds his cattle, chickens, hogs, sheep, and so forth the very best nutrients, their market value will be low, and his income accordingly will suffer. Unfortunately few American farmers have learned to apply this same philosophy to their plant kingdom crops, as they seem to be stuck in the limited nitrogen/phosphorus "fertilizer" cycle, along with the use of hybrids that produce large, healthy appearing vegetation with lopsided nutrient values or without a whole lot of nourishing qualities.

Most religions teach that man is both spirit and animal. And while it is most important to nourish the spirit, this can be increasingly difficult without pesistently buttressing our animal natures with the proper nutrition and nutritional supplements. If not, the spirit may leave the body prematurely.

Everywhere on earth are healthful foods growing wild: insects, worms, nuts, fruits, various vegetation. There's probably more healthful edible foods growing wild on this planet even today than there are unedible, poisonous foods -- but we and you are not about to break our childhood conditioning to seek after it. So, what is left?

Well, the closer we can come to the diet of our foraging ancestors, the more healthy we will become, excepting, of course, unavoidable intake of parasites, bacteria, et. al. In other words, we need organically grown food free of pesticides, herbicides, and chock full of enzymes, vitamins, minerals, and essential fatty acids. If we were to plant and raise our own gardens, insuring that the soils are balanced and mineral-laden, we'd more than likely not need vitamin and mineral supplements.

As it has become increasingly difficult to obtain what our animal natures require, we must do the best we can. After having chosen the very best store products available to us, we must choose wisely in supplementing with various vitamins, minerals, and essential fatty acids -- because our foods no longer contain the proper balance or they lack sufficient quantity of these life substances.

Those are just the general principles. A scientific discourse on the proper food baffles the best of physicians, so don't expect this non-encylopoedic book to provide you with foolproof, complete advice suitable just for you. Each person is genetically different, and each has different requirements, and those are the ingredients that you must learn about with the assistance of a knowledgeable health professional. The "4-food groups" or "6-food groups" recommended by dietitians is nonsense, not even suitable for grade-school children, providing incomplete, misleading information, and leaving out the very varying biochemistry that makes you different, or supports your life.

Derrick Lonsdale, M.D. (*Why I Left Orthodox Medicine*), describes five patients who are non-genetically related. Each of them are clinically diagnosed as having rheumatoid arthritis, each described as having joint inflammation, pain and swelling. Traditional medicine would attempt to treat each and every one of these five patients the same, but on a nutritional basis, each would require a different approach, depending upon their biochemical needs which must be learned by astute biochemical analysis. Dr. Lonsdale's nutritional approach also emphasizes that rheumatoid arthritis and related rheumatoid diseases are not a disease of joints, but a disease of the whole body -- and we wholeheartedly agree.

There are many who achieve wellness from rheumatoid arthritis -- and the other 79 collagen tissue diseases which we call rheumatoid diseases -- simply by improving their nutritional intake to that which best fits them. We would guestimate that about 30% can get well by this means alone.

Chose to remove undue stress, and improve nutrition, and you may very well achieve wellness from rheumatoid disease!

3. Candidasis and Food Allergies.

Candida albicans, a yeast/fungus, is an organism of opportunity, just as many other microorganisms are. Whenever conditions are right these organisms-of-opportunity set up shop in our bodies, particularly the intestinal tract. Right conditions (for them) are provided by the use of antibiotics, hormones (cortisone, birth control pills, etc.) and other chemicals, exposure to stress, and poor nutrition. A particularly virulent form of candidiasis -- the name given to the *Candida albicans* yeast/ fungus infection -- is a fungal form that plants itself in the intestinal mucosal membrane, there to grow inward rootlets that penetrate all the way into the blood stream. (See *The Yeast Connection*, William Crook; *The Yeast Syndrome*, Morton Walker, D.P.M., John Trowbridge, M.D.; others)

Candidiasis, as will most yeasts, produces either acetaldehyde or alcohol, or both. Acetaldehyde is the metabolite of alcohol, the part of drinking liquors that gives you a hang-over the next morning. This persisent production of acetaldehyde in your intestinal tract passes through and into every organ and bodily system day by day, night by night, placing extreme chemical stress on your cells, organs, and systems. In time virtually every degenerative disease condition can be mimicked, including those of rheumatoid arthritis as well as the other 79 so-called "auto-immune" diseases.

Simultaneously, as acetaldehyde is slowly, drastically, affecting your life, the rootlets planted in your mucosa are permitting small molecular particles of food to pass directly into the blood stream without being digested. These particles in your bloodstream are recognized as foreign invaders, and your immune system builds up protection against them, forming what's called an antigen/antibody complex which is the biochemical beginings of a food allergy.

The number of your food allergies increases over time, and they have some peculiar characteristics: (a) Some food allergies can be spotted as soon as you've eaten the substance: headache, nausea, joint pain, depression, lethargy, and so on. (b) Some food allergies require as much as three days from the time you exposed yourself to the food to kick in with headache, nausea, joint pain, depression and lethargy, and so on. This type becomes hard to associate with foods eaten by causal observation, and may require either a valid blood test for allergies or a carefully prepared log of foods eaten compared to daily symptoms (*Dr. Braly's Food Allergy and Nutrition Revolution*, James Braly, M.D.).

Just as infestation by *Candida albicans* can create a huge variety of symptoms, depending upon which tissues are most affected, so can food allergies. And, just as candidiasis can mimic rheumatoid disease, and the other 79 collagen tissue diseases, so can food allergies.

In short, candidiasis produces food allergies, and both of them not only create their own disease symptoms, but both of them can also mimic any of the 80 rheumatoid diseases, including rheumatoid arthritis.

Incidentally, you're probably not going to want to learn that food allergies behave according to the same biochemical rules as does drug addiction.

Health professionals who have had their patients rid themselves of stress, improve nutrition, and conquer candidiasis and food allergies have cured a high percentage of those afflicted with rheumatoid disease.

4. **Mercury Detoxification, Pesticide and Herbicide Detoxification, and Sterilization of Foci of Infection.**

Solving stress may get the arthritic well.

Changing stressful conditions and improving nutrition may get the arthritic well.

Attending to stressful conditions, improving nutrition, reducing candidiasis infestation, and avoiding allergenic foods may get the arthritic well.

-- and any of these life-style changes may be permanent or temporary, depending upon each individual's temperment and situation.

But what will surely work? And what will also come closest to returning your body (and youthful spirit) back to an early period when you were free of disease?

Broad Spectrum Anti-Microorganism Treatment

Two foundations, The ArthritisTrust of America (The Rheumatoid Disease Foundation) and The Road Back Foundation, have historically recommended the use of prescription medicines to halt the progress of rheumatoid arthritis and some osteoarthritis (about 10%). The Road Back Foundation recommends a series of treatments of minicycline, whereas The Arthritis Trust of America has long recommended any one, or combination, of several broad-spectrum anti-microorganism drugs.

Both treatments have resulted in remissions or "cures," from rheumatoid arthritis.

Coupling broad spectrum anti-microorganism treatment with treatment for improper nutrition, candidiasis, and food allergies has consistently resulted in an 80% cure rate since 1982, according to one of us (Gus J. Prosch, Jr., M.D. of Birmingham, Alabama).

According to Lee Cowden, M.D. of Dallas, Texas, (Health Restoration Systems, Inc.) various foci of infection are important to remove, but they will not leave completely until accumulated herbicides and pesticides are removed. Hebicides and pesticides will not go completely until mercury is removed.

We don't want to use this limited space to get involved in a lengthy pro and con as to why each of these factors are so important. That's what The Arthritis Trust of America's recommended books and articles do in some detail. We'll briefly describe the nature of each of the above factors.

Mercury Poisoning

The US Environmental Protection Agency sets no lower limit for the amount of mercury that is dangerous to health. Dentists who handle mercury must do so under guidelines set by the agency for a very dangerous substance, including the need to dispose of mercuric waste scraps in a manner that will not endanger our environment, thus also endanger people.

For some irrational reason, once mercury is placed in fillings of teeth American dentists consider it no longer of danger because, they say, it is in an amalgamated form -- mixed with other metals -- and will not come free. This assumption is demonstrably false, and can be easily shown to be false by measuring the percentage of mercury from removed fillings and plotting percentages of remaining mercury against the time the amalgam spent in the mouth. Mercury disappears from the amalgams in a very predictable (linear) manner. The longer in the mouth, the less mercury contained in the filling.

The Swedish Medical Association, after resisting these claims of danger in the use of mercury fillings and after studying available scientific data, concluded they were wrong, and they publicly apologized to the Swedish public. Sweden, as well as some other European countries, are now phasing mercury from dentistry.

The normally intransigent American Medical Association has declared mercury dangerous, in agreement with the Environmental Protection Association.

The American Dental Association, however, is so blind, so irrationally protective of their trade union, that they and some of their captive
licensing boards have threatened to take the license away from dentists
who remove fillings and replace them with a non-dangerous substance.

When mercury is amalgamated with another metal, the filling is
bathed in either an alkaline or an acid environment, the saliva and food
mixture in your mouth which changes according to what you eat and
when you eat.

Two dissimilar metals in either an alkaline or acid environment
form a small battery which, when activated, produces an electric
current. Such an electric current is easily measured in each and every
metallic filling in your teeth.

The joint effect of all the little batteries in all of your teeth is also
measurable as both a current, and also as a persistent source of
evaporated mercury in your mouth.

Evaporated mercury combines with organic matter in the mouth to
form a mercuric/organic compound, which your body accumulates.
Over time, your body will accumulate a considerable amount of
mercury from your fillings as well as from other sources, such as
consumed fish (which accumulates mercury), herbicides and pesticides, and additional dangerous environmental stressors surrounding us
everywhere.

According to Hal Huggins, D.D.S. (*It's All In Your Head*), and other
health professionals, here's the two major effects of the use of mercury
fillings:

(1) Organic mercury tends to accumulate at nerve ganglion where
it interferes with the proper functioning of nerve signals. Accumulated
mercury in a ganglia in the face -- for example -- may easily affect
performance of a joint in a remote part of the body, causing a form of
"arthritis." The proof is that when the organic mercury is removed from
the ganglion in the face, the pain in the joint stops immediately, and the
joint begins to heal and function properly.

This is but one example among thousands of seemingly unrelated
dysfunctions that might be cited, including that of improper functioning
of the immune system.

(2) Organic mercury forms small pockets or envelopes in various
tissues of the body within which foreign microorganisms set up shop.
These are usually mutated, anaerobic (live without oxygen) forms of
organisms. When our macrophages and leucocytes try to attack these
foreign organisms as they're supposed to do, they are prevented from
entering the pocket by the mercury.

Thus, the foreign organisms continue to thrive, producing toxins
(microbial waste products) which, if our human tissues are not already
sensitive to the toxins, will, for the arthritic-prone, probably become
sensitive to them. The daily production of toxins, and their distribution

throughout the tissues, organs, and systems of our body are what produce the various disease symptoms that are then classified as one of the 80 so-called "auto-immune" diseases, and also many of the "degnerative" diseases.

It greatly surprised one of us (Anthony di Fabio) to learn that the red coloring matter used to produce partial dentures and full dentures consists of a mercuric coloring matter. This mercury also leaches out over time, continuing our accumulation of dangerous mercury. A clear flexite denture is recommended by Lee Cowden, M.D. of Dallas, Texas.

We were shocked to learn from one manufacturer of denture plastic that he used cadmium to help keep the red (mercury) from leaching out.

Yea Gad! Cadmium is as dangerous as the mercury, and a major problem for the Environmental Protection Agency to keep cadmium from leaching into our soils and water systems especially by it's improper disposal.

The problem of obtaining dentures made from a clear flexite material may prove difficult, but, if you insist, can be solved.

Root Canal and Tooth Extraction Foci of Infection

Extracted teeth and root canal surgery are extremely large sources of persistent infections that create degenerative diseases, including the various arthritides. "Arthritides" refers to all forms of arthritis.

George E. Meinig, D.D.S. (*Root Canal Cover-Up*) reports on the work of Weston Price, D.D.S., who, under the auspices of the American Dental Association, headed studies performed by 60 top-ranking medical scientists from very prestigious medical and dental institutions.

Whenever a tooth is extracted, or root canal work has been performed, the muscular tissue in the socket is usually left in place, and the dentist makes an assumption that the use of antibiotics will penetrate this tough tissue killing any microorganisms that may be present after the surgery.

The assumption is demonstrably false.

Steptococus feci, or any one of hundreds of viruses, bacteria or mycoplasmas, will find themselves in these open sockets during surgery. Within the apparently healed gums, microorganisms that thrive in oxygen in the mouth (aerobic) will mutate to a type that thrives without oxygen inside the tooth socket (anaerobic).

Only 10% of those infected in the gums will have sore or sensitive gums, and will ever suspect that something is wrong.

One of us (Anthony di Fabio) had all of his teeth removed 50 years ago, and argued loud and long with those who insisted that the teeth be checked for a focus of infection. After all, "I had no root canals performed, and my gums feel normal!" Burton Goldberg (*Alternative Medicine: The Definitive Guide*) insisted, and so more to oblige him than because of belief, several non-invasive tests were made, and two blood tests.

Two kinds of non-invasive tests are effective in making such a determination: (1) kinesthiology, a method of testing for muscle strength or weakness in the presence of an antigen or allergen; or (2) a computron, or dermatron (Electro-Acupuncture according to Voll), a device that sends a small amount of un-noticeable current along an acupuncture meridian. By reading the resulting effect on a changing electrical measurement one can determine if foreign invaders are involved, often what species.

Each blood test confirmed the presence of a species of mycoplasma, one of them also inferring the presence of an associated virus.

Under the care of a biological dentist, his computron confirmed the presence of both a mycoplasma and a virus throughout the upper and lower gums, also naming their species.

Still there was no belief or acceptance, but permission was granted to cut into a small portion of the gums as a final determination.

Lo! A greyish mass was present. Evidence was found of infestation throughout the top and bottom along the whole gum line -- a fifty year-long unsuspected focus of infection. These were laser sterilized and cleansed with hydrogen peroxide injections.

Later a nerve ganglion that could not be cut into by the biological dentist was also cleansed of infection by a medical doctor with appropriate techniques, as were other nerve ganglia containing mercury in other parts of the body. Still a residual focus of infection remained in the lower right dental quadrant. Toxins from remaining microorganisms affect a finger on the right hand, and will be sterilized further in the future. How does one know for sure that these toxins affect the finger? Because when novocaine is injected in to the lower right dental quadrant, the finger pain disappears, and felxibility returns.

According to Dr. Meinig, so long as the immune system is young, and functioning properly, these toxins and foreign invaders are properly handled. Once we age, as do our systems, the immune functions become slowly overwhelmed, and the various degnerative diseases set in.

By the way. None of this kind of dentistry should be attempted without a <u>Biological Dentist</u>, sometimes called a "detoxification dentist." They are few in number, and not too easy to find. The untrained, normal dentist not only will not believe, but even if willing to remove mercury or cleanse foci of infection, they are likely to leave you worse off than when you began. Especially dangerous is the possibility of accumulating more mercury in your system than you had before amalgam replacement with a neutral filling. <u>Specialized techniques and training are necessary!</u>

There are cases on record where once the mercury has been removed, and the foci of infection cleared up,(by use of the proper procedures) arthritis has totally disappeared without further treatment.

There are also cases where obvious health improvement has been obtained, but the arthritis has not cleared. Reason: Stress, nutrition, candidiasis, food allergies, and additional problems to be discussed in the following.

Adnoidectomies and Tonsilectomies Foci of Infection

Additional foci of infections may result from improper sterilization after adnoidectomies or tonsilectomies, according to Dr. Meinig.

What's Happened to This Important Information?

What has happened to information, about the dangers of mercury, gum infection after extraction of teeth and root canal surgery, and after improperly cleansed adniodectomies and tonsilectomies?

Why hasn't the public -- or the arthritic -- been told of it?

Although the important medical research was initially sponsored by the American Dental Association, when one of us asked his dentist about knowledge of these fantastic, long-term, definitive research works, he shook his head, saying, "No, I've never heard of them! They never taught us this in dentistry school."

We gave him copies of Meinig's and Huggins' books.

Like so many important medical discoveries, the knowledge got buried by mean-spirited, closed-minded, suppressive personalities -- or people with vested interests.

Original research records are stored in the American Dental Association library archives, and copies are also found in the Price-Pottenger Nutrition Foundation (PO Box 2614, La Mesa, California 91943-2614). However, George Meinig, D.D.S. has nicely summarized the work in his book *Root Canal Coverup*.

Pesticides and Herbicides

Pesticides and herbicides surround us everywhere. It's as though we live in a sea of these dangerous, man-made substances. The initial idea was to kill pests (insects, rodents, etc.) or to kill weeds that are undesirable on our farms so that we could produce more and better crops. A similar motivation led to the use of antibiotics which, at first glance, appears to be a miraculous use of nature's own means of limiting undesirable microbes.

However, what has happened is this: Insects, microorganisms, and even so-called weeds adapt -- usually faster than we do. One surviving microbe, for example, can breed a generation of descendents that not only cannot be killed by the chemical or antibiotic that killed its forebearers, but thrives on it instead, and so another chemical or antibiotic must be manufactured against this new generation.

And so it goes, until there is hardly anything that can be used against these adaptable organisms that is not also dangerous to the cells of man.

Dangerous pesticides and herbicides have also become extremely widespread: winds spread the chemicals to our shores as does wave; and even traffic from country to country by car, ship, plane, and feet which all spread these deadly man-made chemicals.

There is little water, whether city conditioned, or farm well-water, stream, ocean, or lake, that does not contain these dangerous substances, just as there is little produce that reaches our markets that does not contain them. Nor are the snows and ices safe. Dangerous herbicides and pesticides can even be found in the arctic and antarctica, carried by wind and wave. Whole eco-systems are dying, and their many varied life-forms are also dying by the tens of thousands from our poisonous incursions.

Harold Buttram, M.D. (*Our Toxic World; Who Is Looking After Our Children?*) reports that "about 70,000 chemicals are now used in commerce, of which several hundred have been tested for neurotoxicity, and among these only a handful have been tested thoroughly. Children have been estimated to be up to 10 times more vulnerable to toxic chemicals than adults."

Generally, these poisons or their dangerous metabolites are accumulated in the parts of the cells of the body called "lipids," or fatty parts of our cells.

Parasites, including infestations of candidiasis, amoebae, mycoplasmas, bacteria, viruses, worms, et. al., will not readily leave the body (especially intestinal tract) until these pesticides and herbicides are driven from the body.

There are many ways to detoxify herbicides, pesticides, and other chemicals from the body, among which are (1) 3-1/2 to 4 weeks of sweat sauna at 140°-180° F, with replacement vitamins, minerals and essential fatty acids (Church of Scientology); (2) use of body soaks with special preparations, including dry scrubbing, et. al. (3) specially prepared herbs and homeopathic remedies, and so on.

Primary, however, and according to Lee Cowden, M.D., is to get rid of the accumulated organic mercury compounds, which permits removal of herbicides and pesticides, which permits removal of parasites.

Parasites

Getting rid of parasites, including yeast, amoebae, mycoplasmas, bacteria, viruses, worms, et. al. may require a number of different treatments over more or lesser time periods.

Nutritionist Ann Louise Gittleman (*Guess What Came to Dinner*) says, "If you think that parasitic diseases happen only to people in Third World countries, think again ... An astounding one out of six people will test positive for parasites," -- those are only counting parasites for which tests are made. Testing for parasites by an established medical professional would most likely result in negative findings. Unfortunately, these standardized tests catch only about 20% of the actual cases, according to Ross Anderson, N.D., D.C., Petersborough, Ontario, Canada, who says, that "Over 1,000 species of parasites can live in your body, but tests for only about 40 or 50 exist. This means doctors are only testing for about 5% of the parasites and missing 80% of these. This brings the ability to clinically find parasites down to 1%."[265]

Lee Cowden, M.D., Dallas, Texas, may recommend ozone colonics, especially the kind that can be used in one's own home. An ozone machine (to prepare ozonated water) is purchased and used in the home to freshly prepare a number of gallons of water, after which, and with the prior layout of a colema board   and training in the method, one injects the prepared ozonated water into the lower colon. Dr. Cowden's rule of thumb is that for each 20 years of life it requires about 1 week of such treatment, twice daily, along with other special dietary factors.

Bernard Jensen, D.C., Ph.D. (*Tissue Cleansing Through Bowel Management*) describes other effective methods, as does Sherry Rogers, M.D. (*Wellness Against All Odds*), and Louis J. Marx, M.D. (*Healing Dimensions of Herbal Medicine*), may provide specific herbal formulations for specific as well as general conditions.

Removing undue stress, satisfying individual nutritional requirements, detoxifying mercury, pesticides and herbicides, treating candidiasis and food allergies, killing undesirable parasites via prescription drugs, herbs and other means, and removing the thickened intestinal lining which harbors parasites, microorganisms, and worms will surely restore health with the vast majority.

5. Necessary Individualized Treatments

There is another level which might be required for optimum health for some individuals, and that is specialized individualized treatments. These are whatever individualized treatments are necessary for the specific person. For example: a person who has diabetes may very well have a type that William H. Philpott, M.D. of Choctaw, Oklahoma has identified as being caused by allergies to certain widely consumed foods. The beta cells in the pancreas swell because of the allergy, thus preventing the body from receiving necessary insulin. We've known folks who, on talking with Dr. Philpott, have tried his allergy recommendations and subsequently have become free of insulin shots thereafter.

Whether or not the type of diabetes is from food allergy, any diabetic can benefit from chelation therapy, a method of improving blood circulation in 80% of the peripheral (extremities) circulation. Such improvement in blood circulation is always accompanied by improved nutritional support for each individual cell, and thus improves ability to heal.

In fact, the use of chelation therapy can very well eliminate the need for by-pass surgery, one of those very costly, mostly ineffective standard, obsolete, medical practices.

As each individual differs greatly from others both in genetics, past nutritional intake, stress, and other important modifiers of our biology, only a trained health professional can determine whether or not Level

Five is necessary, and in most cases, while perhaps not necessary, may be desirable.

Level Four Toward Wellness. and possibly Level 5, are such important steps (especially when combined with levels 1 through 3) there's virtual certainty that when properly implemented every (100%) arthritic will achieve wellness. But this doesn't mean that all of the damage to joints and other body systems will necessarily be reversed. Special treatments may be necessary for damaged, irreversible problems.

Not just those suffering from rheumatoid arthritis, not just those suffering from rheumatoid disease (the whole 80 of them), but also a large portion of any who suffer from many so-called degenerative diseases will achieve wellness.

We knowingly include many forms of cancer among the promised wellnesses accomplished through the directions described.

You see, we've sort of snuck up on you!

We started by describing simple levels of healing strategies just for arthritides, and arrived at a level that will heal almost everything, so common are the causes, and so basic are the common physiological conditions.

The Catch

Implementing the above recommendations can be a serious problem. Although The Arthritis Trust of America's physician list contains many doctors knowledgeable in one or more of the preceding treatment programs, there are few, indeed, knowledgeable or trained in all of them.

Finding a biological dentist in your geographical region, as has been mentioned, can be a pain in the tail. Although this foundation has listed a few in its physician list, the Price-Pottenger Nutrition Foundation has a greater listing of biological dentists.

Finding a compatible physician or dentist may take some time, and may also require you to search throughout the country, or even out of the country. Some procedures can be accomplished only at the risk of the professionals' license in some states, and some medical procedures (such as colonics) can be best done by yourself, in your own home after proper training. Some, of course may be best with your family physician.

Thus it is -- with all the many implementation problems -- that we highly recommend that you begin learning. Learning is what The Arthritis Trust of America's articles and books are about. When you've studied the variety of causes and aspects to getting well, you can decide for yourself how much expenditure of time and effort you'll make to heal yourself.

Some things you'll do yourself, based on the knowledge we've provided you.

Some treatments will require guidance by a knowing health professional.

Some treatments will require full attendance by a knowledgeable health professional.

Some treatments can only be found a long way from your home.

Your best bet is still to begin by ordering books and articles from The Arthritis Trust of America and from elsewhere.

Study, and decide!

Only you can get you well!

References

1. James Braly, M.D., *Dr. Braly's Food Allergy and Nutrition Revolution*, order from The Arthritis Society of America.

2. Harold Buttram, M.D., *Our Toxic World: Who Is Looking After Our Children?* order from The Arthritis Society of America.

3. William Crook, M.D., *The Yeast Connection Handbook*, order from The Arthritis Society of America.

4. Anthony di Fabio, *Rheumatoid Diseases Cured at Last*, 1985 edition, only computer print-out available, The Arthritis Society of America.

5. Ann Louise Gittleman, *Guess What Came to Dinner*, order from The Arthritis Society of America.

6. Burton Goldberg, *Alternative Medicine: The Definitive Guide*, order from The Arthritis Society of America.

7. Hal Huggins, D.D.S., *It's All In Your Head*, order from The Arthritis Society of America.

8. Bernard Jensen, D. C., Ph.D., *Tissue Cleansing Through Bowel Management*, order from The Arthritis Society of America.

10. Derrick Lonsdale, M.D., *Why I Left Orthodox Medicine*, order from The Arthritis Society of America.

11. Louis J. Marx, M.D., *Healing Dimensions Through Bowel Management*, order from The Arthritis Society of America.

12. George Meinig, D.D.S., *Root Canal Coverup*, order from The Arthritis Society of America.

13. John Parks Trowbridge, M.D. & Morton Walker, D.P.M., *The Yeast Syndrome*, order from The Arthritis Society of America.

14. Sherry S. Rogers, M.D., *Wellness Against All Odds*, Pestige Publishing, PO Box 3068, 3500 Brewerton Road, Syracuse, NY 13220.

15. Joe Wallach, D.V.M., N.D., Ma Lan, M.D., *Rare Earths: Forbidden Cures*, Double Happiness Publishing Co., PO Box 1222, Bonita, CA 91908.

16. James P. Carter, M.D., Dr.P.H., *Racketeering in Medicine: The Suppression of Alternatives*, Hampton Roads Publishing Company, Inc., 891 Norfolk Square, Norfolk, VA 23502, 1993.

17. Julian Whitaker, M.D., "Chelation Therapy Under Review by California Medical Board," Townsend Letter for Doctors & Patients, 911 Tyler St., Port Townsend, WA 98368-6541, p. 120.

Non-Profit Nutrition Information and Archives

Price-Pottenger Nutrition Foundation, PO Box 2614, La Mesa, CA 91943-2614; (619) 574-7763.

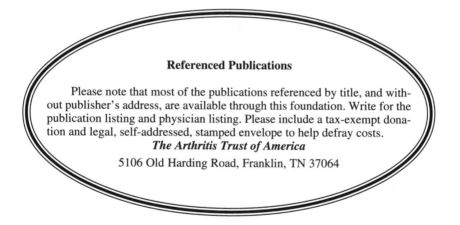

Referenced Publications

Please note that most of the publications referenced by title, and without publisher's address, are available through this foundation. Write for the publication listing and physician listing. Please include a tax-exempt donation and legal, self-addressed, stamped envelope to help defray costs.
The Arthritis Trust of America
5106 Old Harding Road, Franklin, TN 37064

Chapter I
Osteoarthritis
The Case of Jane Trowhouser
The "Incurable Disease"

Jane Trowhouser, seventy-eight year old widow, came to William Kaufman, M.D., Ph.D. at his private medical practice in Bridgeport, Connecticut, seeking help for "uncurable degenerative arthritis." She also had rheumatoid arthritis, two conditions that sometimes appear together.

Dr. Kaufman, was also a medical researcher and instructor at the University of Michigan Medical School as well as at Yale University School of Medicine. Awarded many honors, Dr. Kaufman was recipient of the Tom Spies Memorial Award presented by the International Association of Preventive Medicine.

Now everyone knew (or knows) that "degenerative arthritis" is a natural condition of aging.

Right?

Jane should have been sent home with a package of pain killers and told to "learn to live with it."

Right?

Jane had enjoyed excellent health until 6 months earlier, when her younger sister, aged 75, had a stroke.

Before her sister's illness, Jane had never done much physical work. However, since the sister did not wish to be hospitalized, or to be taken care of by strangers, Jane undertook to give nursing care to her sister at their home.

Bedrooms were on the second floor, and Jane made many extra trips up and down the rather steep flight of stairs, usually carrying her sister's meals to her. She was so busy with her sister's care that she neglected to eat her usual abundant diet, substituting starchy foods for high-protein foods.

After a month Jane became aware of pain, stiffness and swelling in her joints. She took 8-10 aspirin tablets (0.3 G) a day with only slightly increased comfort.

Now she was unable to climb up the stairs without gripping the banister with her left hand and pulling herself upward step by step.

Jane's sister improved over a period of several months, so that workload was lessened, but Jane's high-carbohydrate diet remained the same. Her joints continued to give trouble. She now had constant neck pain, severe low back pain, and painful swelling joints at the knees, ankles, wrists, hands, elbows and shoulder joints. She also had persistent numbness and tingling of her hands, which were so swollen she could not make a fist.

Many of Jane's joints were hot to the touch, and she noticed that she had considerable joint noise on movement (crepitus).

Every morning for several hours she felt stiff, until the aspirin reduced the pain, and then the stiffness recurred toward evening, when it was not at all relieved by the aspirin.

Changes in weather brought about increased joint discomfort. She lost 16 pounds during 3 months, and felt that she was becoming progressively weaker, feeling exhausted most of the time.

When Dr. Kaufman examined Jane, she was in great pain, and she seemed mentally dull, her voice quavery and querulous, and she walked with an extreme slowness and with some loss of sense of balance.

Jane's combined Joint Range Index -- a measure devised by Dr. Kaufman of how far patient's joints could comfortably move -- showed severe joint dysfunction.

Her knees, ankles, wrists, hands, elbows and shoulder joints showed the marked swelling seen in classic rheumatoid arthritis, with prominent venous swelling around the knees, joints hot to touch, and a few nodules below the skin on the ulna and tibia, the two lower arm bones.

Jane's skin was yellow-brown and somewhat wasted. Her gums were swollen, and there were many other physical signs of either osteoarthritis or rheumatoid arthritis, including laboratory findings and also those found on the tongue, liver and by her poor reflexes and loss of tickle sense.

The William Kaufman, M.D., Ph.D. Treatment

Jane was prescribed niacinamide (the amide of niacin) to be taken 150 mg every 3 hours for 6 doses daily (900 mg/24 hours). After 22 days of therapy, much of her joint swelling had disappeared, although she still complained of pain and stiffness. She walked and sat more erectly than on her first visit, and with better balance, and also more rapidly. Her liver tenderness was improved, and her Joint Range Index measurement changed from severe joint dysfunction to that of moderate joint dysfunction.

After 84 days of therapy, her Joint Range Index stabilized. She had slight swelling around the ankle and other joints. Only one aspirin a day now sufficed for her pain, and her voice had lost its quaver; she seemed also to be more mentally alert and more vigorous physically. Her tongue and mucous membrane of the mouth were improved considerably.

In 172 days of treatment her laboratory tests also had improved, and she was emphatic that she was better, no longer requiring aspirin for pain. Her liver was no longer enlarged or tender.

At the end of 280 days of treatment she was able for the first time in a year to go upstairs without either pulling herself up by the banister or climbing up the steps hand over hand, foot over foot.

Her skin had become more elastic and less wasted, and her color improved, the yellow-brown having disappeared.

No evidence of joint swelling could be observed, and even the ulnar and tibial nodules beneath the skin were gone, and further, she had no evidence of liver enlargement or swelling of the liver.

Since the mucous membrane in her mouth had responded slowly, her niacinamide intake was increased to one capsule every 3-1/2 hours for 5 daily doses (900 mg/24 hours).

Jane Trowbridge Is Cured

On the 417th day her Joint Range Index and laboratory tests were further improved.

At this time Jane became euphoric and could not remember when she'd felt so well. She was physically and mentally vigorous, her voice clear, resonant and decisive. She reported a renewed interest in being with people and in entertaining guests.

Jane looked younger than when first seen, appearing to be closer to 60 than to 80 years of age. She was entirely free from bone and joint symptoms and had not taken any aspirin for 8 months. She could walk up and down stairs without difficulty and without any sense of physical impairment or exhaustion. Her carriage was erect, although she still had some moderate curvature of the spine. Her skin was smoother, softer, less wasted and more elastic than when first examined. She had no noticeable joint swellings or deformities, no liver tenderness or enlargement, and the mucous membranes of her mouth were recovering much more rapidly.[13]

Osteoarthritis (and rheumatoid arthritis) is an "uncurable degenerative disease," a natural condition of growing old.

Right?

Wrong!

Had Jane Trowbridge followed the directions recommended by traditional treatments for osteoarthritis (or rheumatoid arthritis) she more than likely would have become crippled. Worse, she'd also be suffering from many of the toxic side-effects that accompany the use of drugs used simply to suppress symptoms without eliminating the cause of the symptoms.

Through familial loyalty and love to her sister, Jane placed herself under severe stress. Her diet laxed, and the quality of her own nutrition became poor while she administered to her beloved sister. In time her body complained and the first signs of osteoarthritis appeared, that of stiffness, and some weakness.

At Jane's age, as has happened to tens of thousands of others, Jane should have resigned herself to a "natural" aging state, but she didn't, fortunately, having sought and found help from a remarkably creative and perceptive doctor.

More than likely what Jane was able to do with the correct advice, you, too, can do.

There are many paths possible for destroying our physical health -- and many paths also for restoring that health. The scope and message of this book will introduce you to some of those wonderful, successful health-building approaches.

What is Osteoarthritis?

Symptoms of Osteoarthritis

The symptoms of osteoarthritis are: bone proliferation at joint margins; deadening of bone beneath cartilage; enlarged, heated joints; grating of bone on bone; joint instability; limitation of joint movements; painful gelatinous cysts; sometimes defective sense of balance; and swollen membranes such as on the tongue and other locations.

Although Jane had some of the symptoms of rheumatoid arthritis, she clearly suffered from osteoarthritis the most common form of joint disease. (The terms "osteoarthritis," "osteoarthrosis," and "degenerative joint disease" are often used interchangeably.)

Osteoarthritis involves loss of joint cartilage, death of cells beneath the cartilage and also cartilage and bone proliferation at the joint margins with bony growth formations. Osteoarthritis often includes inflammation of the tissue around the fluid-filled sacs (bursae) surrounding joints -- which would otherwise be subject to friction without these sacs -- and tendon sheaths (synovium).

Distribution of Osteoarthritis

Estimates of the number of Americans like Jane Trowhouser who suffer from osteoarthritis vary from 20 million to 40 million.

According to Thomas J.A. Lehman, M.D., Chief, Division of Pediatric Rheumatology, The Hospital for Special Surgery, and Associate Professor of Pediatrics, Cornell University Medical Center,[3] one child in every thousand in a given year will be affected by arthritis. . . . one child in every ten thousand will have more severe arthritis that doesn't just go away.

The American College of Rheumatology reports that, "Osteoarthritis accounts for more than seven million doctor visits per year and 36 million work days lost. Annualized costs of treatment for all types of arthritis were estimated to be $17.5 billion in 1987. Osteoarthritis of the knee alone in elderly Americans accounts for at least as much disability as other chronic conditions, including congestive heart failure, diabetes, heart disease, hip fracture, chronic obstructive pulmonary disease or depression."[3]

Perhaps one-half of those who live long enough will suffer from some degree of osteoarthritis.[1,2,3]

Robert M. Giller, M.D. and Kathy Matthews,[62] author of *Natural Prescriptions*, estimate that 80% of those over fifty years of age will have some degree of osteoarthritis.

The large variation in the estimate in numbers who suffer, or will suffer, from osteoarthritis probably stems from how severe the disease must become before it is noticed and tallied.

Although both men and women may suffer from osteoarthritis, and both may suffer in the same body parts, generally men suffer more in the lower spine and hip than do women, who suffer more in the cervical spine and fingers.

The main structural protein of the body is collagen. There are as many as twelve types, the most abundant being that which makes up connective tissue, tendons, bones, and skin. Osteoarthritis is commonly called "degenerative arthritis," because the condition seems to come with the wear and tear that accompanies the aging process. According to this theory, the cumulative affects of decades of joint use lead to degenerative changes by stressing the collagen matrix of the joint cartilage. While this theory may have some merit, the condition is actually much more involved than this simple view presents. Nutritionist Carlton Fredericks, Ph.D., for example, reasonably argued that a correlation between age and osteoarthritis does not necessarily mean that age causes osteoarthritis.[44]

There's more than one kind of osteoarthritis, and subsets within some categories, but, as with other disease classifications, there is chiefly a (1) primary (idiopathic) osteoarthritis, and (2) secondary osteoarthritis.

Genetic Marker

Darwin J. Prockop, M.D. and his co-workers at Jefferson Medical College in Philadelphia, Pennsylvania uncovered one clue to the underlying cause of osteoarthritis. Examining an extended family of 19 spanning three generations, they found that nine members developed osteoarthritis in the fingers, elbows, hips, and knees by their 20s or 30s, an age far younger than the usual onset of the disorder after age 40 or 50.

The researchers discovered a protein called "type II pro-collagen," which forms coils that intertwine in groups of three to build the cartilage that protects bone ends and reduces the friction in joints. A defective gene responsible for instruction to cartilage cells to manufacture collagen causes the triple fibrils in the arthritis sufferers in this family to unravel after 20 to 30 years, causing the cartilage to wear down and therefore no longer providing a protective cushion.[75]

While this genetic marker may apply only to the family studied, it is a clue substantiating the feeling that those suffering from osteoarthritis may do so because they also have a genetic factor involved.

Clinical Symptoms of Primary Osteoarthritis

As pictured in *Figure 1: Names of Joints of Right Hand*, joints most commonly affected are those closest to the fingernails -- the last phalanges of fingers (distal interphalangeal) -- with hard nodules or enlargements of bone (tubercles) called "Heberden's nodes," second joints from the end of the fingers (proximal interphalangeal) with hard nodules or enlargements called "Bouchard's nodes," the second joints of the foot (bunion: metarsophalangeal), spine, hips and knees.

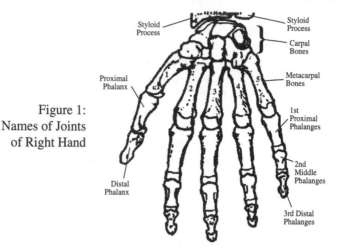

Figure 1:
Names of Joints
of Right Hand

Pain is the principal symptom associated with osteoarthritis. As there are few nerve endings in joint cartilage, pain arises from joint capsules, ligaments, adjacent tendons, or muscles surrounding joints, and from bone, usually when the joints are moved or bear weight.

As the disease progresses, even small motions or weights can produce pain, during which use of the joint becomes limited.

Rest, conversely, relieves the pain.

When pain becomes great, muscle spasms may become continuous, unrelieved by rest. They may awaken the patient at night, or may occur spontaneously even in non-weight bearing situations.

Joint stiffness may occur after periods of rest and it is important to distinguish these from the usual morning stiffness associated with inflammatory joint disease, such as rheumatoid arthritis. Joint stiffness, on arising, is usually of short duration, unless the disease has progressed considerably. (See Chapter II, Rheumatoid Arthritis.)

In an advanced state, pain is often referred from -- for example -- the knee to the hip. Spinal pain may also appear elsewhere, as referred pain, as nerve root compression occurs from bony structures, called "osteophytes," that grow along the spine.

Inflammation of the fluid that surrounds the joint cavity, bursa, or tendon sheath may be associated with osteoarthritis. Usually such inflammation is low-grade unless a form of crystal lodges in the lining of the tendon sheath, the "synovium."

Joint tenderness often occurs, especially over joint margins where bony outgrowths -- osteophytes -- have formed.

In advanced stages, bones will grate on bones, called "crepitus." As joint space narrows, due to loss of cartilage and fluids, pain becomes more frequent, and more severe.

Muscular atrophy, weakness and limitation of range of motion may lead to malalignment of the joints, especially weight-bearing joints, such as the knee, producing a "knock-kneed" or bow-legged stance. There are generally no systemic characteristics associated with osteoarthritis, such as there are in inflammatory joint diseases, like rheumatoid arthritis, although obviously there are enzyme and other metabolic systems affecting the overall functioning of the body. But, there are no symptoms of weight loss or fever, nor will the white blood count or red blood (erythrocyte) sedimentation rate be elevated. ["Sedimentation rate" is simply the rate at which red blood cells drop to the bottom of a test tube. The red blood cell (erythrocyte) sedimentation rate, often signals probability of the presence or absence of an infection.]

In the "nodal" forms of osteoarthritis, bony swellings called, Heberden's or Bouchard's nodes, may appear with early evidence of swelling, redness, localized warmth, and tenderness.

During early growth of outgrowths, or "osteophytes" there can be considerable pain and discomfort. If this pain is also coupled with inflammation, or joint infection, then a great deal of confusion can result between osteoarthritis and an inflammatory form of rheumatoid disease, such as rheumatoid arthritis. See Chapter II, Rheumatoid Arthritis.

By the time X-ray of joint damage is easily viewed, the disease may have progressed considerably, and therefore X-ray plates are relatively insensitive for purposes of early diagnosis.

Patients with abnormal X-ray pictures of the spine may have no symptoms whatsoever, or the symptoms may occur wherever the bony outgrowths; i.e., osteophytes, have compressed a nerve root, and already refer the pain to another location of the body.

Subsets of Osteoarthritis

There are two forms or subsets of osteoarthritis: "nodal" and "non-nodal."

Nodal Osteoarthritis

In primary osteoarthritis, normally the joints affected by bony nodes are those closest to the fingernails (distal), and the second joint from the fingernails (interphalangeal). Woman may show these affects more often than men, and localized inflammatory changes may be pronounced. Activity may become so great as to destroy the joints with the growth of spurs and cysts. Wrist, toe and spinal joints may also become involved, leading to joint deformity and fusing of the joint (ankylosis). (See *Figure 1: Names of Joints of Right Hand*)

As women after menopause are affected most frequently, there is presumed to be a hormonal relationship.

As with any form of osteoarthritis, the hand, wrist, spine and feet may be affected both by deformities and loss of function.

Non-Nodal Osteoarthritis

The non-nodal form of osteoarthritis most often affects men, with hand and wrist most frequently involved.

While the lack of nodes can be distinguished from nodal osteoarthritis, the two subsets of arthritis are probably otherwise indistinguishable.

Chondrocalcinosis

Metabolic or degenerative changes in tissue will sometimes deposit a chemical substance (calcium pyrophosphate dihydrate crystal) which causes a form of crystalline inflammation of the lubricating membrane of the joints, the synovial membrane (synovitis), called "chondrocalcinosis." This is also called "pseudogout," because of resemblance to gouty arthritis, a painful joint condition that is also thought to be of metabolic origin where deposits of uric acid crystals (monosodium urate) drop out of solution from the blood, and deposit in and about joints and tendons. (As causative of gout, the latest research indicts a mycoplasm, a bacteria without a definite cell wall.)

Chondrocalcinosis is determined -- after intermittent attacks of acute arthritis and from X-ray examination -- with the finding of evidence of nodules of calcium salts under the skin, muscles, tendons and nerves (calcinosis) of the joints.

Chondrocalcinosis is frequently associated with other conditions such as osteoarthritis, diabetes mellitus, excess thyroid (hyperparathyroidisim), gout, and a skin condition involving an excess if deposits of iron throughout the body (hemochromatosis).

The disease develops in maturity, and affects both sexes equally. Over 50 years of age the incidence is appreciable. Unexplained acute or subacute attacks of arthritis occur, usually in the peripheral joints: legs, arms, feet, hands.

There is a suggestion that deposits of calcium pyrophosphate dihydrate in the cartilage is secondary to degenerative changes in the joint.

Attacks follow the pattern of uric acid gout, but are less severe, with complete freedom between attacks. At other times, distress persists, with low-grade symptoms similar to rheumatoid arthritis. (See Chapter II, Rheumatoid Arthritis.)

Symptoms may persist intermittently for life.

Other Subsets of Osteoarthritis

There are additional subsets or forms of non-nodal osteoarthritis, but each of them may involve similar affects on the body, or be mixed with previously defined osteoarthritic forms.

Clinical Symptoms of Secondary Osteoarthritis

There are numerous secondary factors that will alter joint surfaces and the functioning of joints, which include mechanical, biologic, biochemical, and enzymatic feedback loops involving seven categories: metabolism, trauma, endocrine imbalances, infectious or other forms of inflammation, mal-functioning nervous system, faulty development of the skeletal structure, and diseased or dying tissues. None of these conditions should be viewed as independent causes for osteoarthritis, as an interrelationship of functions is common, resulting in a complex system of interacting relationships.

These seven categories may lead to seven subsets of secondary osteoarthritis that develop as a secondary complication. Rheumatoid arthritis, for example, which displays with inflammation at the joint, may also affect the joint with manifestations of secondary osteoarthritis. (See Chapter II, Rheumatoid Arthritis.)

Heritable or developmental bone problems may produce mechanical bone stresses unnatural to the design of the skeleton, also resulting in secondary osteoarthritis.

Thus, trauma, disease, diet, metabolic and all the other factors can be involved in producing a form of secondary osteoarthritis.

Traditional Treatments

Traditional treatment involves (1) reassurance to the patient, (2) outlining of management goals; encouraged to participate in self-management programs, (3) advice on the use of canes, crutches or walkers to protect weight-bearing joints, (4) weight reduction where required, (5) relief of pain and muscle spasms by use of hot packs, electric pads or warm soaks for 15 to 30 minutes twice a day, (6) isometric exercises -- placing tension on muscles without changing their length -- to maintain muscle tone and build muscle power two to three times per day, increasing gradually to 10 or 15 repetitions at a time, (7) advice that isotonic exercises -- shortening muscles while applying equal tension on them -- while maintaining range of motion, may damage joints, (8) aspirin or other forms of pain-relieving medicine (analgesics), (9) other kinds of pain-relieving drugs that do not contain corticosteroids (substances derived from adrenaline glands), called non-steroidal anti-inflammatory drugs (often four times a day), such as acetaminophan, ibuprofen (Motrin®, Advil®), naproxen (Naprosyn®), piroxicam (Feldene®), and others, (10) use of corticosteroids inside the joint capsule for symptomatic relief when necessary during acute flare-ups, (11) occasional use of traction, neck (cervical) collars, or back-of-the-loins (lumbodorsal) corsets to relieve cervical and lumbodorsal spinal symptoms.

When the above treatments are no longer effective, then the following treatments may be employed, together or in combinations: (1) removal of foreign material and dead or dying tissue from a joint, (2) surgery on a bone, or partial removal of a bone, (3) fusion of joints, (4) joint replacement, or (5) other forms of surgery.

What's Wrong With Traditional Treatments?

Traditional treatments address only the symptoms of the disease, not its source or cause.

Clearly, where weight reduction is useful, and walkers and canes are necessary, and where management goals and patient reassurance calms and effectively directs the patient, these are all extremely helpful healing tools. Where one kind of exercise is damaging and the other kind helps to maintain tone and muscle strength during the progress of the disease, it would be clearly inadvisable not to follow preferred recommendations.

Dr. William L. Henrich,[95] a member of the National Kidney Foundation scientific advisory board, says, "I think the public has a perception that medicines you can purchase over-the-counter in drugstores and grocery stores are inherently safe. This is clearly not so. . . . Taking an analgesic, or painkiller, daily for as long as three years or in too large a dose can cause inflammation, followed by scarring of the kidney and the loss of kidney function. The usual recommended dosage of a painkiller is two tablets, three or four times a day, for no more than three days.

"As much as 8 to 10 percent of new cases of chronic kidney failure may be related to the misuse of painkillers."

Aspirin and other analgesics are sometimes useful for the purpose of temporarily alleviating joint pain, but their use in the long run simply hides the disease progress, and delays recognition of a system in imbalance that needs serious correction and concentrated attention.

Acetaminophens, a slightly bitter, white, odorless, crystalline powder, non-opiate, non-salicylate chemical, is mixed with many other substances such as Tylenol®, Excedrin®, and other formulations commonly sold over the counter (without prescription) for allergies, sinus, pain relief, cough syrups, and so on. While safer than some other drugs that might be used, acetaminophens have been linked to liver disease in patients who consume excessive amounts of alcohol. Long-term use of both acetaminophens and other drugs used for pain relief not based on cortisone, called non-steroidal anti-inflammatory drugs, can increase the risk of kidney failure.

Prolonged use of non-steroidal anti-inflammatory drugs (NSAIDs) such as acetaminophan, ibuprofen (Motrin®, Advil®), naproxen (Naprosyn®), piroxicam (Feldene®), and others, actually appears to contribute to the progression of osteoarthritis.

According to a report in *The New York Times*, "About 3.4 percent of the 2.2 billion prescriptions written each year are for non-steroidal anti-inflammatory drugs (NSAIDs). Millions more nonprescription NSAIDs are bought as over-the-counter drugs . . . . On any day, 10 to 15 percent of Americans aged 65 and older have a filled prescription for an NSAID. . . . "

An associate commissioner of the FDA, Dr. Stuart Nightingale, cited studies that showed that bleeding ulcers develop in about 1 percent of those who use the drugs for three to six months, and from 2 to 4 percent of those who use them for a year. Other studies have shown that those who use the drugs have a greater risk by a factor of four of developing an ulcer than nonusers in all age groups. Additional complications of this drug usage leads to 30 percent of the hospitalizations and deaths from ulcers in people aged 65 and older in this country. (A bacterium, *Helicobacter pylori*, causes the remaining 70 percent.) "It appears that you are at about the same risk in the first month of taking an NSAID as in the 12th or 24th, not getting any worse or better."

Describing the use of pain-killing medications, Sherry A. Rogers, M.D., Syracuse, New York practitioner and author of many health-oriented books, says, "Studies show that the pain relief effect is greater in the first few weeks of treatment and then gradually wears off. This leads people to explore the use of other pain medications often and waste a lot of money evaluating many types of nonsteroidal anti-inflammatory drugs and other pain medicines." The use of these nonsteroidal anti-inflammatory drugs "actually hasten[s] the deterioration of cartilage, . . . they have many other nasty effects of their own."[102]

Regarding traditional recommendations for joint replacements, Jack M. Blount, M.D., Philadelphia, MS, one of the founders of the non-profit, charitable The Arthritis Trust of America, and also a former victim of rheumatoid arthritis having had hip-joint replacement, feels that "If joint replacement is a necessary lesser evil of two, then joint replacement should be accepted, <u>especially after all other remedies have been researched.</u>"[82]

Besides the clear dangers of traditional treatments, the basic problem, as has already been stated, is that in no instance does the patient perceive advice from traditional practitioners that holds out the hope of slowing down or reversing the progress of the disease. Trying anything else that is safe, although not effective, may, in the long run, be better for the patient's mood, attitude and disposition -- and possibly health -- than accepting hearsay about the "inevitable."

Virtually all of the foregoing traditional treatments strive to suppress pain symptoms while teaching patient endurance through increasingly restrictive ranges of motion and pain. Such traditional treatments say, in effect, "We don't know how to solve your problem. Go home and suffer! Learn to live with your increasing limitations, and especially your pain and degeneration of tissues."

This book will provide you with numerous opportunities to halt or reverse these so-called "inevitable" degenerative processes.

What Causes Osteoarthritis?

As osteoarthritis appears to be caused by a combination of factors -- hormonal deficiencies, faulty nutrition, stress, infection, deficient enzymes -- each of these should be attended to.

According to Louis J. Marx, M.D., after nutrition, chronic infections are the second most important factor in osteoarthritis.

The third factor is body pollution which invites infections, damages the immune system, and generally interferes with regeneration of tissues. These pollutants are chemicals in our food and all sorts of environmental poisons.

"Of course, each person must be individually evaluated to determine what set of causative agents are involved in the person's disorder."[92]   Although there are certain treatments that may help a majority of osteoarthritics, there is no *one* standard treatment modality that will help a majority of arthritics. According to Robert Atkins, M.D., "The flaw in the logic is pigeonholing. The idea of reducing a multifaceted disorder into a single category will not work with arthritis, and many other illnesses, for that matter. To practice medicine well we should understand causation, not diagnosis."[61]

Female hormonal deficiencies -- estrogen (estradiol), testosterone, progesterone and dehydroepiandrosterone (DHEA) -- certainly play their part, as one-third more women suffer from osteoarthritis after menopause than do men.

Thyroid deficiencies can also contribute to osteoarthritis in both men and women because proper systemic thyroid functioning determines our temperature (cellular temperature), which then determines efficient utilization of all important enzymes, chemical catalysts that promote proper functioning of every human system.

Faulty nutrition (including enzyme deficiencies) and stress must also play their fair share, as probably do genetic predisposing factors.

As will be explained in this book, a major cause of osteoarthritis is physical or bio-chemical damage to key nerve tissue that results in nerve signals to muscles around joints becoming overly tense. As cartilage within each joint has very little blood supply of its own, it must receive its nourishment from the sponge-like action of squeezing and expansion which draws up nutrition-filled blood, and squeezes out the blood, along with waste products.

There are many practitioners who look at the nature of arthritis, and its accompanying psycho-emotional state, and conclude that such individuals derive their increasingly frozen joints from the chronic condition of anger, or even suppressed hostility.

L. Ron Hubbard, founder of the philosophy of The Church of Scientology, author of numerous books and articles containing 40,000,000 words on mind/emotion/body phenomena, in *Science of Survival*,[104] for example, classifies arthritis as a depository disease associated with emotions of violent and expressed anger or unexpressed resentment and fear. Such a person will hold onto motion from his environment, freeze it, and the result will be a crystalization of immovable joint structures.

Those with some form of arthritis suffer considerably, and the very act of moving creates pain and consequent depression and lethargy.

With freedom from pain, whether temporarily or permanently, temperament vastly improves. To argue that psychological traits have induced arthritis may be quite valid, as thought determines emotion, which determines the body's physical ability to move. But it may be equally valid to argue that a body unable to function properly due to biochemical constraints will also produce emotion of expressed or unexpressed hostility.

There is never but one path to wellness as with the question of which comes first, the chicken or the egg, one must look inside for truth and answer for one's self whether to tackle the body, the mind, or both aspects to insure wellness.

As already mentioned, prevailing general medical theory suggests that osteoarthritis may be divided into two categories, primary and secondary.

In primary osteoarthritis, the degenerative 'wear-and-tear' process occurs after ages fifty to sixty with no, or little, apparent abnormalities, and with no known predisposing factors. According to traditional views, the invisible cumulative effects of years of use leads to the degenerative changes by stressing the collagen matrix of the cartilage. As with all evidence of aging, the rate at which we repair or replace damaged or worn out cells does not quite keep up with the rate at which worn out cells are discarded. Damage to the cartilage also results in the release of enzymes that destroy collagen components. With aging, the ability to restore and synthesize normal collagen structures is decreased.

While the 'wear-and-tear' view contains some truth, it does not explain how some octagenerians retain pain-free fluidity of joints, or how some actually restore normal functioning after what appears to be one-way permanent changes.

Secondary osteoarthritis is associated with some predisposing factor which is responsible for the degenerative changes including: congenital abnormalities in joint structure or function (hypermobility and abnormally shaped joint surfaces); trauma (obesity, fractures along joint surfaces, surgery, etc.); crystal deposition; presence of abnormal cartilage; and previous inflammatory disease of joints (rheumatoid arthritis, gout, infectious (septic) arthritis, etc.)

In the view of traditional medicine, many forms of secondary arthritis may also be irreversible. This determination can only be made on an individual basis, and surely should not be made without thought to the broad range of new and effective treatments available, once the dogmas of tradition are refused.

Causation of Arthritis According to F. Batmanghelidj, M.D.

Water Treatment and Body Thirst Signals

As a result of many years of clinical and scientific research, F. Batmanghelidj, M.D., who received his training at St. Mary's Hospital

Medical School of London University, developed an elegantly simple explanation and hypotheses for prevention and cure of arthritic pains and many other common diseases. (See Dr. Batmanghelidj's *Your Body's Many Cries for Water* & *Prevent Arthritis and Cure Back Pain.*)

Dr. Batmanghelidj holds that "The separation of low back pain from rheumatoid joint pains elsewhere in the body is inaccurate. The mechanisms of pain producing in these joint conditions seems to be the same. They denote the same physiological phenomenon in the body . . . For the one, one goes to a rheumatologist and for the other to an orthopedic surgeon or a chiropractor. The outcome is the same in both, pain management rather than its cure. Basically both conditions have the same pathology, except they are in different locations."[40]

According to Dr. Batmanghelidj, chronic recurring pain of the lower spine and joints of the hand and legs "is a signal of water deficiency in the area where the pain is felt."[40,41] A deficiency in water circulation prohibits the acidity and toxic substances to wash out from the affected area, and the pain is a cry from part of your body for more water.

Low back pain is composed of a muscle spasm and disc cartilage degeneration. The muscle spasm is very much like that described by Roger Wyburn-Mason, M.D., Ph.D. and Dr. Paul K. Pybus as a reflex arc from the spinal column to the joint, which creates the tension in joints leading to insufficient cartilage nourishment. The degeneration of cartilage is a secondary effect of the lack of appropriate nourishment, in this case, water. (See this chapter on Structure.)

Cartilage consists of large components of water, and water is necessary in joints for padding, and to provide a smooth, frictionless gliding surface upon which joints can operate. Lack of sufficient water intake leads to prolonged dehydration in the cartilage, which creates friction and sheering stress at the joint's points of contact.

The joint environment is normally alkaline, but under dehydration, becomes acidic, and the acidity sensitizes nerve endings that will register pain. Lack of water at the joint cartilage not only decreases gliding ability, but sends out a signal of alarm -- pain -- otherwise the cartilage would die and peel off from contact surfaces.

During the process of "shunting more circulation to the joint through its outer capsule, for its lubrication and repair process, pain is also produced. This joint pain is an indicator of local dehydration and the inability of the joints to cope with the extra demands for its movement."[40]

Salt -- sodium chloride -- helps to wash out the acidity in the cells of joint cartilage, and such activity is a continuous process, and so, therefore, both water and salt are essential for treatment and reduction of joint pain, whether the pain has been labeled as osteoarthritis, or rheumatoid arthritis.

When joint cartilage begins to decompose through high acidity and abrasive action, the body's ability to repair is accompanied by the secretion of powerful hormones to stimulate repair activity. According to Dr. Batmanghelidj, Several things happen when these hormones are secreted.

1. The dying tissue is broken up from inside the cells and the broken fragments are extruded only to be ingested by the "garbage collectors" and to be recycled.

2. More blood circulation is brought to the area, even if it has to come to the nearest sites in the fibrous capsule covering the joint. It is the swelling and stretch in the joint capsule that causes stiffness and eventually added pain.

3. There is an associated protein breakdown and more amino acids are mobilized for the "pool" that may be needed for the repair of the damage.

4. In the inflammatory environment inside the joint, some white cells begin to manufacture hydrogen peroxide and ozone for two obvious purposes. One, to keep the joint space sterilized and prevent bacteria from infecting the joint cavity. Two, to supply with adequate oxygen to the cells that are engaged in the repair process and, because of their local isolation and the stagnant nature of the inflammatory exudates, have less of an access to the blood oxygen.

5. There is a local 'remodeling growth factor' that promotes the growth of tissue along the line of greater force.

6. Knowledge gained from its on-going experience by the brain is put to use for the rest of the body. The remodeling and 'fortification' of the other similarly structured joints will also be carried out. This seems to be the reason why rheumatoid joints of the hands will often show a mirror image inflammation and eventual deviation of the actual joints on both sides.[40]

Dr. Batmanghelidj reports that seventy-five percent of the weight on bearing surfaces of each joint vertebrae is held up by the hydraulic properties of the discs between them. When not drinking sufficient water on a regular basis, the body mass squeezes the vertebral discs, they become less supportive, less easy to move, and, in their dehydrated condition, can shift so that they press on local nerves. "This pain is called sciatic pain and is far more serious than the local pain in the back. It means the spinal joint structure has become so disorganized that one of the discs that have to shock absorb for the spine -- 95% of cases the lowest lumbar disc . . . is now out of its normal position and is pressing on the nerve."[40]

When dehydration becomes more severe, facet joints, "four small vertically positioned joints, two on either side of the back of each vertebra," become weight-bearing, contrary to their design intent.

Osteoarthritis results when "cartilage in the joint dies, the bone to bone contact begins, be it in the back, the legs, or the hands. Whereas the cartilage cells had a water-given resilience and survived the trauma of movement against one another, the hardened bone surfaces produce an inflammatory process that destroys the bone surfaces. Thus osteoarthritis of the joint will establish a second stage process to dehydration that first destroyed the cartilage surfaces."[40]

Dr. Batmanghelidj recommends at least two quarts of water daily. This daily intake does not include "caffeine-containing fluids and alcoholic beverages that further dehydrate the body."

"Water should be taken at regular intervals. Its intake should become a habit. One cannot rely on the thirst perception to recognize the urgency to drink water. As we grow older, we lose our thirst perception. . . . My rule of thumb: for every ten 8-ounce glasses of water one should add about 1/2-1/4 teaspoon of salt to the daily diet; if the food is already salty, the lesser amount. If the food is bland, the full measure. Frequent cramps in the leg muscles should be taken to mean salt shortage in the body.

"With the new information about the emergency calls of the body for water -- and the role of water and salt in the integrity of joint functions -- I can predict a virtual disappearance of back pain and rheumatoid joint pains as we enter the 21st Century."[40]

Alternative Treatments for Osteoarthritis

In addition to Dr. Batmanghelidj's recommendations, treatment and prevention for osteoarthritis -- or osteoarthritis-like symptoms -- can be divided into five general components: treatment for (1) nutritional deficiencies (and water), (2) defective skeletal structure, (3) pain, (4) hormonal imbalances, and (5) mind/body influences.

There are -- apparently -- four major aspects to treatment of osteoarthritis: restore proper nutrition (and water), relieve stress, detoxify, and replace hormones.

The Case of Robert "Bob" Kelley

When Robert Atkins, M.D. was asked for medical help by sixty-six-year-old Bob Kelley, Bob had already been a patient of a highly competent alternative physician with complaints of severe "shooting pains" in both knees.

Bob's diet was satisfactory, and his health otherwise excellent, in part because of the vitamin and mineral supplementation treatments he'd already received, but his pain had not disappeared. However, he'd had serious medical problems in the past, including coronary bypass surgery.

Bob Kelley had been told to exercise, so he'd taken up walking, doing two miles each day, but now walking had become painful, which frightened and concerned him. The lack of exercise would adversely affect his heart, whereas, the walking adversely affected his knees.

Bob received the Atkins Center standard evaluation, which included a glucose tolerance test that indicated hypoglycemia, a condition of low blood sugar. It was also discovered that he was sensitive to nightshades, yeast, cheese, wheat, mushrooms, broccoli, carrots, oranges, and vinegar. (See Chapter II, "General Dietary Recommendations for the Rheumatoid Arthritic," Rheumatoid Arthritis.)

Dr. Atkins used his Center's anti-arthritic nutritional formula -- a combination of nutrients that combine B_6, niacinamide, pantothentic acid, para-aminobenzoic acid (PABA), bioflavonoids, zinc, and copper -- adding in Vitamin C, extra vitamin E and cod-liver oil, but he also took Bob Kelley off of the foods to which Kelley had shown a sensitivity. (Later Dr. Atkins added selenium and L-cysteine, and manganese, to his Center's arthritic formula.)

In a week after the food allergies had been identified, Bob was walking with but mild discomfort. When he tested the foods again, his pains returned.

By the second week of removal from foods to which he'd become sensitive, Bob Kelley's pains had totally disappeared, and they have not returned.

Bob walks long distances, and has added bicycling and gardening to his exercise program. Dr. Atkins reports that "If you didn't know that Bob had undergone serious cardiac surgery, you would probably guess he was a good ten to fifteen years younger than his sixty-six years. I can't honestly say now whether what I've done for Bob constituted a cure or a remission, but he is still well."[61]

Like Bob Kelley, you want relief from pain, and freedom once again to move. In the treatments that follow will be one or more that will most likely provide you with the relief desired. We've categorized these treatments into (1) proper diet and nutrition, (2) useful botanicals, (3) body energy medicine practices, (4) body structure problems, (5) and stress.

Nutrition and Supplements
Boron

One mineral that may be of great importance in the treatment and prevention of osteoarthritis is boron. Dr. Rex E. Newnham, Ph.D., D.O., N.D. of Leeds, England, teacher, naturopath, nutritionist, osteopath and homeopath, demonstrated through the uneven distribution of boron in different regions of the world, and later clinical trials, demographic and clinical evidence for the usefulness of Boron in preventing and treating osteoarthritis and some forms of rheumatoid disease, including rheumatoid arthritis.[12]

According to Dr. Newnham, clinical trials at Royal Melbourne Hospital demonstrated that 70% of those who completed the trial received much help from boron tablets; and the U.S. Human Nutrition Research Center in North Dakota showed that boron works through the parathyroid to stop or reduce calcium loss in woman who suffer from osteoporosis, that is, weakened bone structure. "Boron also helps to increase the natural hormones in older women, to normal." Bone fractures also heal in about half normal time.

Flouridated water, besides contributing to osteoporosis, and other degenerative diseases, including skeletal fluorosis (which many doctors wrongly call "arthritis"), without in any way helping the teeth or bones, also is a natural antagonist to boron, and so Dr. Newnham recommends removing the flouride from your water if you are to get benefit from boron. If you make tea with flouridated water, there will be much more fluoride in your tea than the cold water alone.[12,45]

For arthritis, rheumatism and osteoporosis, Dr. Newnham recommends the use of tablets containing boron (sodium tetraborate) and other vitamins, minerals and supplements. Such a mixture he has patented under the name of Osteo Trace™ and B-Alive™ .

The exact formulations for Osteo Trace and B-Alive are the following:

Osteo Trace:

Magnesium ascorbate	200 mg
Calcium ascorbate	100 mg
Sodium tetraborate	27 mg (boron = 3 mg)
Vitamin B_6	20 mg (pyridoxine)
Nictoinamide	10 mg
Vitamin B_5	10 mg (calcium pantothenate)
Devil's Claw	5 mg (*Harpagophytum procumbens*)
Kelp	5 mg
Zinc gluconate	15 mg (zinc = 2.2mg)
Manganese gluconate	15 mg (manganese = 1.2mg)
Copper gluconate	2 mg (copper = 0.3mg)
Selenium	30 mcg (sodium selenite)
Molybdenum	25 mcg (sodium molybdenate)
Vitamin B_{12}	3 mcg (cyanocobalamin)

Inert ingredients (excipients) are di-calcium phosphate, cellulose, magnesium stearate, and silica. Silica may also be an active ingredient.

B-Alive: This is the same as above, except that 300 mg of vitamin C (ascorbates), magnesite or magnesium carbonate is used, as younger people have more stomach acid and can handle the magnesium carbonate well, but older people have less acid, in which case the Osteo-Trace is better.

Calcium fluoride, 1 mcg, on the label is a homeopathic remedy (6X) chiefly to help remove fluorides from the body.

Dr. Newnham sells Osteo-Trace in the United States, but not B-Alive, although the latter can be ordered from England.

Osteo Trace™ can be obtained through: Dr. Don Breen, 2427 East High St., Springfield, OH 45505; (513) 324-1110; Joe Gibbs, NRG Products Ltd., PO Box 264, Webb City, MO 64870; (417) 673-5414; Rex Newnham, D.O., Ph.D., N.D., Cracoe House Cottage, Cracoe,

Skifton, North Yorkshire, England BD23 6LB.

Dr. Newnham recommends 3 tablets a day, one with each meal, if under 168 pounds, 4 tablets a day if over 168 pounds but under 210 pounds, and 5 tablets a day if over 210 pounds. For children between 50 and 100 pounds weight, he recommends 2 tablets per day, and infants under 20 pounds only half a tablet per day. Dr. Newnham advises 1 tablet for every 25 kilograms or 60 pounds of body weight, or part thereof. "Those who drink fluoridated water could well add another tablet per day because fluoride and boron are natural antagonists."[12] (See Chapter II, "Boron," Rheumatoid Arthritis.)

Dr. Newnham's[12] follow-up of numerous patients shows that many are improved through the use of boron:

The Case of Iris Anderson

Iris Anderson was aged eighty-one. Because of arthritis, she could not get up steps without help. After a course of Osteo-Trace™ she could move freely up and down steps, and she could even bend down and touch the floor with the palm of her hands.

The Case of Mary Lamb

Polymyalgia rheumatica is a chronic, generalized inflammatory rheumatic disease of the large arteries. Mary Lamb, seventy, had polymyalgia rheumatica and was given high doses of steroids that relieved some pain, but when she reduced the dose, the pain returned. Now, with the use of boron, her pain is gone.

The Case of Tom Boyd

Tom Boyd, forties, had arthritis in both hands for a period of eighteen months, which made it difficult to work. He used boron and had a complete cure.

The Case of Mrs. Brooks

Mrs. Brooks had arthritis for nine years, with degeneration of both back and hips. Pain when walking or climbing steps went from extreme to severe, to moderate, to mild, to none, when she took boron. She could then take her weight on both legs and could walk or climb steps freely. A very satisfied user.

The Case of Bert Clare

Bert Clare, sixty-eight, had been a pilot during World War II. During a crash he sustained a broken neck. This largely incapacitated him for many years. He developed arthritis that gave much pain. It took him half an hour to get out of bed at night for the toilet, the pain was so intense. After a few boron tablets, he was able to get out of bed and back again in three or four minutes and there was no pain. This remedy helped him where others had failed completely.

Dr. Newnham reports many other cases with swollen, heated and painful joints that were miraculously cured through the use of the proper mixture of boron and, sometimes, other minerals and vitamins.[12]

Testimonials[73]

Mrs. L.J. O'Neil: "I am feeling so much better since taking boron, the arthritic pain is not so bad as before. In fact, I've not been so well in years."

Joyce Cheetham, age 74: "I had very bad arthritis in my knee. I have been completely cured for over a year."

Mr. K.G. Pounder: "For the past four years I've been using your mineral supplementas a treatment with great success. In fact, it is the only treatment that works."

Mrs. J. Philip: "I noticed that the awful ache in my feet had miraculously gone!"

E.M.F. Swabey: "Incidentally, a friend who is a fruit farmer says that our soil is boron deficient, and they have to add boron to it or their fruit won't store well."

"Generally," Dr. Newnham says, "those under 60-years-of-age get better within a month; those in their sixties take up to two months; and those in their seventies or over take about three months. If they had the osteoarthritis for many years, it sometimes takes longer to correct the problem."[12]

Calcium, Vitamin D_3 and Sunshine
Origin of Research

Over 40 years ago, Carl J. Reich. M.D.,[53,54,55] Ottawa, Canada, discovered the principle that many of the symptoms and diseases of civilization, including various forms of arthritis, could be accounted for on the basis of chronic calcium, vitamin D, and sunshine deficiencies created by specific defects in lifestyle, including diet.

In the beginning of Dr. Reich's private practice in the 1950s, Dr. Reich saw patients exhibiting all the physical signs and symptoms of an overstimulated autonomic nervous system that all too often had been relegated to psychosomatic or all-in-the-head complaints: chronic fatigue, physical weakness, anxiety, sleep disturbances, headaches, cramping of toe, foot, and calf muscles, muscular aches, restless legs, pins and needles sensations of the hands at night time or hands and legs during the day time, bloating and indigestion, chronic diarrhea or chronic constipation, night sweats, and chronic allergic nasal congestion.

An example of the interrelationship of those findings, and their relationship to osteoarthritis and rheumatoid arthritis, may be seen in patients complaining of chronic fatigue and chronic anxiety who also frequently show a pattern of physical signs that sometimes involve irritable and spastic skeletal muscle and intestinal muscle, ridged, or soft, or easily broken fingernails, coated tongues, and an acidic saliva.

To Carl Reich, M.D., a lifestyle pattern of nutritional and sunlight deficiency began to be recognized in patients who experience health problems. Whether or not this pattern was unique to his Canadian climate has not been fully explored. However, his patient's diets were high in meats and starches containing excesses of the acidic minerals sulfur and phosphorus and were low in vegetables, fruits, and milk products containing alkaline minerals of calcium, magnesium, and potassium. Diets were also low in milk and butter that contained natural vitamin D_3 or had been fortified with synthetic vitamin D_2 or natural vitamin D_3. Some other sources of vitamin D are animal liver, egg yolk, and fish.

Modern civilized patterns of working, living, and playing in indoor environments and the wearing of modern clothing that covers everything but hands and face were also recognized as creating vitamin D deficiency by preventing sunlight exposure to large areas of skin. Too much indoor living and dietary deficiencies were part of the pattern of ill health. Modern indoor living had far removed humankind from its heritage of distant ancestors who wore only a loin cloth exposing large areas of the skin to sunlight. Even our immediate ancestors exposed one-and-a-half to two square feet of skin over long periods of working and living outdoors. Modern society, on the other hand, all too often limits the exposure of skin to daylight and sunshine to no more than a half square foot for five minutes as people walk from their cars to work or home.

Dr. Reich knew that some vegetation cells used the ultra violet rays of the sun to photosynthesize a limited amount of vitamin D_2 (ergocalciferol) and that the living cells in the skin and coverings of humans, animals, birds, and fish synthesized vitamin D_3 (cholecalciferol). Vitamin D_3 is metabolized in the liver and then in the kidneys to create vitamin D analogs that assist in intestinal and kidney absorption of calcium, and maintain a balance of calcium stores in bone and an important balance of highly functional free ionic calcium of cells. It is this cellular balancing role of vitamin D that Dr. Reich claims is so critical to health.

In Dr. Reich's words, vitamin D makes calcium "biologically active," through ionization, to be soluble and usable for the body's needs. Dr. Reich theorized that, because of such activity of vitamin D during the early evolution of man, calcium which had been ionized by vitamin D was essential to transfer energy -- liberated by the oxidative process -- for the 1000 or more enzymatic processes scattered throughout each cell.

On that basis, Dr. Reich proposed that chronic ionic calcium deficiency would create energy starvation in the body's cells to create symptoms such as anxiety, fatigue, depression, diarrhea, leg cramps, constipation, asthma, and allergies. Many other disease-states, such as cancer, prostate problems, and arthritis of various kinds would, according to Dr. Reich, reflect a single underlying physical "maladaptative state." Direct physical signs showed up in ridged, layered, softened or cracked finger nails, muscle tenderness and irritability when firmly squeezed or the body tapped (percussed).

Biochemical Inheritance

According to Dr. Reich, a calcium and vitamin D well-nourished parent living in the southern latitudes, where sunshine is more frequent, who complemented their vitamin D by spending significant time outdoors, would experience no physical signs and symptoms of ionic calcium deficiency. A second generation child deprived of outdoor living and sunlight, moving to northern latitudes, where sunshine is less frequent, and deprived of dietary sources of either calcium or vitamin D, might begin to show symptoms. By a third or fourth generation, complaints, physical signs and disease arising because of deficiency, energy starvation -- organ adaptation to that starvation -- might well be in evidence.

Other Factors

According to Dr. Reich, other factors, such as genetic change, other deficiencies and excesses -- and a combination of these factors -- may play an important secondary role in the precipitation of many diseases, including osteoarthritis. Therefore, these many other different factors may dictate which tissue or organ is to be affected by the underlying deficiency diseases.

Moreover, the treatment of one of these secondary factors may induce moderate resolution of the disease in many cases while the primary cause of ionic calcium deficiency is untreated.

Despite such resolution one must not ignore the indications of the existence of an underlying ionic calcium deficiency, creating a disease-prone state.

Case Histories[55]

In 1954-55, case studies led Dr. Reich to see that common diet and lifestyle patterns might account for apparently different diseases among which would be those called "arthritis." Such a pattern indicates that many differently named diseases may, in fact, have the same underlying source-causation.

The Case of Katie Duvain

A dairy-man's wife, Katie Duvain, complained of chronic allergic nasal congestion and diarrhea that became aggravated during the spring. Assuming an allergy association, she was placed on a milk free diet, only to find that leg cramping in a polio-damaged leg became worse. Ten cubic centimeters of calcium gluconate injections were then given intravenously to correct the calcium deficiency created by elimination of dairy products in her diet.

Within days the leg cramping was resolved. At the same time Katie's bowel activity, nasal congestion, and sneezing were unexpectedly and markedly improved. Resolving calcium deficiency easily explained the relief of leg cramping, but improvements in apparently allergy-related nasal problems was puzzling to Dr. Reich. It was clear, though, that calcium had altered the "allergic" reaction.

Warren Levin, M.D., reported that Theron Randolph, M.D., a pioneer in clinical ecological, has observed that, "allergic reactions produce acidity and relief of symptoms requires alkalization." See Chapter II, "Calcium, Vitamin D$_3$, and Sunshine," Rheumatoid Arthritis.)

The Case of Janis Semple

Janis Semple, an 18-year-old female bank clerk who subsisted on a very greasy and milk-poor diet complained of chronic constipation. Using his experience of relieving Katie Duvain's overstimulated muscle spasms creating diarrhea, Dr. Reich attempted the same calcium injections on the bank clerk to find that in only a few days, her constipation was greatly relieved.

The Case of Nora Handle

Dr. Reich had been treating Nora Handle, a middle-aged woman who experienced chronic asthma, with bronchial relaxant and antihistamine drugs and hoped to repeat his success with irritable bowel and leg muscle groups on what he now suspected to be irritable bronchial muscle spasms brought on by calcium deficiency. Within several days of giving her the same injections the chronic asthmatic patient was vastly improved.

The Case of Tom Crosol

A similar pattern of irritable intestinal and skeletal muscle spasms was found in Tom Crosol, a 9-year-old boy subject to chronic asthma since he was two years of age. Irritable muscles of the body and bronchial muscle spasms suggested one pattern. With the boy, Dr. Reich tried supplements of calcium combined with halibut liver oil capsules 3 times a day. The boy experienced a dramatic 80% improvement in his symptoms.

The Case of Mary van Vogt

On Mary van Vogt's first visit to Dr. Reich, she had severe pain in her knees, but prior to that she'd had various joint pains, and she was hospitalized for intravertebral lumbar disc degeneration causing sciatic pain down the left leg, and pain in her shoulders. She walked with great difficulty using a cane. Her knees were moderately swollen and flexion was limited.

Mary had occasional leg cramps, had drunk no milk for years, but recently was drinking 3 glasses each day.

She was taking 25 mg of a non-steroidal anti-inflammatory suppository drug -- a pain-killer taken through absorption in the lower colon -- 2 times daily and diuretics -- a medicine that promotes the secretion of urine -- and potassium supplements. Nutritionally, she was taking some wheat germ, vitamin E, calcium supplements, alfalfa, kelp, and B and C complex 3 times daily.

Dr. Reich advised adding 2 halibut liver oil capsules and 6 drops of Aquasol A & D 3 times daily.

Within six weeks Mary's knees were just as painful, but she felt stronger and healthier. She was instructed to increase her calcium supplements and add 400 units of vitamin E 3 times daily.

Within 3 months Mary discontinued use of her cane, and all inflammation was gone from her knees, but she couldn't kneel. Her shoulders were less painful, and she still experienced weakness in the muscles of her legs.

Within 6 months Mary was able to work in her garden, although she still had some residual knee, shoulder and neck pains.

After 8 months she had no pain in her legs, but they felt weak. Her neck was perfect but her shoulders were slightly to moderately painful.

After 2 years and 2 months of therapy, she visited Holland on an extensive holiday, with only the slightest pain in her legs. She no longer required her anti-inflammatory suppositories and her current therapy consisted of 5 drops of Aquasol A & D, 1 halibut liver oil capsule, 2 tablets of calcium supplements and 1 brewer's yeast 3 times daily, with 100 mg of a non-steroidal anti-inflammatory 2 times daily.

Four years later she had no recurrence of arthritic pains and was reported by another patient, one of her friends, that she'd been seen carrying heavy trays during a Dutch ethnic club dinner!

The Case of Deak Williams

Deak Williams, 70 years of age, complained of constant back pain for years, and also considerable pain in left hip and knees. He had occasional finger cramps, his legs tired easily and he had frequent gas. He drank no milk and did not eat margarine. He'd had a colon surgery (resection) for carcinoma.

In therapy Deak was provided with 2 halibut liver oil capsules, 1 cod liver oil capsule, 6 drops of Aquasol A & D 3 times daily, 1/2 gram of calcium supplement 3 times daily, and 400 units of vitamin E 1 time daily.

Within 4 months Deak Williams' pains were less. He was given a B_{12} injection.

Seven months later he stated that he was fifty percent relieved and that his energy was good.

One year later Deak stated that he rarely had knee, hip or back pain, and that he now only rarely experiences finger cramps, and that his legs are stronger. Each time he received a B_{12} injection, his energy was improved, although Dr. Carl Reich's therapy was actually aimed at relieving calcium and vitamin A & D deficiency.

In osteoarthritis, Reich agreed that the thyroid gland, which produces hormones that control the metabolism of each cell, and parathyroid gland, which controls utilization of calcium, were intimately involved in the generalized drain made on the bone's mineral reserves. As the bones weaken, Reich sees the growth of bone spurs as an attempt to form a bridge between two joints to protect weakened bone. This may be an example of a second adaptive mechanism creating spongy (cancellous) bony spurs trying to rectify a primary deficiency mal-adaptive disease. (Chapter II, "Calcium, Vitamin D_3, and Sunshine," Rheumatoid Arthritis.)

The Litmus Test, Dosages, and Results

In his clinical studies of ionic calcium, vitamin D_3, and sunshine deficiencies, Reich developed a simple test which could easily be used by any arthritic. Based on the results of a saliva alkaline/acid test, one could monitor the progress of his or her own nutrtional treatments. All that is required is litmus paper available through any chemical or drug supply source. Along with the litmus paper will be a color chart. When the saliva placed on the litmus paper is orange, it is acidic. When the saliva produces dark purple, it is alkaline. Testing small children will usually produce dark purple, but as age increases, the purple shades gradually into lighter colors, until, at last, with the elderly arthritic, the shade is orange or light yellow. A healthy body will produce a dark litmus color.

There will also be a number chart, indicating concentration of acid or alkaline fluids in the saliva. The concentration of ionized hydrogen is measured with the litmus paper by a pH (concentration of hydrogen ion) scale that ranges from 4.5 to 7.5. Reich found that his healthy patients had neutral to alkaline saliva readings on litmus paper of 7.5 to 7 pH (almost black to dark purple) that he believes faithfully represents blood and tissue pH.

Unhealthy patients, on the other hand, have acidic saliva readings showing evidence of acidic blood pH at or below 6.5 (greenish, brown, tan, orange, and yellow).

The best time for taking the litmus test is 11am just before eating. At least 1-2 hours should pass since eating, drinking, or chewing anything.

Within a few weeks or months of diet and supplement changes, the acidic saliva pH may return to a more normal neutral to an alkaline reading of 7 to 7.5 (almost black to purple) accompanied by a disappearance of arthritic symptoms.

In chronic asthma of children under five years of age, Reich found that his vitamin D and calcium therapy provided 93% with a moderate to excellent resolution of their diseases within one to three weeks.

In adults, within a few weeks or months of dietary therapy with alkaline producing foods, calcium-magnesium, and A and D vitamin supplements, Reich noted that, with gradual resolution of asthma, other deficiency complaints, such as joint pains, also resolved. Also, acidic saliva pH tests began to approach the more normal neutral to alkaline state (almost black to purple). As normalization of ionic calcium levels in the body's cells signals the autonomic nervous system that adaption to deficiency is no longer required, bronchial muscles and cellular secretions relax, ending the lung's excessive retention of carbon dioxide and normalizing acid-base balance.

Reich's therapy included calcium and magnesium, A and D vitamins in halibut liver oil (containing natural A and D_3 vitamins) or Aquasol A and D (providing natural A and synthetic D_2).

The results of prescribing dietary and calcium-vitamin D supplement changes for thousands of patients over 32 years of Dr. Reich's practice are given in the Table 1, below:

Table 1: Patients Treated with Vitamins and Minerals

Type of Disease	Number of Patients	Good to Excellent Resolution
Osteoarthritis	2,000	60%
Rheumatoid Arthritis	100	60%
Adult Chronic Asthma	5,000	67%
Very Young Chronic Asthma	1,000	93%
Older Child Chronic Asthma	4,000	85%

Table 2, Schedule of Initial Daily Doses of Vitamins and Minerals, summarizes Dr. Reich's treatment protocol by age group. Treatment is maintained for several weeks or months, then reduced to one half or one third.

Table 2: Schedule of Initial Daily Doses of Vitamins and Minerals

Patient (Age)	Vitamin A (I.U.)		Vitamin D (I.U.)	Calcium (Mg)
3-6	5-8,000	1-2,400	250-500	
15	30,000		4,800	750
Adult (160 lbs)	54,000		7,200	1,250

Although these dosages seem high to many doctors, the FDA (as of April 1989) reported only 11 Adverse Reaction Reports to "high" dosages of vitamin A and vitamin D.

The 1980s *Special Report on the Recommendations of the National Research Council's Committee on Diet and Health, Regarding Dietary Supplements* states the minimum toxic dose for vitamin A ranges from 25,000 IUs-50,000 IUs. For vitamin D, the minimum toxic dose was believed to be 50,000 IUs. Despite those exceptionally high initial toxic figures the The National Research Council's recommended adult intake presumed for safety is only 5000 IUs of A and 400 IUs of D.

Dr. Reich's dosages of vitamin D are one fourth to one sixth of that which is known to create toxic effects, but vitamin A dosages are above the National Research Council's extremely low presumption of a toxic level.

Dr. Reich proposes that the National Research Council's level of initial toxic vitamin A toxicity is too low and that, instead, the toxic level is in the 50,000 to 100,000 IU range.

According to a 1986 *Nutrition News* report, vitamin D toxicity only takes place at massive *daily* doses of 25,000 IUs, where calcification of soft tissues has been noticed.

The Merck Manual (1992) states: "Frequent determinations of serum calcium (weekly at first and then monthly) should be made in patients receiving large doses of vitamin D." Normal values are considered to be 8.5 to 10.5 mg/dL; elevated levels to be 12 to 16 mg/dL.

Early signs of vitamin A toxicity include dry skin, sparse coarse hair, cracked lips, and swelling of the optic disc of the retina (papilledema). Symptoms are headache and dizziness together with symptoms of "false brain tumor" (psuedo-tumor).

Symptoms of acute vitamin D toxicity include headache, nausea, anorexia, diarrhoea and growth retardation in children.

Signs of chronic toxicity that arise because of tissue calcification include urine indications of kidney damage.

Toxic symptoms of both vitamin A and D disappear within 1 to 4 weeks when vitamin doses are reduced or discontinued and fatalities have not been a result of high doses (*Merck Manual* 1992).

Dr. Reich reported finding only rare instances of elevated blood serum calcium levels as a result of his supplement therapy. Reducing vitamin D dosages quickly took care of the problem.

On looking back at his 32 years of successful practice, Dr. Reich feels that whatever the theoretical explanation, supplementation with vitamins D_3 in halibut liver oil, or cod liver oil, sometimes combined with vitamin D_2 in Aquasol A and D, had good results in the vast majority of patients.[55]

Diet and Proper Nutrtion

Nutrition must be designed to fit each individual, of course, but there are always broad outlines that are safe and helpful for each of us. Since our human bodies evolved through a varying diet of grains, nuts, berries, fish, meats and other food substances, proper nutrition is the eating of <u>fresh</u> fruits and vegetables, whole grains, nuts, animal protein, non-farmed cold water fish and other sources of essential fatty acids.

It's generally accepted that degenerative changes appear first in that part of the joint cartilage which receives the greatest wear and tear and has the poorest nutrition. Furthermore, most osteoarthritis patients are elderly and inactive, with many of them suffering from blood circulation problems, especially in the poorly fed tissues surrounding and inside the joints. This leads directly to linking poor blood supply and poor nutrition to degenerative cellular functions of cells in and around the joints.

From these known and accepted medical facts, and through studies by nutritionist Luke Bucci, Ph.D., it's easily concluded that those wishing to improve osteoarthritis should, "Feed The Chondrocytes!, the cartilage cells. . . .   How does one go about feeding chondrocytes?

Fortunately, the   state of research on chondrocyte needs   is sufficiently advanced to be able to list specific nutrients which play very important roles in chondrocyte function.

Most osteoarthritis patients consistently show deficiencies of vitamins A, C, D and E along with insufficient intakes of calcium, iron, copper, zinc and selenium.

Some of these deficiencies may be caused or exacerbated by the pain-killing medications commonly used by these patients. For example:

• Aspirin use can lead to gastro-intestinal bleeding, resulting in 'anemia of arthritis.' This condition would worsen deficiencies of iron, copper and vitamin C.

• Non-steroidal   anti-inflammatory drugs (NSAIDS) such as acetaminophan, ibuprofen (Motrin®, Advil®), naproxen (Naprosyn®), piroxicam (Feldene®), and others, make the gut more permeable, which at first glance sounds desirable. However, at least a third of arthritis sufferers are "very low" in stomach acid (achlorhydric), with more being just "low" in stomach acid (hypochlorhydric), meaning mineral absorption is compromised and protein digestion is suboptimal. Poor protein digestion and increased gut permeability means absorption of large molecular weight pieces of proteins leading to collagen tissue and   autoimmune diseases, arteriosclerosis, rheumatoid   diseases, osteoarthritis, and neurological changes.

Forty percent   of arthritis patients have mixed degenerative [osteoarthritis] and rheumatoid arthritis. (See Chapter II, Rheumatoid Arthritis.)

Returning stomach acidity to normal levels greatly improves protein digestion. Dietary supplementation can quite easily increase stomach acidity to normal levels. The only contraindication is an active gastric or peptic ulcer.

For digestive aids, Jonathan V. Wright, M.D., Kent, Washington, frequently recommends hydrochloric acid-pepsin capsules, pancreative enzymes, and vitamin B injections.[104]

Other general dietary guidelines include decreasing sugar and refined foods, and removing fried foods, margarine and preserved meats.

Adding more whole grain products, fresh vegetables and fruits is recommended.

Replacement of most red meats with fish, poultry and wild game has the advantage of reducing consumption of proinflammatory fats and increasing intake of anti-inflammatory fats.[9] If at all possible, raise your own poultry. Rex Newnham, Ph.D., D.O., N.D. of Leeds, England cautions that "If hormones are used in the growing of poultry in the U.S.A., it should not be recommended to anybody. These hormones, at least in Australia and New Zealand, do inhibit the menstrual cycle in women and sometimes men develop swollen breasts, [and the hormones placed in poultry] interfere with the normal [human] hormone balance and can upset calcium retention."[12]

If there is difficulty in procuring or preparing fish, fish oil supplements are available. Oils and supplements containing significant amounts of linolenic acids (GLA and ALA) [from foods such as linseed or flax oil, walnuts and beans, whole grains, chestnuts, soybeans and pumpkin seeds] are also available to fortify a return to dietary intake of polyunsaturated anti-inflammatory fats. (See Chapter II, Rheumatoid Arthritis.)

The following is a general dietary guideline that is recommended to osteoarthritis patients by many medical doctors well-versed in nutrition:

General Guidelines

1. Improve gastric acidity by use of digestive aids such as hydrochloric acid-pepsin capsules, pancreative enzymes and B-vitamin injections.

2. Eliminate refined sugars, corn syrups, fried foods, margarine, preserved meats from your diet.

3. Decrease consumption of refined foods, replace with whole grains, fresh vegetables and fruit.

4. Replace most red meats with fish, lean poultry (hormone free, if possible) or wild game.

5. Keep total fat intake below 30% of total calories.

6. Reduce consumption of white potatoes, tomatoes, green peppers, eggplant, chili peppers, and use of tobacco if osteoarthritis or rheumatoid arthritis symptoms also are apparent. These "nightshade" plants produce a saponic-like glycoalkoloid, which can cause many symptoms in man, including the most common effects of chronic or low-level poisoning which is pain and stiffness in joints and their related muscles.

Nightshade plants are white potatoes, tomatoes, green peppers, eggplant, chili peppers, and tobacco. Dr. Norman F. Childers originally described arthritics' sensitivity to nightshade plants which contain solanines, a glycoalkoloid that causes arthritic symptoms, reporting that nightshade's toxic chemical interferred with the neuromuscular chemistry which vitamin therapy is intended to improve.[44]

Tobacco, besides being a member of the solanines, carries toxic substances into the blood and tissues, damaging to muscle and nerve metabolism.[24] Some of these toxic substances are added by the tobacco manufacturer to "improve" taste.

According to orthopedic surgeon Robert Bingham, M.D., 1/3 to 1/2 of rheumatoid disease victims are sensitive to the chemicals in nightshade plants. Carleton Fredericks, Ph.D. suspects an even higher percentage are affected by solanines, and both osteoarthritis and rheumatoid disease victims should consider avoidance of these substances.[44]

Vitamins and Minerals

Since dietary deficiencies of vitamins and minerals are usually found in osteoarthrits patients. A multiple vitamin/mineral product should help prevent gross deficiencies from occurring.

Modest doses of B vitamins are sufficient for [ordinary] supplemental purposes (1-10 mg B_1, B_2, B_6; 20-50 mg for B_3 and B_5; 6-25 mcg for B_{12}).

High doses of B vitamins (over 500% of RDA) have not been useful for osteoarthritis, according to several studies, but there is one significant exception demonstrated by William Kaufman, M.D., who describes the way in which niacinamide deficiencies can be repaired by the use of relatively large dosages spread out over a 10 hour daily intake period, and also the use of other vitamin B supplements.[13,44] (See "Niacinamide," this Chapter.)

Another exception is the use of high doses of folic acid combined with high doses of vitamin B_{12} (cobalamin) which have shown beneficial effects on osteoarthritic hands by Margaret A. Flynn, Ph.D., RD.,[101] University of Missouri-Columbia School of Medicine, Columbia, Missouri. Two hundred times the Recommended Dietary Allowance (RDA) of cobalamin (B_{12}) (20 mcg) and folic acid (6,400 mcg) were injected into an experimental group drawn from 26 osteoarthritic patients in a double-blind study over 6 months. Neither the folic acid, or the cobalamin or the placebo pain control of acetaminophen Tylenol®, proved as beneficial as did the combined injections of B_{12} and folic acid.

Vitamins A, D and E are oil-soluble, which means that the most efficient forms of supplementation are emulsified forms[7]. For vitamins A and D, supplemental amounts of 100-200% of RDA are sufficient. Higher doses seem to be unnecessary and may possibly lead to toxicities if very large amounts are ingested for very long times. As an antioxidant, vitamin E is important, and larger amounts may be supplemented (400-1200 IU daily if nonemulsified; 90 IU or more if emulsified[6]).

Vitamin C (ascorbate) plays a major role in cartilage metabolism. Osteoarthritis is worsened by deficiencies of vitamin C. Vitamin C is a growth factor for cartilage construction, the chondrocyte cells. One to two grams daily (preferably buffered) is sufficient to raise blood levels of vitamin C. Nobelist Linus Pauling, Ph.D., however, recommended a maintenance dosage of 4 to 6 grams per day.[50]

Bioflavonoids are a group of nutritional plant compounds which includes citrus bioflavonoids rutin, hesperidin and herperidon chalcone. All of these factors reduce excessive permeability of the walls of blood vessels and strengthen the vessels, a problem that is suffered by many elderly arthritics. Excessive permeability is also responsible for the loss of fluid which creates watery eyes and water-laden nose marked by allergies.

Bioflavonoids taken together with vitamin C help to preserve the vitamin C and   add   their   own   antioxidant   anti-inflammatory characteristics.

Citrus bioflavonoids are commonly used, usually in amounts 1/10 to 1/2 the amount of supplemental vitamin C.

Researchers at Boston University Medical Center, as reported in *Arthritis & Rheumatism*, link antioxidant nutrient intake with a decrease by three-fold in the progression of loss of joint cartilage which accompanies osteoarthritis. Pain was also reduced. These nutrients included vitamin C, vitamin E, and beta carotene, although not as dramatically or consistently as with the use of vitamin C.

Several minerals are of vital importance to cartilage metabolism and are also deficient in those suffering from osteoarthritis patients. Of primary concern are calcium, magnesium, zinc, iron, copper, manganese and selenium. Daily supplemental amounts of these minerals should reach 100% of RDA amounts, as recorded below:

Vitamins:

B vitamins — 100-500% of RDA [Except that niacinamide might be required temporarily in higher dosages spread out evenly over a ten hour period.[13,44]]

A — 5,000-10,000 IU

D — 400-800 IU

E — 30-1,200 IU

C — 1-2 grams [Many physicians recommend 4 to 6 grams daily.[50]]

Minerals:

Calcium, magnesium, iron, zinc, copper, selenium all 100% RDA; manganese -- 5-50mg.

In addition to the above, Dr. Newnham recommends 8-10mg of boron and cobalt in vitamin B_{12}.[12]

According to Louis J. Marx, M.D.,[92] Ventura, California, "Osteoarthritis has three causes. The most important cause is nutritional deficiency, mainly mineral deficiency. The treatment is similar to that of osteoporosis, and it is likely that both conditions coexist. The most important mineral is magnesium followed by calcium, potassium, manganese, boron, and silica. These minerals need to be in *organic* form [calcium ascorbate, magnesium ascorbate, etc.] to be useful."

Along with appropriate minerals, vitamin D is needed, and the thyroid and parathyroid need to be evaluated. The thyroid hormone is necessary to deposit the minerals in the bones and joints. The Epstein-Barr virus is almost always the cause of low thyroid. The chicken pox virus can produce an inflammation of the parathyroid gland resulting in loss of calcium in the bones and joints.

Oils:

Fish oils — 3-9 capsules

Evening Primrose Oil Capsules [Gamma linolenic acid (GLA) oils] — 3-6 capsules (Caution: Not all in the United States labeled as "Primrose Oil" is.)

Enzymes:

Enzymes are fundamental to all living processes. They're necessary for every chemical reaction and thus for the normal functioning of cells and fluids, tissues and organs. There are, quite literally, hundreds of thousands of necessary enzymes pervasive throughout every form of life.

All vitamins and minerals which we intake require enzymes, of which there are three kinds: (1) plant or food enzymes found in all raw foods; (2) digestive enzymes, secreted by the pancreas; (3) metabolic enzymes produced by the body to run all body processees.

Hector Solorazano del Rio, M.D., D.Sc., Universidad de Guadalajara, Guadalajara, Mexico, writes, "You must know that without enzymes, there is no possibility of life, in animals, plants or persons. Enzymes are essential for each and every reaction in a living organism."

Enzymes are catalysts, or rather we should say, 'biolcatalysts.' We are dealing with determined substances whose presence causes the transformation of an organic substance and it also accelerates it, just as a catalyst would do it. Today we know what these enzymes are and how they act, now known to number better than 2,700. Made of 20 different amino acids, each enzyme is specific in its effect.

Dr. Solorazano del Rio may recommend proteolytic enzymes which affect the digestion of proteins — 2-8 tablets 3 times daily -- and anti-oxidant enzymes which enhance the quenching of free radicals — 2-6 tablets 3 times daily.

Lita Lee, Ph.D., licensed clinical nutritionist, is an enzyme therapist who has helped a large population of varying types of illnesses to wellness based on a method developed by Howard Loomis, D.C. using a 24-hour urine analysis test plus physical evaluation test and an extensive patient history to determine what enzymes and nutrients are missing from the patient.

Food enzyme programs were developed that consist of a large variety of enzymes. Taken alone, or together with other formulations, the enzymes found in Dr. Lee's programs could be matched for nearly any condition discovered by the earlier analysis. For example: Those who suffer from sugar intolerance can take *Chirozyme DGST* which contains protease, amylase, lipase, cellulase plus sugar digesting enzymes.

Osteoarthritis as well as rheumatoid arthritis have nutritional components, thus enzyme components, and these may involve every system in the body. [Lita Lee, Ph.D. may be contacted at 2852 Willamette St, #397, Eugene, OR 97405; tel (541)-746-7621; fax: (541) 741-0354.]

Plant Compounds:

Yucca saponins are natural, non-toxic plant substances extracted from the yucca plant which flourishes in Southwestern deserts and Mexico. It improves blood circulation, lowers blood pressure, cholesterol and triglycerides (when abnormal). It also acts like a natural form of cortisone (without dangerous side-effects), reducing and eliminating pain, swelling and joint stiffness. Robert Bingham, M.D. recommends 300 mg of yucca plant extract daily.

Gamma oryzanol/ferulic Acid (FRAC) is a fatty acid derived from rice bran, is a protective antioxidant and also affects cholesterol levels.

Bioflavonoids — 10-1,000 mg

Antioxidants: Antioxidants quench "free-radicals," chemical substances that, when in excess, damage tissues, destroying their function, and known to be a major factor in degeneration of cartilage in osteoarthritis. Lack of oxygen from poor circulation increases free radical damage. Whenever an antioxidant reaches moderate to high levels in the body, reductions in cartilage degeneration and improvements in healing have been seen.

Beta carotene — 5,000-25,000 IU

Vitamin C[7] (ascorbate) — 1-2 grams [Many physicians recommend 4-6 grams daily.[50]]

Bioflavonoids — 10-1,000mg

Vitamin E[6] (tocopherol) — 30-1,200 IU

Coenzyme Q_{10} is a vitamin-like compound that occurs naturally in our body. It is an essential component for converting fuel into energy, functioning as a catalyst in the production of energy (ATP) and its storage. Deficiencies can lead to a wide range of illnesses or health problems — 1-100mg

Selenium — 25-200mcg: Low blood levels of selenium have been found in those with various forms of arthritis, cancer and arteriosclerosis. In a British Arthritic Association three-month study with a formulation of selenium, plus vitamins A, C and E, "The trial included the worst cases, and yet 64 percent reported considerable reduction in pain within the three months."

Selenium deficiency is common, usually triggered by, or the result of, alcoholism, smog, ozone exposure, heavy metal poisoning, and processed/cooked foods. Deficiency symptoms result in free radical damage leading to sclerosis (hardening) and loss of elasticity in many tissues, and resulting in arthritis and premature aging, muscle degeneration, some cancers, hair and nail loss, heart problems (including heart disease, stroke, high cholesterol levels, hypertension, and heart attack), as well as other problems.

Selenium, like other antioxidants, can be taken in too little as well as in too large a quantity. The likelihood is greater that the individual will be short of selenium rather than long in it, but to be safe, tests should be monitored by a physician specially trained in this area of nutritional supplements.

Superoxide dismutase (SOD) and glutathione peroxidase (GP) are protective antioxidant enzymes useful for maintaining maximum health requirements

Plant phenolic acids and derivatives: Dietary phenolic acids and their derivatives (one example is curcumin, a component of turmeric) are found in plants and frequently account for medicinal properties seen for herbs. Recently, one of these compounds, the fatty acid gamma oryzanol derived from rice bran, has been shown to be a potent antioxidant. Its water-soluble active component, ferulic acid, is available in supplemental form as FRAC (Ferulic Acid).

Mixtures of antioxidants usually work better than a single antioxidant. Many such products abound. For use in osteoarthritis, the manufacturer's suggested usage should be doubled or tripled. Fortunately, antioxidants are quite safe, except for massive doses of selenium.

Calcium/Magnesium Aspartate or Chelate: Usually, a calcium and magnesium supplement (but not carbonate or phosphate forms) is required to reach RDA levels for these minerals, unless a very high calorie diet is eaten. Soluble, organic forms of minerals are always preferred such as the orotates. However, as the orotates have been removed from the American market by the FDA, calcium or magnesium chelate or aspartates are recommended.

Glucosamine; Chondoitin Sulfate: According to Julian Whitaker, M.D.,[16] editor of *Health & Healing*, "If the mechanism of the body to make cartilage and other connective tissues is intact, osteoarthritis will sometimes stabilize and actually begin to reverse itself. This results in 'joint space recovery,' which can happen even if the entire joint space has been lost." Glucosamine can stimulate the body to heal osteoarthritis. Glucosamine is an amino derivative of glucose, the form of sugar that is found in our bodies. It is the starting point for the synthesis of many important large molecules, called muccopolysaccharides (carbohydrates that form chemical bonds with water), that help to repair and maintain tissue found in joints such as synovial fluid, mucous membranes in the digestive and respiratory tracts, and blood vessels and heart valves. It can be used as glucosamine, as glucosamine hydrochloride, guclosamine sulfate, or some other salt of an equally suitable acid.

Joint connective tissue regenerates by the production and modification of large quantities of collagen tissue and proteoglycans, both major components of connective tissue. When the joint is injured, manufacture of connective tissue, synovial fluid, collagen and proteoglycans all dramatically increase. The composition of proteoglycans consists primarily of glycosaminoglycans (GAGs), long molecular chain sugars. Glucosamine is the key building block for these large and complex proteoglycans which results in new connective tissues. Sherry A. Rogers, M.D., private practitioner and author in Syracuse, New York writes, "There is a treatment for pain that is safer and does not have side effects: It doesn't make osteoarthritis worse; is cheaper; does not require a prescription; and helps to restore the proper chemistry and rebuild or heal the osteoarthritic cartilage. Glucosamine sulfate -- an amino-monosaccharide naturally present in cartilage -- is the substance that can do all this."[60]

According to Michael T. Murray, N.D.,[145] a leading natural medicine researcher, glucosamine sulfate has an absorption rate when orally administered as high as 98 percent, and that once absorbed it is then distributed primarily to joint tissues where it is incorporated into the connective tissue matrix of cartilage, ligaments, and tendons.

Cartilage needs sulfur to regenerate properly. Both inorganic and organic sources of sulfur can be utilized, but organic forms (such as the amino acids cysteine, taurine and methionine) are closer to the final product, glycosaminoglycans (GAGs). Glucosamine is a key regulator of glycosaminoglycans (GAGs) synthesis which produces the necessary proteoglycans for tissue repair.

Nutritionist Luke Bucci, Ph.D. draws special attention to chondroitin sulfates and antioxidants for the repair of osteoarthritis. Glycosaminoglycans (GAGs), a fundamental building block for repair of joint tissue, contains chondroitin sulfates made up of sulfated sugars. Up to several grams per day of each sulfur amino acid may be supplemented for long periods of time.

One form of injectable glycosaminoglycans (GAGs) [glycosaminoglycan polysulfuric acid (GAGPS)] was used in a 1 year double-blind, randomized, placebo-controlled study of 80 patients with osteoarthritis of the knee by Associate Professor Karel Pavelka, M.D., Ph.D.,[100] Director of Institute of Rheumatology Prague, Czech Republic, "the index of severity of knee osteoarthritis decreased after the end of the injection period by 34% from baseline, and this effect persisted to 26 weeks. . . . The same results were shown by other assessment criteria," including pain and knee function, although the significance measured was somewhat lower for these last two.

Richard A. Kunin, M.D. writes that "N-acetyl glucosamine and glucosamine sulfate have also proved beneficial in treating cartilage, tendon and joint inflammation, including both rheumatoid and osteoarthritic conditions. Usually it takes a couple of weeks before the tenderness abates, but once it is gone it tends not to come back. Golfers are particularly grateful to find their hip pain fading away.

Several products have now been marketed which contain beneficial mixtures of glucosamine sulfate and chondroitin sulfate, compounds which occur naturally in joint cartilage. These mixtures may or may not be fortified with Vitamin C, calcium citrate, and zinc gluconate, all of which aid in tissue repair, and also bromelain (a mixture of enzymes found in pineapples) to help joint flexibility, *Boswellia serrata* (from a large branching tree native to India), supplying 60% boswellic acids, and *Curcuma longa* (the yellow pigment of turmeric), supplying 90-95% curcumin.

A chemical fraction of curcuma oil extracted from *Curcoma longa*, has been shown to have anti-inflammatory and antiarthritic activity. There are many medicinal plants of great therapeutic value referred to in the ancient treatment systems of Ayurveda practiced in India over five thousand years, combining natural therapies with emphasis on body, mind, and spirit. According to studies, *Boswellia serrata* appears to act by mechanisms similar to non-steroidal groups of anti-arthritic drugs, but free of side effects and gastric irritation.[89]

Available in Europe and some non-European countries, Arteparon®, glycosaminoglycan polysulfate, called GAGPS, is a mixture of sulfated glycoaminoglycans from bovine trachea and lung. It is administered by intramuscular (IM) injections, usually as a series of ten to 15 injections, 2 injections per week.[143]

"In two double-blind, randomized, short-term trials, some significant improvement in pain and joint mobility was recorded during a 6-month follow-up period in 120 and 74 patients, respectively, after ten intrarticular (IA) injections of 50 mg," of glycosaminoglycan polysulfate, the patients suffering from osteoarthritis of the knee or hip. Pain and mobility was significantly improved in 140 patients with patients who had at least a possible narrowing of joint space in the knee or hip. Other studies confirmed these results.

Rumalon® contains a glycosaminoglycan-peptide complex, called GP-C from bovine cartilage and bone marrow. This preparation has been used excluisvely in the form of a series of intramuscular injections, a series of 25 injections of 1ml each and generally 15 injections of 2ml each, two to three injections weekly.[143]

Double-blind trials in patients with different forms of osteoarthritis demonstrated that the symptoms in 99 patients were significantly improved by 20 injections. These findings were confirmed in additional studies of 1,704 patients with osteoarthritis of the knee, hip, and fingers conducted in rheumatology clinics in five European countries. Other studies including 10,000 patients have also confirmed these results on patients having little to virtually no cartilage; that is those having determinable open space between the joints.[143]

According to German Professor Werner Scheidl,[144] consultant to Instituto Medico Biologico, Tijuana, Mexico, Sulconar® is an Argentina substance very similar to Rumalon®, consisting of cartilage 33%, bone marrow 33%, hepato (liver) catalase enzyme 33%, and tumor necrosis factor (TNF). It is successfully used to halt joint destruction when administered as intramuscular injections, 1 ampoule per day for 10 days. One week after the last injection good results should be noted.

Sulconar is used as an anti-cancer agent, to decrease inflammation in osteoarthritis, against streptococcus, and against mycoplasm.

Sulconar can be obtained through Alfonso Garcia, Instituto Medico Biologico, Tijuana, Mexico, U.S. business office phone, (619) 482-1686; fax (619) 482-4394; Mexico phone (011+526) 682-4230 or (011)+526) 682-4030.

Shark   Cartilage

Shark cartilage contains large amounts of muccopolysaccharides (carbohydrates that form chemical bonds with water) just as does the cartilage from cattle or animals. In either powdered or capsule form, it is the latest substance to become widely used among those with osteoarthritis, rheumatoid arthritis, or cancer.

Shark cartilage has the ability to halt the growth of blood vessels, a process called "anti-angiogenesis," apparently having more of the growth-halting agent than of any substance known. Halting the growth of blood vessels can be very important for halting the progress of cancerous tumors, and may also be effective in stemming the growth of unwanted blood vessels that reach into joint areas where cartilage has thinned, or disappeared, subsequently causing calcification of the joint.

Mucopolysaccharides contained in the shark cartilage also stimulate the immune system and reduce pain and inflammation of arthritis. According to I. William Lane, Ph.D., an independent consultant on marine resources, oral dosages are believed to actually help repair damaged human cartilage.[5] This would be true if for no other reason than the high content of chondroitin sulfates contained in shark cartilage which would be available as a simple nutritional supplement.

"Jose Orcasita of the University of Miami School of Medicine gave six elderly patients suffering from 'significant-to-unbearable' osteoarthritis doses of dry shark cartilage for a period of three weeks. In all cases, each patient reported that pain was grealy reduced and quality of life was vastly improved."[64]

Eighty percent of osteoarthritis patients at Comprehensive Medical Clinic in Southern California responded well. The percentage of response for rheumatoid arthritis patients studied in other research was 50 to 60 percent.[5]

Usually, after two to three weeks of therapy, improvement should be noted, but if not, then this treatment probably won't help.

A daily dose is taken 3 times daily in equal amounts about 15 to 30 minutes before meals. One gram of dry powdered shark cartilage is to be taken for every three to five pounds of body weight. A 120 pound person would take between 40 and 60 grams, 3 times daily.

There have been a few reports of allergy reactions to shark cartilage, but normally it's non-toxic and so you can't overdose. Best, (for reasons of taste), that you blend the substance with fruit juices or water, or take it in capsule form.[64]

Bovine Cartilage

In contrast to the above, one of us (Gus Prosch, Jr., M.D., Birmingham, Alabama) has found clinical successes better with bovine cartilage than with shark cartilage. There are more than 40 years of significant scientific research verifying the effectiveness of bovine cartilage.

As much as $10,000,000 has been invested in clinical research directed by John F. Prudden, M.D., Med.Sc.D., Chairman of the Foundation for Cartilage and Immunology Research, who also discovered the use of bovine cartilage in 1954 while experimenting with methods to improve wound healing. He published in 1974 (*Seminars in Arthritis and Rheumatism*) studies showing that of 28 patients, over a period of 3 to 8 weeks receiving daily subcutaneous injections of 50 cc of bovine cartilage solution, 19 were classified as "excellent," 6 were "good," and 2 noted "some" benefit. No toxicity was reported, and the pain relief lasted an average of 7 months after completion of the study.

Dr. Prudden later tested the effects of orally ingested bovine cartilage, 9 grams daily. Of 700 cases of osteoarthritis treated with bovine cartilage, 59 percent experienced "excellent" results and 26 percent experienced "good" results for a total amelioration rate of 85 percent. The average length of remission was 6 to 8 weeks.

In the early 1970s Dr. Prudden began long-term clinical trials and his studies, since then, have involved more than 1,000 patients, some of whom have more than 18 years of follow-up history.

A long term, double-blind study in 1987 at Charles University in Prague, Czechoslovokia confirmed Dr. Prudden's results. Pain scores dropped an average of 50 percent in 194 participants. (See Chapter II, "Shark Cartilage" and "Bovine Cartilage," Rheumatoid Arthritis.)

Chicken Cartilage

Joel Wallach, D.V.M., M.D.,[139] author of *Rare Earths: Forbidden Cures*, reports on an arthritis research program conducted at Harvard Medical School and the Boston VA Hospital. Twenty nine people who had failed to respond to traditional medical treatment using aspirin, prednisone, cortisone, gold shots, methotrexate, and physical therapy were preparing for hip surgery. They were asked to delay for 90 days during which period they were fed heaping teaspoons of ground-up dried chicken cartliage in orange juice each morning. In ten days all their pain and inflammation was gone. In thirty days they could open new pickle jars, and in ninety days they had return of their natural joint function.

Summary

The general dietary guidelines   for   specific nutrients should allow useful concentrations of nutrients   to reach cartilage cells (chondrocytes). When chondrocytes are fed, they are   more able to perform their function — repair cartilage. Combined with   other treatment modalities to reduce the wear on cartilage, optimal nutrition allows the cartilage cells (chondrocytes) to perform to their capabilities, meaning a net result of healing. The most important single nutrient for cartilage cells (chondrocytes) is chondroitin sulfates.

One of the advantages of nutrition is that all body cells are affected, and there can be improvements in the growth of new blood vessels where needed, and the halting of such growth where inappropriate. Thus many factors contributing to osteoarthritis can be favorably modified by judicious use in diet and specific nutrients.

Botanicals

Recommended Herbs

The cases of deaths caused by the use of herbs in the United States can be counted on your fingers, whereas there are reported from 10,000 to 20,000 deaths per year from gastric hemorrhages from non-steroidal anti-inflammatory drugs used for arthritis.[147]

Dr. Louis J. Marx, M.D., Ventura, California, reminds us that the proper use of herbals is in the preparation of a specific formulation that is needed by a particular person at that time; "others with the same symptoms may need very different formulas."

Various herbs[16] have been useful for treating arthritics, especially in treating inflammation without the serious side-affects attributed to aspirin and non-steroidal anti-inflammatories (NSAIDS). These are licorice *(Glycyrrhiza glabra)*, alfalfa *(Medicago sativa)*, devil's claw *(Harpagophytum procumbens)*, and the proanthocyanidins, cherries, hawthorn berries and blueberries[17,18]

CF Randall[103] reports in the *British Journal of General Paractitioners* beneficial effects of two elderly people who used stinging nettle (*Urtica dioica*). One, an 81 year-old man with confirmed unilateral hip (one hip) osteoarthritis, "found great relief where ibuprofen had previously failed. He had to apply the leaves only once every few days to maintain the effect.

"An elderly woman of unidentified age had similar benefits for inflamed, arthritic fingers."

Michael T. Murray, N.D., Bellevue, WA, author of many medical articles and books on the use of natural healing methods, also recommends the use of sulfur-containing foods such as garlic, onions, Brussels sprouts, and cabbage, as these will increase the sulfur content in sufferers who are often deficient in sulfur.[47]

According to Dr. Murray, feverfew (*Chyrsanthemum parthenium*), long in folk history for the treatment of arthritis and migraine, acts to inhibit inflammation and fever better than does aspirin, also inhibiting the synthesis of many pro-inflammatory compounds. A related herb, *Tanacetum parthenium*, also decreases the pain of headache as well as arthritic pains. The active ingredient, parthenolide, must be present in sufficient concentration, which is not always the case with various species or as presented for sale at the marketplace.[85]

Reported in the *Alternative Medicine Digest*[96] are new (1995) clinical studies from Sun Yet Sen University of Medical Sciences in China demonstrating that devil's claw root (*Harpagophytum procumbens*) extract can bring some relief to osteoarthritis. In that study, a total of 40 patients, aged 38-52, received daily dosages of Pagosid™, a standardized water-based extract of devil's claw root, for 4 weeks at the dosage rate of 500 mg daily.

Doctors rated effectiveness of the herb at 85%, while the patients rated it 90%.

A parallel study (1995) consisting of 38 patients at China's First Military Medical University gave arthritis patients one gram of Pagosid every day for 4 weeks. Doctors rated it 79% effective as patients reported relief from their general arthritic conditions, including joint swelling, morning stiffness, and lowered grip strength. Effectiveness for Osteoarthritis was 85%.

Dr. Michael T. Murray describes the gum exudate from *Boswellia serrata*, a large branching tree native to India, as containing boswellic acids which have an effect on the inflammation of osteoarthritis and rheumatoid arthritis. "The standard dosage for boswellic acids is 400 mgs, 3 times daily." There are no side effects from its use.

Kombucha Tea is grown from a Manchurian mushroom in one's own refrigerator. The fungus is placed in a tea base where complicated biochemical processes take place. Author of "Kombucha Tea," Debbie Carson,[71] reports that, "Fermentation produces a small amount of alcohol (0.5%), carbon dioxide, B vitamins, Vitamin C and various organic acids that are essential to human metabolism." Its most important products are said to be glucuronic acid and polysaccharides.

The glucouronic acid has the property of bonding to harmful substances in the body, rendering over 200 substances harmless, and also helping to "form connective tissues, cartilage, gastric mucous membranes and the vitrious body of the eye."

The polysaccharides "strengthen the body's immunity responses to pathogenic bacteria, yeasts, viruses, and increases the body's resistance to these diseases."

Energy Medicine
Background

Until the last half of this century there has been but sparse attention to the application of physics to the practice of medicine. Pharmaceutical industries had long promoted chemicals (drugs) almost exclusively for treatment of symptoms. With the growth of physics applications in medicine, more and more new therapies are being discovered that utilize electrical, magnetic, sonic, acoustic, microwave, infrared or other light frequencies that have beneficial effects on the body when they're correctly utilized .

Energy medicine can be as simple and inexpensive as the transfer of energy by touch to another, or as complex and costly as some of the newly developed hospital equipment whose function is to form accurate images inside the body's soft tissues. In the early dawn of our history, the physics of medicine was first -- and perhaps unknowingly -- applied when a loving touch or comforting voice aided another human being through painful moments. Massage therapy, therapeutic touch and other forms of energy transfer have assumed such an important role that they often have their own special chapters, and are seldom described as a "transfer of energy" or even as similar to the utilization of portions of the electromagnetic spectrum on the human body which we now define as "the physics of medicine."

Seldom, if ever, does a natural therapy operate independently from one another, and in this section we will see that several forms of therapies operate together to reduce pain and restore health for the arthritic.

According to Yang Jwing-Ming, Ph.D., Jamaica Plain, Massachusetts, author of numerous books, physicist and master of Chinese qigong -- an ancient healing discipline -- writings in *Oracle-Bone Scripture (Jia gu Wen)* show evidence that from 2690 B.C. to 1154 B.C. "stone probes" pre-dated the discovery and use of acupuncture, specific body points connected by energy flow lines called "meridians."

Until 1026 A.D. there was much disagreement about acupuncture theory until Dr. Wang Wei-Yi wrote on its principles and techniques in *Illustration of the Brass Man Acupuncture and Moxibustion (Tong Ren Yu Xue Zhen Jiu tu)*. Although the concept of bio-electricity was unknown, Dr. Wang Wei-Yi also cast a famous brass human figure which illustrated for the first time many of the important acupuncture points and energy flow lines -- meridians -- that were important bio-electrical connections to all parts inside and outside the body.

Dr. Wang Wei-Yi's acupuncture points and meridians have been verified during modern times using modern physics equipment, and they have been added to until now we know of over two thousand that have a specific relationship to internal organs.

In the 1940s Reinhold Voll, M.D. was able to measure changes in electrical conductivity of each of the body's acupuncture points, discovering that electrical resistance of the skin decreases dramatically at these points when compared to surrounding skin areas. Dr. Voll also found that each point had a standard measurement for anyone who is in good health. The energy flow along meridians was called by the Chinese "qi" (pronounced "chi"). The measure of this bioenergy -- Chi -- deteriorates as the health deteriorates.

Based upon these early Chinese discoveries and later discoveries of Dr. Voll and colleagues along with Japanese researchers, modern energy medicine has rapidly matured, becoming an accurate, safe, and effective means for both assessment and treatment of health conditions.

Acupuncture and various forms of massage therapy have become so well known in their own right that energy medicine is now more restrictively defined as the application to healing of safe and appropriate frequencies in the electromagnetic spectrum.

Some of the important applications of these frequencies for arthritis, including osteoarthritis, follow:

The TENS Unit

TENS is an acronym for Transcutaneous Electrical Nerve Stimulator, which is used in doctors' offices, physiotherapy clinics, and homes. By applying a light electrical current to affected nerves and muscles, the TENS unit causes a blockage of electrical conduction, hence pain, along that particular nerve.

It's believed that TENS units also stimulate the production of endorphins, the body's natural painkillers.

Although the TENS unit provides great relief for many arthritics, it does not, as a rule, address itself to the causation of pains, but rather to symptoms, and therefore does not solve the initial causation of the pain signal, nor promote self-healing.

The MORA

Based on further discoveries of his colleague, Dr. Voll, the MORA was invented by Franz Morrel, M.D. Dr. Morrell believed that disease is primarily the body's production of the wrong electromagnetic information. The MORA reads the information which the patient produces, and the MORA corrects it. No artificial signal is introduced into the body, thus the MORA is considered a "natural" therapy.

The MORA is being successfully used for treatment of many conditions, including aches and pains of the body that are, or appears to be similar to, osteoarthritis.

The Electro-Acuscope

The Electro-Acuscope reduces pain by stimulating tissue to repair itself. Using current that is much less than TENS current, the current is constantly adjusted to match the resistance of damaged tissue.

Operator training is quite important as during use of the Electro-Acuscope information that is reported to the therapist by the unit can be used to adjust the instrument so that it will perform its best work.

According to Mark Kana, physical therapist, supervisor of physical therapy for Southwest General hospital and its Sports West Clinic in Middleburg Heights, Ohio, "the best response depends not on the specific diagnosis, but on the skill of the user. The modality's applications are limited only when the user is not employing the full spectrum of treatment."[47]

Over the the past three years, Mark Kana, P.T. uses the Electro-Acuscope system to treat a variety of pain and arthritic conditions involving the neck, back, hip, knee, ankle, and shoulder. The Electro-Acuscope requires about 3 minutes to treat a sprained ankle, with reduction of swelling, inflammation and pain.

Joan Shrum-Brown, Physical Therapist, owner and director of the Marguerite Physical Therapy Clinic, Mission Viejo, California, feels that any condition involving nerve or muscle tissue can be improved, especially in conjunction with "therapeutic exercise, body mechanics, and especially mobilization."

Shrum-Brown uses the system most frequently for patients with muscle spasms, temporomandibular joint disorders (jaw), bursitis (soft tissue arthritis), other forms of arthritis, surgical incisions, sprains and strains that can lead to osteoarthritis, herpes zoster infections (virus), dysmenorrhea (painful and difficult menstruation) and hematomas (a tumor containing blood)."[76]

As sports injuries often lead to stretched or torn tendons and ligaments which, in turn, may result in classically described osteoarthritis, the improved ability of the body to repair itself is also important for preventing future osteoarthritis. An arthritis diagnosis is quite often a 'catch-all' diagnosis. The doctors use this diagnosis when there is pain around a joint and they don't know the cause. In most cases, the pain is soft tissue inflammation or muscle injury that can be treated with the Electro-Acuscope. It is very common for one or two treatments to completely solve the pain. In conditions where it may actually be arthritis, such as pain in finger joints, it is usually just as easy to treat. Even when heat can be felt in the painful joint, you can feel the temperature return to normal in a few minutes of treatment and the pain will go away at the same time.[48]

Herm Schneider, A.T.C., Head Athletic Trainer for the Chicago White Sox, says that "We have just about excluded ice and the routine treatments for sprains and bruises, and we treat players immediately as they come out of the game."

The Case of Bo Jackson

Bo Jackson was signed by the White Sox as a free agent before the 1991 season after he was released by the Kansas City Royals.

Gary Emerson, D.C., Santa Ana, California, consultant for many well-known sports figures, at the request of White Sox's Herm Schneider, A.T.C., used the Electro-Acuscope as part of Jackson's rehabilitation, and Bo appeared in 23 games with the White Sox. After undergoing hip replacement surgery in 1992, Bo was treated with the Electro-Acuscope immediately afterward to speed recovery.

The Case of Paul Asmuth

In a condition that is often reported as "osteoarthritis," marathon swimmer Paul Asmuth sought aid for inflammation of the muscle and the capsule of the shoulder only days before a 21-mile marathon swim that included a punishing final stretch against the tide. "After five Electro-Acuscope treatments Asmuth was able to outdistance a swimmer ten years his junior, finishing second and providing how rapidly his shoulder condition had improved."

Electro-Acuscope's Range of Uses

The Electro-Acuscope can be used for acute and chronic pain mainly of musculoskeletal origin: automobile accidents, lumbrosacral sprains, shoulder strains, rotator cuff tears, and sports injuries -- all of which can lead to osteoarthrits. Others have used it for various forms of arthritis, herpes zoster neuralgia, local skin infections, bedsores, spasticity, chronic fatigue syndrome, migraine and other headaches, and also for relief of the pain of carpal tunnel syndrome, a condition of the hand and thumb resulting from repetitive tasks and nutritional deficiencies.

The Case of Cassie Summers

Stephen Center, M.D.[22] of San Diego, CA, reports on 15 year-old, ninth grader, Cassie Summers', whose Achilles tendon pain was worse on the right which was associated with hip joint pain, both conditions of which have been described as "arthritis."

The hip pain had begun eight months earlier, and the ankle pain had begun a month earlier. As Cassie was a member of her high school track team, competing in one to two mile races, and also ran cross country, this kind of pain was a real disturbance.

She was found on examination to have chronic muscle contraction headaches with possibly a vascular component, a condition consistent with her ankle/hip diagnosis.

Dr. Center started Cassie on a course of therapy using the Electro-Acuscope instrument applied locally, directly related to one of the bursae sacs surrounding a joint and the achilles tendon. Similar treatment was used on a muscle and also on four points on the kidney and bladder (acupuncture) meridians that also traverse the heel bone region. This treatment was applied to both ankles and the right thigh.

"Within two treatments the ankle symptoms were largely abated. The patient received a total of seven treatments . . . . [and] at that time she was entirely asymptomatic and discharged."

Cassie returned again eleven months later complaining of pain in her muscles immediately after her heel struck the ground during running, a condition called "shin splints," Although a stress fracture was suspected, Dr. Center found x-rays negative. "We decided to see how she responded to a course of electrical stimulation. She received five treatments over a period of two weeks and was discharged without symptoms."

"Cassie continued to run cross-country and track, and reported no further symptoms in the last seven months."

The Case of Jerrie Armstrong

Jerrie Armstrong, 22 year-old tennis player, complained to Stephen Center, M.D., of a right ankle in pain for three months in four locations. This kind of condition when treated by mere suppression of the pain through use of drugs will often lead to osteoarthritic complaints in the future.

Jerrie didn't recall any specific injury, but played tennis regularly, and also frequently exercised on a stair-climbing machine.

Three years previously she'd sprained her ankle on the same side that she occasionally experienced pain when walking, but especially when sprinting. The onset of her symptoms was gradual.

X-ray examination was negative, and examination of the appropriate parts of the anatomy of her foot showed no ligament instability and no tenderness, fluid leakage or swelling.

Prior to visiting Dr. Center, Jerrie had been started on a non-inflammatory drug and advised to avoid tennis. After referral to an orthopaedic surgeon (and another for a second opinion) exercises were recommended with follow-up x-rays. She was given exercises to strengthen certain muscles of her leg.

Because Jerrie continued to report persistent pain symptoms, further diagnostic testing revealed chronic ankle instability, and she underwent a tendon transfer procedure to correct this instability.

After the operation Jerrie experienced pain and stiffness, and other problems. Now she was diagnosed as having nerve and stiffness problems resulting from the operation, "post-operative neuralgia and post-immobilization stiffness," physicians called it.

Dr. Center diagnosed Jerrie as having inflammation of the membrane surrounding a tendon, arthritis, or inflamation of both bone and cartilage. She was started on therapy in Dr. Center's office using the Electro-Acuscope applied to her ankle and to associated acupuncture trigger points along appropriate meridian conduction paths where bioelectrical energy flows.

Jerrie received three treatments the first week and her incisions became less tender.

By the next week she was walking without a limp for the first time, and she was seen at weekly intervals for five weeks thereafter.

After one month, "during which she was doing quite well," she returned with residual tendon discomfort.

Jerrie received six treatments over the next two weeks, with only slight residual heel (achilles) pain after walking for over a mile.

"She received three additional treatments over the next month, with complete cessation of all symptoms," and was released from treatment, having no residual pain or stiffness in the ankle or foot.

Jerrie resumed playing tennis and her other aerobic activities without further problems.

Light Beam Generator and the Lymph System

As described by Thomas Gervais, certified masseur, appropriate application of portions of the electro-magnetic spectrum can easily reduce or eliminate pain which will stay gone provided the body does not continue to reconstruct the pain. Beyond this, one of the important mechanisms which assists self-healing has been worked out through better understanding of our lymph systems.

The Importance of Lymph

Lymph is an integral part of the body's circulatory system, being the connecting medium between enclosed arteries/capillaries/veins, and the cells and tissues outside of those blood vessels. It is composed of water, inorganic mineral salts, and white blood cells. To this base constituency is added the food nutrients and oxygen which it carries to cells, the waste products which it transports from cells, and a variety of other wastes (dead cells, particulate/environmental pollutants, post-infection debris, etc.). In general, the veins absorb the smaller proteins and most of the fluid present in the lymph, and then return these to the heart. The slow-moving lymphatic system (it functions against gravity and without the assistance of a strong heart pump) returns the larger proteins, excess fluid, and remaining wastes to the kidneys (by way of the heart) for processing and elimination.

To summarize, the lymphatic system includes the following functions: carries food and oxygen to the body's cells and tissues; carries wastes from the body's cells and tissues; removes larger protein wastes from the body's regions between or inside of organs (interstitial regions); maintains fluid balance in the connective tissue; removes excess protein from many sources (antigen-antibody complexes, dead cells, androgens, estrogen, enzymes, lipoproteins); removes foreign particulate and environmental toxins; transports long-chain fatty acids (in food) from the small intestine to the liver; provides the medium in which the immune system functions, and intimately assists with that function

In short, the lymph is an indispensible part of the human cleansing, self-balancing (homeostatic), and defense systems.

Lymph has the characteristic that when placed under pressure from forces external to the body, it congeals, forming loosely bound protein-like clumps. When pressure is released, these clumps are supposed to return to a more fluid state. When clumps form in the lymph system, and do not restore to a fluid state, the lymph system becomes blocked which then prevents cells from being properly nourished, and prevents cellular waste products from being properly eliminated from the body. Just as blockage of the arterial system can be an extremely important contributor to any disease-state, blockage of the lymph system contributes to, or causes, many disease-states, including that of osteoarthritis and osteoarthritis-like pains.

Importance of the Vodder Manual Lymph Massage (VMLM)

The Vodder method of Manual Lymph Draining (MLD) is a European massage tool for gently stimulating movement of the lymphatic vessels, and increasing the drainage of connective tissues. Masseurs are taught to gently stroke along lymph flow channels with the natural flow of lymph, but in increments that begins with the lowest down-stream section, and work backward. It has been successfully used to treat post-mastectomy patients who subsequently develop severe disease of the lymph nodes (lymphadenopathy). Among dozens of other massage techniques, the MLD massage seems superior in its ability to effectively move lymph from a given area of the body back to the heart and kidneys for waste processing and elimination, but used by itself it gets results slowly.

From the initial discovery of the presence of "milky veins" in 1622 by Gaspard Asselli additional discoveries were made by John Pecquet (1622-1674), Olauf Rudbeck (1630-1708), Alexander of Winiwarter (1848-1910), E.P. Millard, Canadian founder of the International Lymphatic Society, through Emil Vodder (1896-1986), the last major advance was made by Bruno Chikly, M.D., formerly of France, now resident of San Gregorio, CA. Dr. Chikly was able to demonstrate a specific rhythm of the lymphatic flow, and to teach how to attune with it while massaging manually. This improvement decreases massage time by several orders of magnitude, also increasing the effectiveness of lymph drainage.[148] [For information on workshops call International Alliance of Healthcare Educators; (800) 233-5880, extension 9320].

The Light Beam Generator (LBG)

The Light Beam Generator (LBG) radiates photons of light that help restore the normal energy state of cells, permitting the body to more rapidly heal itself. It can be used anywhere on the body and, because of its deep penetration, can help heal organs and structures deep within the body. There are no adverse effects from its use.

Of special importance for its successful use is temporary unclogging of lymph circulation, a most important part of our system for bringing nourishment to cells and eliminating cellular wastes.

The application end of the Light Beam Generator -- a glass tube -- is about the size of a medium-sized flashlight, with wires at one end that are attached to a carrying-case. Inside this case are electronic circuits which, when plugged into the wall circuit, sends pulsed electromagnetic radio frequencies through the tube filled with a mixture of argon, neon and xenon.

This hand-held device emits an intermittent pulse of light and a stream of (negative) electrons which temporarily disorganize the electrical bonds of non-functional protein chains, lumps, and accumulations, especially in the lymph system. These waste protein chains can result from a breakdown in the normal operation of the lymph system, and, as they are poorly bound electrically, they disassociate under gentle influence of these negative electrons, whence, liquified, the breakdown products -- waste -- pass out through the lymph system.

The masseur, who may or may not be under the directions of a physician, holds the glass-tube end directly on the skin of the patient, either along key lymph channels or over the pain.

In the case of applications for pain, it is considered safe to hold the bulb directly on the pain for 20 or 30 minutes, or even longer. Pain will definitely reduce, or disappear completely. If the body is restoring the pain in some biochemical or physical manner, such as a pinched nerve, pain will return. Such an event is also diagnostic in that one knows immediately whether or not inflammation and pain is the result of a primary condition that should be sought and attended to, or whether the source-causation of the inflammation and pain is due to lymph blockage.

In its use with Vodder massage therapy (or the newer Chikly method), the Light Beam Generator is held for ten minutes or so at key lymph nodes, and slowly moved along the lymph channel in the directions specified by the Vodder Manual Lymph Massage. Immediately thereafter, techniques of the Vodder Manual Lymph Massage are employed to sweep out the now-fluid lymph, thus opening up fresh nourishment to the cells, and removal of cellular wastes which can be quite toxic.

To some extent, immunocomplexes -- combinations of antigen/ antibody compounds that result from allergies, invading micro-organisms, pollutants and so forth that are always found as localized irritants which produce inflammation, pain and swelling in arthritic tissues -- are also swept out by clearing out the lymph system. [Workshops in Vodder Lymph Massage, coupled with a type of light beam generator device is offered by Sky David, 1933, Kiva Rd., Santa Fe, NM 87501; (505) 989-4416]

Importance of the Light Beam Generator

The Light Beam Generator (LBG) and similar instruments seem unique in their ability to safely soften nodules of accumulated wastes clogging the lymph system. For a short time following LBG application, a previously undesirable, tightly-bonded, molecular congestion will exist in a now electrically un-bonded, or fluid state. If the lymph obstruction is massaged out, the lymph system will clear up. If not immediately removed, however, most of the lymphatic material will likely re-bond in place, once again plugging up the lymph system.

Just as the use of Vodder Massage techniques by themself are slow, (and the Chikly method faster) improvement through the individual use of the Light Beam Generator will also be slow. Applying any method alone greatly reduces the benefits which can be experienced.

When combining the two in clinical practice, a massage therapist can achieve in just one session what previously took eight sessions when working with massage alone. However, any individual can use either the Vodder massage, Chikly Lymph Drainage, or the LBG on themself safely and effectively, although perhaps not with the speed and success that a trained therapist can.

Under a trained therapist, when the Light Beam Generator (LBG) and Manual Lymph Drainage (MLD) or Chikly Lymph Drainage (CLD) are combined, a client may notice some improvement after one session, usually shows marked improvement after six weeks and is normally finished after three months.

Although the Light Beam Generator swiftly reduces osteoarthritic pain -- which may stay gone provided the body is not reproducing it again -- the focus of this method is on cleansing the body of unneeded, obstructing wastes by improving lymph flow. When this occurs, a broad range of health improvements may follow.

Any medical ailment demands appropriate attention by a qualified physician, but the following conditions have been frequently found to improve or to be favorably influenced by, the LBG/MLD or LBG/CLD method of lymph therapy: stored environmental pollutant levels; general inflammation, including those of arthritis; inflammation of cellular or connective tissue including "soft tissue" arthritis; cysts and fibrosis; immune function by optimizing it; cellular nourishment and cleansing (self-balancing systems); healing of many bruises and injuries by accelerating healing; arteriosclerosis (prevention); breast/ prostate cancer (prevention); skin scar tissue; lymph node swelling.

As the manufacturers of the Light Beam Generator were proud of its ability to reduce or eliminate pain, one of us (Perry A. Chapdelaine, Sr.), demonstrated an "osteoarthritic" finger that was stiff and sore, and had been inflamed for at least a full year for reasons that had never been diagnosed. No traditional medicine, or -- up until then -- no non-traditional medicine, had been able to solve the problem.

Representatives challenged their visitor to hold the Light Beam Generator on the inflammed finger while we talked around their conference table. Skeptically, this was done, and lo! -- twenty minutes later the sore finger was no longer sore, and the inflammation was gone, and also the stiffness.

The finger is still well after four years. However, another finger on the other hand which became sore but a year ago does not respond in the same manner, and there is some evidence supporting the belief that this finger is "osteoarthritic" because of deadly toxins stemming from remaining gum infections yet to be sterilized.

A classic illustration of the Light Beam Generator's effect   on swollen lymph glands when a sore throat is beginning to form was also seen by the experience of another visitor who held the Light Beam Generator on each of her swollen glands, and the swelling visibly reduced to normal within minutes.

The other one of us (Gus J. Prosch, Jr., M.D.) -- along with other knowledgeable healers and therapists -- believe that the combined use of the Light Beam Generator (LBG) with the Vodder Method of Manual Lymph Drainage Massage helps to increase circulation of lymph and is yet another effective means for sustaining general good health. Working together, these techniques powerfully aid the lymph system in cleansing the body of accumulated protein wastes when buildup of the latter has occurred.   Though the primary focus of the Light Beam Generator, Chikly Manual Lymph Drainage, and the Vodder Lymph Massage is to simply clean out the lymph system and restore its natural circulation, this improved condition leads to a variety of pain-reducing and health benefits for the osteoarthritic.

Other Means for Moving Lymph

Two other approaches can be helpful adjuncts for effectively moving lymph -- gently exercising on a high-quality mini-trampoline, or lying down with legs and feet slightly elevated, as on a slant board, which causes the lymph to move with gravity instead of against it -- but these do not replace the core combination of LBG/MLD or LBG/CLD.

The Sound Probe

There is some evidence that various kinds of arthritis have a source-causation of micro-organisms. While this is not always demonstrable for osteoarthritis, perhaps one in ten will respond with beneficial results to an anti-microorganism treatment.

The Sound Probe emits a pulsed tone of three frequencies that, when in resonance with bacteria, viruses, and fungus, will destroy them without harming human tissue. Connected to the device is a sound-emitting pad which is placed anywhere on the body where there is a problem, or pain. Alternation of frequencies guarantees that the body does not adjust to the frequency, so that the treatment is beneficial over a time period. After microorganisms have been killed, the Light Beam Generator, or a similar instrument, is used to assist the lymph system in cleaning out the debris.

The Light Beam Generator and the Sound Probe can be used together, as is described in The Photon Sound Beam below.

The Photon Sound Beam

This instrument utilizes gas tube technology similar to that of the Light Beam Generator or Electro-Acuscope, and also affects the lymph system in a similar manner. Inert or noble gases contained in round glass tubes are evacuated of air and filled under pressure with Argon and Xenon. A high voltage at low current ionizes the gases to a plasma state which emit safe electromagnetic radiation.

Two glass photon tubes with insulated handles are included in each unit. A high voltage energy is produced by an electronic circuit that drives the energy by means of a pulse repetition rate in the audio spectrum. In addition, a sound probe is attached, so that one can use the photon and sound outputs indvidually or together.

The Omega Ray

The Omega Ray operates very much like the Light Beam Generator and the Electro-Acuscope with the additional ability of generating a random pattern or varying cycle of frequencies. The advantage of this randomness is that the body will find only those frequencies most effective for it. Because of this variability, it is believed that the body will be less likely to accomodate or become resistant to the energy. It is also said to work in a gentler manner.

[The Light Beam Generator, ELF Laboratories, RR #1, Box 21, St. Francisville, IL 62460, (618) 948-2393; the Photon Sound Beam, (801) 782-5552; Omega Ray from Energize! Products, Inc., PO Box 286, Hastings, MI 49058 (616) 948-9732, Fax (616) 948-8703; Electro-Acuscope, Electro-Medical Incorporated, 18433, Foundation Valley, CA 92708; (800) 422-8726; (714) 964-6776; Sky David, 1933 Kiva Rd., Santa Fe, NM 87501; (505) 989-4416 produces a variable intensity device, with settings for different tissue depths.]

Magnetic Therapy
Background on Magnets

The use of magnetic fields is important for diagnoses, pain relief, and healing. Many arthritis victims, physicians and researchers are now exploring physics in relation to the body.[37,38]

Magnetic electric fields surround us everywhere: power lines, computers, electric motors, household electrical appliances, office equipment and even from the electric wiring in our homes.

Magnetic electric fields are produced by each living cell in our bodies, and they also accompany the movement of current through our nervous system.

Magnetic resonance imaging (MRI), which reaches live tissue not observed by   X-rays, relies on the use of an exceptionally strong magnetic field which interacts with the magnetic fields that make up the atoms and molecules of our cells and tissues.

Orthopedic surgeon and researcher Robert Becker, M.D., author of numerous scientific articles and books, found that weak electric currents will promote the healing of broken bones. Dr. Becker also pointed to the danger of living within the electromagnetic influence of power grids that criss-cross our nation, as "abnormal electromagnetic fields results in significant abnormalities in physiology and function."[5]

Wolfgang Ludwig, Sc.D., Ph.D., Director of the Institute for Biophysics in Horb, Germany, believes that magnetic field therapy can influence every organ in the body. Magnetics has therefore been used for treatment of a wide variety of conditions, including, but not limited to, arthritis, cancer, infections and inflammations, headaches and migraines, insomnia and sleep disorders, circulatory problems, fractures and pain, and environmental stress.

There are two kinds of magnetic sources: pulsating magnetic fields generated by electrical devices already described, and static magnetic fields generated by stationary ferro-magnetic materials, such as manufactured from iron and certain modern ceramics. Magnetic fields from either source penetrate tissues of the body and influence responding magnetic materials, such as the iron contained in red blood cells, oxygen, and the transmission of nerve impulses. William H. Philpott, M.D., Choctaw, Oklahoma, author and researcher of biomagnetic fields, diabetes, and other diseases, has found that magnetic fields can stimulate metabolism and increase oxygen delivered to cells.

As magnetic fields can interfere with the natural magnetic field of the cells of the body, one must be very careful not to use these magnets indiscriminately. Researcher Albert Roy Davis, M.D. discovered in 1974 that positive and negative magnetic polarities have different effects upon the biological systems of human beings, finding that "magnets could be used to arrest and kill cancer cells in animals, and could also be used in the treatment of arthritis, glaucoma, infertility, and diseases related to aging?"[5]

Industrial magnets often have different positive and negative pole identifications than the magnets used in medicine and therapy. Use a magnetometer or a compass to confirm proper identification.

William H. Philpot, M.D. reports that "The human body functions on a direct current circuit and thus references to positive and negative are most appropriate. A positive electric field produces a positive magnetic field. This parallel makes it possible to appropriately use the electric terms of polarity.

"The brain makes a pulsing response to the magnetic field it receives. When increasing the positive magnetic field the brain [bioelectrical] frequency increases and the amplitude decreases. When the brain is exposed to a negative magnetic field the brain frequency decreases and the amplitude decreases.

How to Use Magnets

Many people have learned that strong, permanent magnets can reduce localized pain. The North seeking side of a permanent magnet produces a positive magnetic field (and is attracted to a negative field), and the South seeking side of a magnet produces a negative magnetic field (and is attracted to a positive field).

If you wish to reduce local pain, and also to assist cellular metabolism, use the South seeking, or negative, pole of the magnet.

If you wish to tear down cellular structure, as with a wart or unwanted growth, use the North seeking end of a permanent magnet.

In Japan small *tai-ki* magnets have been designed to stimulate acupuncture points.

Simple magnets may be used, or specially designed ceramic, plastiform, and neodymium (a rare earth element), used individually, or placed in clusters above pain sites, organs, lymph nodes or on the head.

Large machines capable of generating high magnitudes of field strength are used to treat pseudoarthritis, a joint affliction caused by nerve breakdown. In some cases, after a Magnetic Resonance Imaging (MRI) diagnosis, which uses a very strong electromagnetic field for imaging molecules, individuals will report exceptional relief from pain from the strong magnetic field that has been applied during the diagnosis.

To use a permanent magnet, place it directly over the pain site. The pain may disappear in a few minutes, or take several hours, or perhaps as long as all night. In serious disease conditions, Dr. Philpott will advise using very strong magnets strapped to the body, or placed in a specially sown sack in the clothing, so that the body will be continuously exposed to the magnetic field.

Some physicians use large electromagnetic loops within which they will place the head, trunk, hip, or knees of a person, exposing them to the magnetic field for lengths of time that depend on severity of the problem. A chronic sinus infection or cold, for example, will dissipate in about 20 to 30 minutes of rest within the magnetic field. Again, repeated exposures may be required, depending upon severity of the condition.

By promoting oxygenation and decreasing the body's acidity, "A negative magnetic field can function like an antibiotic in helping to destroy bacterial, fungal, and viral infections," reports Dr. Philpott.

Metabolic functions are normalized also decreasing swelling that accompanies many arthritic conditions.

Combining magnetic therapies with other therapies is acceptable, and should serve to assist in the healing of all types of inflammatory reactions for joints, muscles, tendons, nerves, skin, internal organs, and so forth, no matter what the initiating cause may be, according to Dr. Philpott. However, "magnetic therapy cannot replace adequate nutrition, and therefore nutritional supplementation based on laboratory assessment is always in order."[10]

The Role of Exogenous Energy Sources

Physiologists figure that no more than 70% of human biological life energy comes from the food digested. Energy is required to process this food and therefore the net gain of energy is about 70%. Where does the 30% extra (exogenous) energy come from and what can we do to enhance this 30%?

Dr. Philpott explains that humans live in a magnetic field and become ill if not in a magnetic field. Astronauts are provided an artificial magnetic field to prevent illness. A fluid passing through the friction of a magnetic field produces electromotive energy. This known fact is used industrially. Blood flowing in the human body, which is flowing through the earth's magnetic field in which the human lives, will provide the production of some electromotive energy. This energy production can be enhanced by placing a magnet over the heart.

Using the negative magnetic pole also keeps the cellular elements properly magnetically poled so they do not stick together.

Hector Solorzano del Rio, M.D., Ph.D., D.Sc., University of Guadaljara, Guadalajara, Mexico, reports that adjoining bones must be of the same magnetic polarity so that they will push away from one another, thus creating space for growth of essential cartilage. Osteoarthritics who've lost cartilage between any two joints should therefore use the same magnetic polarity across the joint. Those suffering from Ankylosing Spondilitis, a condition where the spine bends, causing great misery and stooped walking, apparently have developed opposite polarities in their adjacent spinal vertebrae, thus causing uneven shrinkage of cartilage. Dr. Solorzano has helped such victims by, among other therapies, placing properly poled magnets along their spinal vertebrae.

Also, oxygen and water have an ability to be influenced by magnetic fields and can carry this magnetic energy throughout the entire body with blood circulation.

According to Dr. Philpott, the earth's magnetic field is waning and therefore humans are living in a magnetic deficient environment. This can be corrected by sleeping on a negative poled magnetic bed pad and/ or with the head in a negative magnetic field.

Many people purchase and use magnetic mattresses, seat cushions and so on without regard to whether there is a mixture of magnetic polarities inside, or if the polarity is the kind that heals or tears down.

It is very important, according to William H. Philpott, M.D., that the correct polarity be used for either healing or destruction of tissue. A mixed polarity mattress, for example, instructs the body to both heal and to tear down simultaneously, which is certainly not what most people want. One woman on learning that her magnets may be of mixed polarity in her mattress and seat cushions, took them apart and aligned them properly, using a standardized magnet that she obtained from Dr. Philpott. (A catalog of various kinds of magnets as well as experimental treatment protocols may be obtained from William H. Philpott, M.D., Chairman, Bio-Electro-Magnetics Institute, Institutional Review Board, 17171 SE 29, Choctaw, OK 73020.)

Wearing the negative pole of a magnet on the heart will help correct the magnetic deficient environment.

Any treatment of the body with a magnetic field will to some degree have a systemic energy increase since the oxygen and water passing through the magnetic field become magnetized, which then goes to the entire body

It is of interest to note that insects and sharks obtain 90% of their energy from external magnetic (exogenous) sources whereas humans receive only 30% of their energy from external (exogenous) sources.

There have been excellent reports from many sources regarding the beneficial effects of the use of magnets on a wide assortment of diseases. As strong, flexible magnets can now be obtained for a reasonable price that will wrap around a leg or arm, or heavy, rigid ones that can be placed at the top of the head up against the headboard at night, there is a great deal of anecdotal clinical case history available.

The Case of Lori Humboldt

Lori Humboldt,[80] 58-years-of-age, housewife in Murfreesboro, Tennessee, had two problems. One problem was a persistent back ache that no other form of treatment had helped. She'd tried chiropractic, homeopathy, rheumatology, internal medicine practitioners, osteopathy, and herbs. None had given her the relief that she sought for the back pain.

Lori's second problem was pain in her feet, especially when she walked.

However, lacking any other recourse, she rather gingerly investigated the use of magnets, not being sure whether this was or was not just another form of quackery.

She purchased a large magnet for her mattress upon which she laid at night, and also smaller, pliable magnets to fit over the pain of her feet, being careful to use the negative (South seeking) polarity as according to William II. Philpott, M.D. who has researched and clinically applied magnetics for many years, it's very important that the correct polarity be used for either healing or destruction of tissue. "the South seeking pole of a magnet heals, while the North seeking pole breaks down tissues."

Within a day Lori's pains in both back and feet had eased. Within several days, they disappeared altogether, and they stay gone so long as she uses the magnets.

The Case of William H. Philpott, M.D.

William H. Philpott, M.D. began his quest for information on the healing powers of magnetics through his own personal experience.

At age of 54 Dr. Philpott found that he had diabetes, discovering that cereal grains containing glutens -- protein contained in wheat and other grains which gives dough its elastic character -- produced high blood sugar, and that when he drank milk he suffered from bursitis, tender elbows, and a tender wrist.

Bouts of arthritic elbow pain developed into carpal tunnel syndrome and a contracture of the wrist and hand called Dupuytren contracture. Dr. Philpott successfully used a four-day diversified rotation diet which freed him of diabetes, bursitis, arthritis, tenosynovitis and the Dupuytren contracture.

Later he discovered the beneficial use of the negative magnetic field and started sleeping on a negatively poled magnetic bed pad with magnets at the crown of his head. He found he slept more soundly, and had more energy the next day, and also lost his dry eye problem. He says, "At 54 I was falling apart with aches and pains, high blood sugar, and I had lost all my molars due to infection over a three year period before I discovered I had diabetes. I have not lost a tooth in the last 21 years."[38]

The Physiological Effects of Positive and Negative Magnetic Fields

According to many researchers, negative magnetic fields seem to affect all the metabolic processes involved in growth, healing, immune defense, nonimmune microorganism defense, and detoxification. The following chart as reported in *Alternative Medicine, The Definitive Guide,*[5] was prepared by William H. Philpott, M.D. and is based on his clinical observations of the effects that positive and negative magnetic fields have upon living organisms.

Biological Response to Antistressful Negative Static Magnetic Fields	**Biological Repsonse to Stressful Positive Static Magnetic Fields**
pH normalzing	Acid producing
Oxygenating	Oxygen deficit producing
Resolves cellular edema	Evokes cellular edema
Usually reduces symptoms	Often evokes or exacerbates existing symptoms
Can relieve addictive withdrawal symptoms	Stress evokes endorphin production and symptoms can therefore be addicting
Inhibits microorganism replication	Accelerates microorganism replication
Biologically normalizing	Biologically disorganizing
Governs rest, relaxation, and sleep	Governs wakefulness and action
Evokes anabolic hormone production-- melatonin and growth hormone	Evokes catabolic hormone production inhibits anabolic hormone production
Counters and processes metabolically-produced toxins out of the body	Produces toxic end products of metabolism and does not counter or process these toxins out of the body
Cancels out free radicals	Produces free radicals

Mineral Infrared Therapy

Historically natural sunlight, a broad range of electromagnetic frequencies, has been used for many disease conditions. Sunlight, for example, is necessary for the utilization of vitamin D, which is necessary in turn for the proper utilization of calcium without which our cells would not function properly.

We are truly a creature of our planet and its energizing sun because proper light frequencies govern our body's inner clock, the timing of sleep, hormone production, metabolic body temperature and many other biological functions.

Since all of the above named functions are vital for healthy cells -- hence organs and systems -- it shouldn't be surprising to learn that every kind of disease condition, including osteoarthritis and other aches and pains identified as osteoarthritis, can respond favorably with the proper use of full-spectrum sunlight. Should a person, for example, lack sufficient sunlight to utilize vitamin D, then the mineral calcium will not be able to enter into cells and perform its metabolic function. The body, according to Carl Reich, M.D., Calgary, Canada, then maladapts, causing any one of several kinds of diseases such as osteoarthritis, asthma, heart problems, and so on. If lack of sufficient sunlight is the cause, its cure is simple: add full-spectrum sunlight, vitamin D, calcium, and other appropriate nourishment and the osteoarthritis disappears. (See "Diet and Nutrition," this Chapter.)

Selected frequencies from full-spectrum sunlight have also been used therapeutically ranging from ultra-violet (UV) to infrared wavelengths. A specialized application of infrared wavelengths produced by coated ceramic materials containing trace amounts of minerals like iron, selenium, manganese, zinc, cobalt, nickel, copper, cadmium and so forth has been therapeutically beneficial, and is called "mineral infrared therapy."

A heated surface no larger than a dinner plate, and about the same shape, is coated with ceramic minerals containing many trace elements required by the human body. The frequency range of infrared used is between 2 and 25 micrometers which is easily absorbed by human tissues consisting chiefly of hydrogen-oxygen and carbon-hydrogen-oxygen bonds that absorb the radiation easily between 3 to 4 micrometer wavelengths. The operating surface is held about 11 inches from the skin producing a surface temperature at the skin of about 102^0 F.

In addition to the beneficial effects of the infrared spectrum, there is broadcast ionic minerals from the surface of the disk that benefit those who lack these trace minerals. According to biochemist Tsu-Tsair Chi, N.M.D., Ph.D., more than 30 million people in China, Australia, Japan and Mexico have effectively used Mineral Infrared Therapy, which, he says, "has the ability to alleviate inflammation, tranquilize pain and improve micro-circulation, as well as stabilize metabolism." He also says that undisputed evidence was gathered substantiating that the use of Mineral Infrared Therapy was conducive to cell-growth, multiplication and restoration, along with promotion of specific types of enzyme activity and immunity levels, and has been successfully used "to treat over 30 different human and animal diseases and disorders,"[69] including various forms of arthritis. According to studies made by scientists and physicians, effects of Mineral Infrared Therapy may be due to a combination of trace element effects, enzyme effects, acupuncture stimulation effects, and general heat effects.

A list of health professionals, representing every one of the American states who utilize the Mineral Infrared Therapy (MIT) can be obtained through Chi's Enterprise, Inc., 5465 E. Estate Ridge Rd., Anaheim, CA 92807; (714) 921-1957. A tabletop model is available for $599, the professional for $1299.

The Case of Gene Dunkin[69]

Rhode Islander Gene Dunkin, 40-years-of-age, had been on a business trip for seven days when the recurrence of his lower back pain prevented him from sitting, so he wasn't able to return home on an airplane. Diathermy -- which is the application of radio frequency electromagnetic energy to the body to cause a temperature rise -- and ultra sound treatments -- also a means of raising body temperature through sound electromagnetic frequencies as a result of molecular level friction -- and ordinary heat were all tried on Gene without effect.

To treat Gene, Dr. Stuart Golden of Orlando, Florida, used Mineral Infrared Therapy for 20 minutes, after which Gene was relieved sufficiently so that he could sit down, and so he was able to return to Rhode Island on the next available flight.

The Case of Frederick Balleny

Frederick Balleny was 5'8" tall and weighed 200 pounds. He went to Las Vegas, Nevada to see Dr. George Ritter for his "degenerative" osteoarthritis in his neck, middle and lower back.

Dr. Ritter treated Frederick for about 40 minutes 3 times a week for 2 months getting very good results.

The Case of Katherine Casey

For years Katherine Casey had had severe osteoarthritis in both knees, and could only move about with the use of a cane. She was 60-years-of-age, 5'2" tall and weighed 140 pounds.

After 15 days of use with the Mineral Infrared Therapy under reflexologist Hal Camp, Bellflower, California, Katherine was able to throw away her cane, and her pain was considerably reduced.

Structure

Those of us who've acquired sufficient age will remember when our grade-school teachers demanded strict compliance with a "proper posture" while sitting, walking and -- yes -- even when using our pens and pencils. Since the body was designed to stretch and restore, move and stay, run and lay, it would have been an interesting study had any-one during those early twenties subjected our school marms' theories to the rigors of modern studies.

Does the habitual, conscious conditioning of a particular postural pattern, such as demanded of military ranks, also produce a better functioning mind and body?

It's clear from what follows that disease states can start from ill-formed structuring of the body, and that these states can be enhanced or sustained by ill-formed structuring including that caused by persistent poor posture. It hardly appears that lack of strict adherence to a particular military or school-advised posture is universally the source-causation for arthritic states.

The actual source-causation of problems seems to stem from stretched or torn tendons and ligaments, however achieved, "sticky" fascia -- the otherwise slippery material that surrounds bundles of muscles -- inflammed nerve sites, and other kinds of physical/mental relationships. A few therapies designed to solve the structural problems that lead to osteoarthritis, or solve the problem of osteoarthritis, are presented in the following.

Neural and Reconstructive Therapy
Neural Therapy

Reconstructive Therapy is labeled "Sclerotherapy" by D.O.s, and "Proliferative Therapy" (or "Prolo Therapy") by M.D.s. The term "Reconstructive Therapy," is preferred by William J. Faber, D.O., Director of the Milwaukee Pain Clinic, Milwaukee, Wisconsin. As this name is growing in popularity we will use "Reconstructive Therapy."

Usually those physicians who practice reconstructive therapy must study beyond courses offered in medical school, also refreshing themselves on detailed anatomy. Since those who practice reconstructive therapy usually combine it with another treatment known as "Neural Therapy," the two subjects are included together in this section.

Strangely enough, and little known to many physicians, scar tissue from past penetrations of the skin can also cause skeletal mis-alignment problems, and these are usually treated at the same time as the use of Reconstructive Therapy using Neural/FascialTherapy,[29] a treatment developed by German physicians, and especially Ferdinand Huenke, M.D. and Walter Huenke, M.D.[30]

In the Huenke Neural Therapy, an anesthetic such as procaine or lidocaine is injected into nerve sites of the autonomic (independent) nervous system, acupuncture points, scars, glands, and other tissues. Through the pathways of the autonomic nervous system, energy to cells short-circuits the disease or injury and serves to regulate biological energy.

Although an individual injection can relieve pain, it is a series of injections that follow along a key physiological pattern that serves to provide the most relief.

Premised on the idea that illness begins when the normal flow of biological energy is disrupted, Neural Therapy seeks to release these energy blockages, and sometimes the results are quite spectacular, providing an almost instantaneous "miracle" cure.

Any part of the body that has been damaged or traumatized can cause these energy blockages, thus the injections may follow old wounds, surgical scars, past body blows, "stored" illnesses, and so forth.

Neural Therapy can also assist in unblocking the lymph system.

Conditions that normally respond to Neural Therapy include: arthritis, allergies,   back pain, and about thirty more .[5,29]

Dietrich Klinghardt, M.D., Ph.D. of Santa Fe, New Mexico adds that "In my experience, between one and six treatments, given twice weekly, are all that's needed."[5,29]

Reconstructive Therapy

Many physicians who use Reconstructive Therapy, such as William Faber, D.O., Milwaukee, WI, have seen such speedy results from conditions of osteoarthritis, or osteoarthritis-like pains, that they recommend reconstructive therapy as a second, and next, trial treatment if osteopathic or chiropractic manipulations are not successful in handling the problem.

Using natural substances injected in key positions, growth of connective tissue is stimulated in such a manner that weak or damaged tendons or ligaments are strengthened. By tightening up these structural defects pains often remotely located from the source of damage disappear.

Arthritic spurs that occur along the spinal column which press on nerves creating "referred" pain in the hip, leg, or foot are thought to be the body's attempts to compensate from the result of skeletal misalignment caused by damaged tendons or ligaments. Although these spurs are more likely to resolve with proper nutritional support than from the use of reconstructive therapy, this form of treatment can usually readjust -- that is, balance -- the body's structure in such a manner that the pain will totally disappear.[27]

In 1950 surgeon George Hackett, M.D. treated 1,600 patients with severe sacroiliac sprain by means of reconstructive therapy. Examined by independent physicians 2 to 12 years later, 82 percent remained free of pain or recurrences.

By 1955 demonstrations on rabbits had shown that loosened, stretched or torn tendons and ligaments could be tightened up by means of inserting just beneath the skin, in the proper location, a natural bodily substance purified from cod liver oil, sodium morrhuate, which promotes the growth of fibrous collagen tissue and bone growth, making the weld between tendons and bones or ligaments at the ends of muscles that attach to bone up to 30% stronger and up to 40% larger. Other natural substances besides sodium morrhuate are also used, such as dextrose, a sugar.

The University of Iowa's Department of Orthopedic Research repeated Dr. Hackett's studies in 1983 and 1985. Both studies found that treated tendons and ligaments were firmly attached, and that structural strength was increased by 30 to 40 percent.

As we age, our tendons and ligaments tend to stretch or can be torn from their connections to fascia -- the band of tissue that surrounds or binds muscle -- through sports or accidents, or can be weakened through poor nutrition, disease or unbalanced chemistries. As the body's skeletal posture is held together by means of tendons and ligaments — not the muscles which provide power applied to tendons and ligaments — an undesireable lengthening of one set of tendons or ligaments will be unconsciously compensated for by other pulley and lever/fulcrum mechanisms that affect   remote parts of the body.

Tendons are muscle ends. Fascia apparently gives ligaments and bones their proper place and structure. The fascial connective tissue thickens and becomes most rigid at places of greatest and most frequent use and demand. Osteoarthritis, also an 'ossification' process of fascia, makes a return to good posture difficult.

One   compensatory mechanism, as already described,   is the production of osteoarthritic spurs in the spine. Although the body's problem is lax or torn ligaments or tendons elsewhere, the body's chemistry attempts to compensate by creating calcium spurs along the spinal column or at other locations. Were these calcium spurs cut out (as is often done for relief of symptoms through surgery), the body's tendon   and/or ligament problems will persist, and the body will continue to attempt to compensate for the tendon or ligament laxness.

To illustrate: James A. Carlson, D.O. of Knoxville, Tennessee was asked to look at the right index finger-joint nearest to the fingernail (between the distal phalanx and the middle phalanx) of one of us (Perry A. Chapdelaine, Sr.). The joint had been inflamed for months and was deforming. After study Dr. Carlson deduced that the cause was a left-foot heel-bone out of alignment. This may sound peculiar until one is versed with the manner in which the skeleton is held together, and the means by which the human body compensates. A bone out of position at one location places undesireable stress on related tendons while also causing an abnormal laxness in other related tendons. The end result is a series of unconscious bodily adaptations that sequentially affect tendon and bone structures remotely connected, and from which the appearance of osteoarthritic pain can result. Using osteopathic manipu-lation -- a series of manipulations that normalizes the position of the structures -- Dr. Carlson placed the heel bone back as well as affected joints at the base of the thumb at the palm of the right hand. He then used reconstructive therapy, placing dextrose injections near appropriate tendons and ligaments and which promoted the body's ability to keep the proper tendons taut, and the heel and other palm bones in place.The finger immediately ceased its pain and deformation stopped.[32]

For the same person, and in a similar experience, the finger nearest the small one on the left hand was unable to touch the palm of the hand, as with many who suffer from osteoarthritis. It was very stiff and often hurt. Dr. Carlson determined that the cause was an arch-bone in the left foot out of alignment. Again he manipulated the bone to its proper location and then used reconstructive therapy injections to strengthen tendons and ligaments which would keep the bone and other structural features permanently where they belonged. The pain immediately disappeared and the patient had restored ability.

In the following chart, many other instances -- much more spectacular[27,29] -- can be described for all parts of the body where so-called "incurable" osteoarthritis is presumed but in fact it is the slackness or over-tautness of a tendon or ligament or torn connective tissue that slowly creates the painful symptoms according to William Faber, D.O. of Milwaukee, Wisconsin and Morton Walker, D.P.M., medical journalist and author of many medical books.[27]

**Chart of Painful Conditions Improved or
Cured by Proliferative Therapy***

Ankle: ankle weakness

Back: generalized back weakness, herniated disks, mid-level backache, low back pain, compression fractures of the vertebrae, ankylosing spondylitis (deformation of backbone), spondylolisthesis (5th lumbar slippage)

Elbows: tennis elbow

Finger: finger dysfunctions, Heberden nodes (according to James O. Carlson, D.O., Knoxville, Tennessee)

Foot: bunions, heel difficulties

Head: migraine headache

Heart: pain after stroke

Hip: dysfunctional hip joint

Jaw: temporomandibular joint (TMJ) syndrome (jaw joint)

Knee: knee (patellar) problems, chronic and acute knee disability

Legs: tennis leg

Muscles and Fascia: fibrositis, fascitis

Neck: neck pain

Other: many other kinds of disabilities, including most forms of arthritis.

Shoulder: chronic shoulder dislocation, shoulder (rotator cuff) tears

Surgery post-pain: post-orthopedic surgery pain

Tendons: Tendonitis, synovitis, pain after severe injury,

Wrist: wrist pain, carpal-tunnel syndrome

* For physician referral contact William J. Faber, D.O., Milwaukee Pain Clinic, 6529 W. Fond du Lac Ave., Milwaukee, WI 53218; (414) 464-7680 or The Arthritis Trust of America, 5106 Old Harding Road, Franklin, TN 37064. Send in stamped, self-addressed envelope and tax-exempt donation for service from the latter organization.

When chiropractic or osteopathic manipulations do not work, Reconstructive Therapy is a treatment of choice for osteoarthritis, and it is often a more effective medical alternative to orthopedic, hand, or podiatric surgery and other traditional techniques of musculo-skeletal repair."[27]

The Case of Diana Beachamp

Diana Beachamp, 40-years-of-age, came to Ross Hauser, M.D. of the Caring Medical & Rehabilitation Services, Oak Park Illinois, for severe back pain with radiation down the left leg. Dr. Hauser says, "Diana could not work and was having difficulty walking. She did have a history of back pain in the past laying her up for weeks at a time."

A previous magnetic resonance imaging (MRI) -- a picture made with a strong magnetic field interacting with the magnetic fields of atoms in tissues -- 3-1/2 years earlier had revealed degenerative disc disease in the lumbar and sacrum, as well as mild disc bulges. There was also a mild narrowing of nerve passages (stenosis) in portions of the lumbar region. A physical examination revealed marked spasm in the lower back with tenderness in this area as well as the sacroiliac joints. There was also some evidence of a pinched nerve.

Reconstructive therapy was administered to Diana's lower back and sacroiliac joints. Neural therapy was also used in two of the lumbar regions.

Diana felt great after this first treatment.

The treatment was repeated 18 days later and again 11 days after the second treatment. When seen again, Dr. Hauser reports that "Diana's previous numbness was gone, her flexibility better, and she was smiling again.

"Follow-up a month later found Diana with increased energy and feeling great. She was given some stretching exercises and told to come back when needed."

The Case of Terry Woodworth

Terry Woodworth, 36-years-of-age, came to the clinic of Ross Hauser, M.D. with severe tempomandibular joint syndrome (TMJ), a condition of the joints of the jaw which can lead to osteoarthritis. According to Dr. Hauser, "Terry could dislocate his tempomandibular joint at will, and also had severe grinding of the joint which could be heard as well as felt."

Dr. Hauser used reconstructive therapy injections on both joints.

Three weeks later Terry was improved, but there was still the clicking of joints many osteoarthritics know so well, and so he was treated again.

Five weeks after his second treatment Terry reported that he had not noticed any clicking of these joints except once when he yawned widely. "Physical examination of the joints revealed them as completely normal. Even Terry's dentist was amazed that the joints remained normal."

The Case of Kenneth Plumer

Kenneth Plumer is a 30-year-old recreational volley ball player who noted his right shoulder popping out of joint when doing a slam. On physical examination Dr. Hauser noted shoulder instability which can lead to osteoarthritis.

Reconstructive therapy was administered and on follow-up visit Kenneth's shoulder was completely normal and the joint stable without any recurrence of dislocation.

The Case of Julia Merrywhether

Julia Merrywhether, 64-years-of-age, suffered from a diffuse body aching, and she also had documented osteoarthritis in many joints (polyarticular osteoarthritis), which affected her spine, knees and hands. On her initial visit she also had disabling back pain with radiation of pain into the left leg. Physical examination showed tenderness over the iliac crest, lumbosacral junction and sacroiliac joints.

Dr. Hauser treated Julia's low back and knees with reconstructive therapy.

On follow-up four months later, Julia reported 95% improvement in her pain. "A few tender spots remained around her lateral collateral ligaments of her knee and these were treated. No additional treatments were required on her lower back."

The Case of Carrie Johnston

Carrie Johnston was a 42-year-old who had had 14 surgeries on her left knee, and was still having difficulty walking because of the pain. She'd had cartilage removed and was getting arthritis in that joint.

Dr. Hauser reported that "After four series of reconstruction therapy injections Carrie became essentially pain-free, except when she underwent extreme exertion. Overall she was 95% pain relieved."

The Case of Bessie Woody

Bessie Woody, 35-years-of-age, had had severe pain in the elbow, neck and back since her second child was born. On physical examination Dr. Hauser found that she had "hypermobility syndrome" a condition which caused many ligaments and tendons to stretch in some after pregnancies and which can lead to osteoarthritis. Bessie was not going to have any more children because of her intense pain.

Injections were started on neck, shoulders, elbows, hips and lower back regions.

A month later, Bessie noted that she felt 90-95% better, and she stated "I don't know if I need a second series of injections."

When she was seen four months later, she noticed some neck pain, but essentially the rest of her pain was gone.

A year and three months later, Bessie gave birth to her third child.

The Case of Sonny Wentworth

One type of joint pain that disturbs some of us greatly cannot be attributed to active rheumatoid disease or gout. Often this kind of pain is the result of having had rheumatoid disease or is traditionally identified as osteoarthritis, and stems from the absence of cartilage, the friction of bone (clicking joints as we move them), or weakened tendons, ligatures and muscles   where   they should attach to bone surfaces through tearing, stretching or physical damage. For example, like Terry Woodworth,   forty-five year-old Sonny Wentworth had severe tempomandibular joint syndrome (TMJ), with numerous surgeries in the past, including implants.

> For those who can't afford to pay, Dr. Hauser offers a free alternative medicine clinic on appointment sponsored by Thebes First Baptist Church of Thebes, Illinois, Ross A. Hauser, M.D. and Marion Hauser, registered dietitian, can be reached at (618) 764-2323; Along with   Dr. Hemwall, Dr. Hauser practices at Caring Medical & Rehabilitation Services, S.C, 715 Lake Street Street, Suite 600, Oak Park, Illinois 60301; Telephones (800) RX-PROLO; (708) 848-7789; Fax (708) 848-7763.

When he first visited Dr. Hauser, his clicks were noticeable and the joints were extremely painful.

After one reconstructive therapy session Sonny was 20-30% better.

Seven weeks later Sonny described his condition as better, the clicking down significantly, with some pain on the right side of his jaw.

Three months later, with the cumulative effect of his treatments, Sonny noticed that the syndrome bothered him only when he was tense. Dr. Hauser said that "No further TMJ treatments was necessary or done, as the patient feels 90-95% better."

How is it that traditional diagnoses and treatments result in such a poor outcome as experienced by Sonny Wentworth and others?

Dr. Faber[27,29] explains: "X-rays cannot show anything but bones, and do not show torn ligaments which stabilize joints by holding bones in place. When ligaments are torn they are unable to effectively function to hold bones in place which then causes friction as bone rubs against one.

According to William Fabor, D.O., the body's structure and form is held together by the ligaments and tendons, not the muscles, which simply provide power across the equivalent of pulleys and lever/fulcrums in the body.

"The body attempts to correct this problem caused by the torn ligaments by creating 'arthritis'. In this instance 'arthritis' [including calcium spurs which also create pain] is the body's attempt to compensate for the torn ligament's inability to hold the bones in place.

"This," says Faber, "explains why anti-inflammatory drugs and cortisone are often not effective. Excess friction, not inflammation, is the cause of the joint pain. Reducing inflammation will not eliminate the problem nor provide long-term relief. Only strengthening the ligaments will correct the problem." [Underlining added.]

Since ligaments contain no muscle fibers, exercise also will not correct the problem or provide long-term relief.

When Should Reconstructive Therapy Be Considered?

According to Drs. Faber and Walker, under the following conditions:

1. When ligaments are either lax or torn, then the ligaments can be strengthened.

2. When any joint has pain lasting longer than six weeks. A healthy body should be able to heal torn or lax ligaments within six weeks. If joint pain persists beyond six weeks, it is an indication that the body has not been able to handle it on its own and that the joint is unstable from lax or torn ligaments.

3. Any joint that is helped by a support or brace. A brace or support functions as ligaments do. That is, they function to stabilize the joint. If a support brace helps, proliferative therapy is indicated as it strengthens the ligaments, enabling the necessary support.

4. Any joint that fails to respond to [chiropractic or osteopathic] manipulation or adjustments. Many joint problems can be resolved with manipulations/adjustments and often manipulation/adjustment is the treatment of choice. Manipulation is highly effective when bones are out of alignment as a result of bad posture or injury. When manipulation or adjustment doesn't provide lasting relief it is because the ligaments are lax or torn and can't hold the joint in place.

5. Any joint that is worse after surgery. When injured joint spacers are removed in surgery (discs, cartilage) this causes the ligaments to become lax. This laxity causes the joint to become unstable and eventually form arthritis.

6. Any joint that is better with rest and worse with exercise. Rest allows the body to heal itself and also reduces friction which is caused by a torn or lax ligament in a weakened joint. Exercise of an unstable joint makes it hurt more as it creates increased friction. Because of the decreased blood supply in ligaments, rest alone is often not sufficient for the body to heal itself. And, because ligaments and tendons do not contain muscle fiber, exercise will not heal an injured ligament or tendon.

7. Any popping, snapping or clicking joint. A joint that is unstable snaps, clicks or pops. Proliferative therapy causes strengthening of the ligaments and thus stabilizes the joint thus eliminating the popping, snapping and/or clicking.

8. Any torn tendon or tendonitis that does not resolve after six weeks. Tendons are like ligaments in that they are fibrous tissue and they attach to the bone. They also have a lack of blood supply like ligaments, and therefore have a poor healing ability. Proliferative therapy causes a permanent strengthening of torn or lax tendons just as

it does for torn or lax ligaments.[27] (See *Pain, Pain Go Away*, Morton Walker, D.P.M., William J. Faber, D.O.; *Do What You Want To Do*, William J. Faber, D.O., John Parks Trowbridge, M.D.)

Intraneural Injections

The Nature of Joint Pain

Reconstructive therapy normalizes and balances the structure of the whole body through the tightening up of lax or torn ligaments and tendons powered by muscles. Keeping in mind that it is the ligaments and tendons, together with bones, that provides the body's overall structural shape, nonetheless prolonged unevenly applied muscles contribute to osteoarthritis and rheumatoid arthritis by creating prolonged, uneven   stress at   specific joints. This prolonged, uneven application of muscle power applied through perfectly normal tendons and ligaments has its ultimate source-causation from specific nerve centers that usually lie very close to the skin.

English Professor Roger Wyburn-Mason, M.D., Ph.D., nerve specialist, demonstrated more than 50 years ago that the source-causation of joint pain in both osteoarthritis and rheumatoid arthritis began with disturbances in the cells of nerve centers called "ganglia."

South African Dr. Paul Pybus, surgeon and acupuncturist, demonstrated that these disturbed nerve ganglia usually corresponded to traditional acupuncture points normally found along the nerve paths of uninsulated nerve fibers that lay close to the surface of the skin (called unmyelinated C-fibers), unlike the deeper, insulated fibers that carried larger electric signals throughout the body. One key nerve center -- ganglion -- for example, is protected by the bony protubance at the base of the small finger of each hand at the back of the wrist. At the base of that bump, on the little finger side, will be found a special nerve from which signals flow to specific parts of the fingers. If that nerve is pressed and there is no pain it is not inflamed or creating problems with the fingers under its "command." However, if pain is experienced when pressing that point, then one has found a key source of finger joint pain.

Another major nerve center, or ganglion, is found at the elbow's "crazy bone," also somewhat protected by a bony protrubance. Between the elbow and the wrist, between the two bony sites described, there are many smaller nerve centers that also may be painful when pressed. Each one of these when inflamed and painful on touch is the source-causation of pain which appears to stem from the joints, and which is traditionally called "joint pain."

Dr. Paul Pybus and one of us (Gus Prosch, Jr., M.D.) traced out a large number of these especially critical nerve centers throughout the body as related to both osteoarthritis and rheumatoid arthritis, as well as other forms of rheumatoid diseases such as ankylosing spondilitis, fibromyalgia, and so on. In almost every instance the center of joint disturbance follows known acupuncture points.

As shown in Figure 2(a): "Normal Joint Position" and 2(b): "Arthritic Joint Position," the arthritic's inflammed nerve center sends out two sets of signals. One set goes directly to the spinal column to form a reflex arc, transmitting directly back to the muscles surrounding the involved joint. The other set goes to the brain where the returning signal to the joint returns as pain at the joint, from which swelling and heat arise. Although the painful joint may be most uncomfortable, the major portion of damage is done by the signal that has passed as a reflex arc to the spinal column and back to the muscles surrounding the involved joint.

A clue to understanding this condition was provided in 1960 by Drs. Robert Salter and Paul Field, Toronto, Canada, Antoni Trias, Oxford, England, and Drs. Crelin and Southwick, Cambridge, Massachusetts. All of them performed experiments on the knee joints of monkeys or rabbits. They clamped one leg of an animal with a device, called a "Charnley clamp," which maintained continuous pressure on the leg joint. See Figure 3(a): "Charnley's Clamp and Figure" 3(b):" Charnley's Clamp on One Leg." The other leg was left unclamped to act as a control. At the end of 3 days, progression of joint degeneration had begun in the clamped leg. After 14 days the condition was well established. After 6 weeks degeneration was in its final stages, the cartilage being worn away and a bone-against-bone polishing called "eburnation" had begun.

Two other scientists, Drs. R.A. Calandruccio and Gilmer W. Scott were able to demonstrate that if this fixation-compression was released from the joint, the condition was reversible, and cartilage showed signs of regeneration.

Corresponding observations have been made in man, especially in the "well tractioned leg" after fracture of a leg. The result is often the start of osteoarthritis in the knee in the unfractured side due to the pressure on that knee exerted by the tractioning apparatus.

As shown in Figure 4: "Sponge Action of Articular Cartilage for Nutrition," unlike other body tissues, essential cartilage between the bones in joints have very little blood supply by means of veins, arteries, and capillaries. Cartilage, just like other tissues, breaks down and rebuilds, but to do so requires that it be continually nourished. Nourishment comes about through a necessary squeezing out of old blood and cellular waste products, and expansion of the tissue to bring in fresh supplies of nutrients, including oxygen. This action, much like squeezing and expanding a sponge, is a necessary one for the health of cartilage tissue.

Below our level of awareness, the spinal arc signals to the muscles surrounding a joint telling the muscles to squeeze more than to expand, and so there is a net loss of the balance between incoming nutrients and outgoing waste products. The consequence is a combination of toxic cellular waste products and "free radical pathology," a condition caused

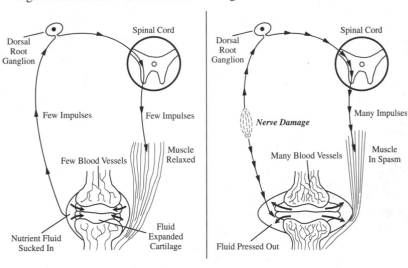

Figure 2a: Normal Joint Position

Figure 2b: Arthritic Joint Position

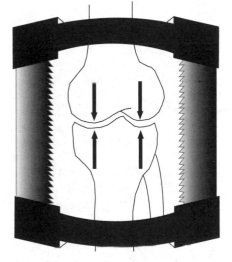

Figure 3a:
Charnley's Clamp

Figure 3b:
Charnley's Clamp on One Leg

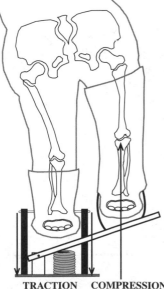

TRACTION   COMPRESSION

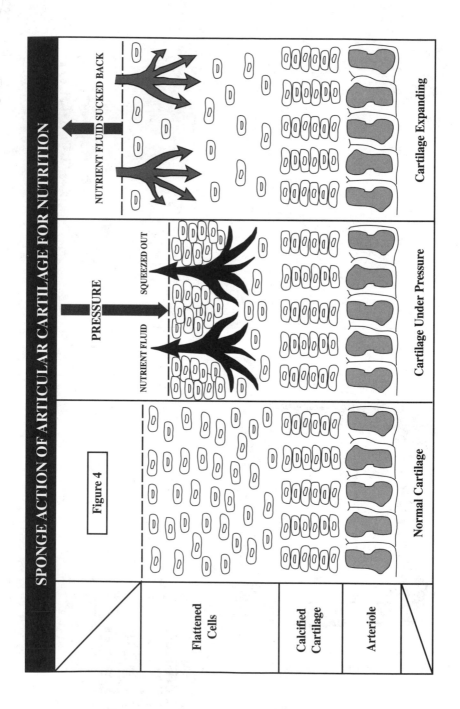

SPONGE ACTION OF ARTICULAR CARTILAGE FOR NUTRITION

Figure 4

Flattened Cells

Calcified Cartilage

Arteriole

NUTRIENT FLUID SUCKED BACK

Cartilage Expanding

PRESSURE

SQUEEZED OUT

NUTRIENT FLUID

Cartilage Under Pressure

Normal Cartilage

by highly reactive, destructive molecules resulting from decomposition of cartilage and some of the toxic cellular waste. It is this over-all, over-looked nerve/muscle process that finally creates heated and swollen joints and eventually permanently damages joints that become distorted and useless.

When the arthritic joint is treated by traditional drugs -- even though pain may temporarily disappear for the time being -- the controlling, inflamed nerve centers continue firing inappropriate signals to muscles that surround the involved joint communicating to them that there should be more muscle compression at the joint than there is expansion. This is the principal reason why traditional drug therapy does not work and why the arthritic joint continues to deteriorate even though the joint pain has been temporarily eliminated by drugs. The wrong target has been selected for pain relief, and therefore the pain function continues to operate, although the sense of pain has diminished. [77]

But what causes these particular nerve centers to be disturbed?

The reasons are many, just as there are many "causes" for arthritis such as faulty nutrition, bio-chemical imbalances, and mechanical and structural problems. There can be as many initiating causes for disturbed nerve centers as there are ways to create faulty nutrition, bio-chemical imbalances, or mechanical and structural problems.

Although osteoarthritis and rheumatoid arthritis have different reasons for manifesting, the joint pain in each stems from the same basic source -- key nerve centers.

Key, inflamed nerve centers as a source-causation of arthritic joint pain also explains why saturation by strong anti-oxidants, such as dimethylsulfoxide (DMSO), intravenous vitamin C and others will quickly dampen pain in the joint, and may from time to time also act as a curative agent on the inflamed nerves that are the source of the problem, in which case, of course, and coincidentally, the joint disease may disappear.

If the reason for unstable nerve impulses from these key nerve centers is nutritional deficiencies, then again, of course, supplying the proper nutritional needs will stabilize the nerve cells, halt the firing of damaging nerve impulses, and act as a curative agent to the painful joint.

If the cause of the damaged nerve cells is the activity of a microbial agent, then halting the proliferation of these microbes, and permitting the body to clean up the toxins and cellular damage, will be curative.

If the cause is physical or surgical injury, or uneven stress from mechanical appliances used in healing bones or other tissues, removal of the stress, massage, chiropractic or osteopathic adjustments, or neural and/ or reconstructive therapy may relieve the problem.

How the Integrity of Nerve Conduction is Lost

As shown in Figures 5(a): "Normal and Diseased Electrical Flow of Nerves" and 5(b): "How Acupuncture Needles Drain Off Negative Current" the integrity of nerve conduction relies on the fact that the inside of the nerve is of negative polarity, while the outside membrane is of positive polarity. When the nerve tissues surrounding a nerve fiber are damaged,   leakage of negative electrons occurs from inside the nerve conduction pathway through the external membrane, thus losing nerve conduction integrity. Excess negative electrons will have an affinity for other molecules in adjacent tissues, most probably creating an additional load of undesireable chemical reactions in the tissue surrounding the nerve membrane damage. See Figure 6(a): "Normal Electrical Flow of Nerve," Figure 6(b): "Disruption of Normal Electrical Nerve Flow," and Figure 6(c): "Resulting Inflammation from Disrupted Nerve Flow."

When acupuncture needles are inserted into acupuncture points, excess electrons are bled off, thus acting as a temporary relief gateway for the mis-directed electron flow, according to Dr. Paul K. Pybus. Patients responded better to his acupuncture therapy when he administered the needles in barefeet, thus better grounding the excess electrons. This may explain why acupuncture provides relief for arthritics to some extent for localized pain, but, as observed by Arabinda Das, M.D., has not by itself found chronic degenerative diseases responsive,[26] although in all fairness, traditional Chinese medicine considers personalized herbs and diet equally important companions to acupuncture.

From the foregoing it's clear that in many cases of osteoarthritis and in many different forms of arthritis, more than one causation factor is operating simultaneously to generate unstable nerve impulses which are also the source-cause of joint pain.

The Case of Bessie M'butu

Dr. Paul K. Pybus, Pietermaritzburg, South Africa, described his discovery of clinical applications of Professor Roger Wyburn-Mason's teachings, that arthritic joint pain stemmed from disturbed nerve cells leading to painful joints.

"A 68-year-old crippled, overweight lady, Bessie M'butu, came to my office, hobbling in on two sticks and complaining of severe pain in her right knee, from which she had suffered for the last 10 years. The knee was swollen and very painful and kept her awake at night. She was quite unable to get around to any extent, and had to have a stick for every step she took. Examination showed her to have a marked degree of knock-knee and there was an escape of fluid present.

"She had come asking for her repeat supply of pills for sleeping, and for hypertension, from which she also suffered, and anti-inflammatory drugs. I proceeded to write her prescription, and as I was doing this

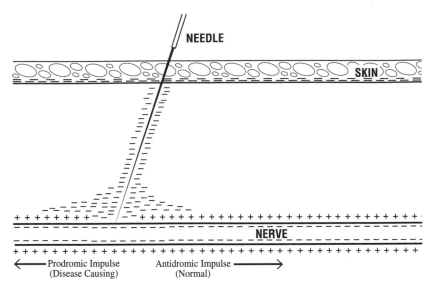

Figure 5a: Normal and Diseased Electrical Flow of Nerves

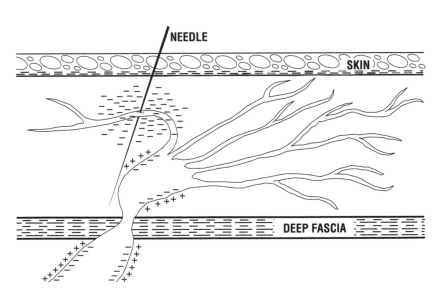

Figure 5b: How Acupuncture Needles Drain Off Negative Current

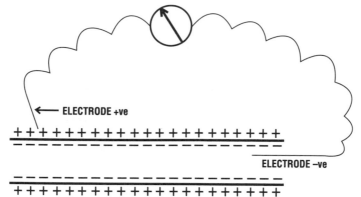

ELECTRODE +ve

ELECTRODE −ve

Figure 6a: Normal Electrical Flow of Nerve

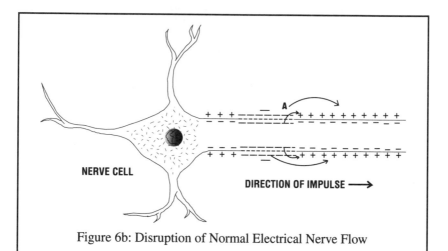

NERVE CELL

DIRECTION OF IMPULSE ⟶

Figure 6b: Disruption of Normal Electrical Nerve Flow

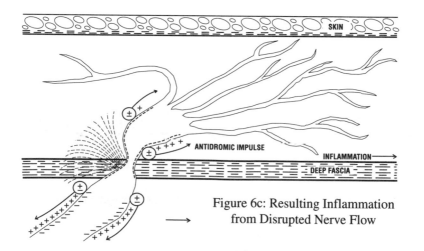

SKIN

ANTIDROMIC IMPULSE

INFLAMMATION ⟶

DEEP FASCIA

Figure 6c: Resulting Inflammation
from Disrupted Nerve Flow

Bessie said to me, 'You know, Doctor, I'm sure if you put something in just here' (pointing to a place below and back of her knee) 'I am sure you would help me a great deal.'

Dr. Pybus agreed to view her problem from the patient's perspective, and he, having in his office several substances that he thought might be useful, injected Bessie where she desired it, creating a small bleb with this mixture. During the injection,"The old lady winced a little, but made no fuss, saying it was just a little painful."

When Dr. Pybus had completed the injection, he felt the joint and tried to bend it. To his great surprise "a miracle had occurred." Instead of the patient experiencing severe pain and resistance to movement as had occurred previously, the knee flexed with the greatest of ease to full opening, and her expression changed from one of painful anticipation to one of satisfied pleasure, an ecstacy in her face, and tears into her eyes. "It was difficult to tell who was the most suprised, the patient, or myself."

Dr. Pybus asked her to stand up, and this she did and there was still no pain. Bessie then pointed to her sticks saying, "I don't want these sticks anymore, I am better now," and with that, walked to the other end of the room and back with a smile of satisfaction.

The next day Bessie returned, saying she still had no pain, and she remained pain-free for five years, on follow-up, as has another patient with osteoarthritis.[25]

The Method of Applying Intraneural Injections

One of us (Gus J. Prosch, Jr., M.D.) has taught the theory and practice of Intraneural Injections techniques to more than 600 physicians on osteoarthritis, rheumatoid arthritis and as many as 79 other rheumatoid and other diseases, but many physicians are afraid to use these wonderful techniques for fear of criticism by orthodox physicians since medical schools do not teach them. He has also treated more than 12,000 patients using the techniques of Intraneural Injections. (See *Intraneural Injections for Rheumatoid Arthritis and Osteoarthritis and The Control of Pain in aRthritis of the Knee*, Dr. Paul K. Pybus.)

Knowing the underlying structure of the nerve network leading to each joint, the physician presses with his thumb, finger, or pen (palpates) over points of expected tenderness. The tender points will be known by observing the patient wince, or the patient will respond in some manner saying, " Right there! It hurts."

Each tender point is marked with a skin pencil.

A very small amount, called a "bleb," of local anaesthetic is injected just beneath the skin using a Dermjet®, Mada-jet®, or equivalent type of power gun. These power guns are usually spring-loaded compression instruments that when held directly over the skin site to be injected will blast fluids directly through the skin without the necessity of using a needle, and are usually relatively painless.

Next a mixture of anaesthetic and a form of cortisone that does not act systemically -- that is, throughout the body -- is injected into the disturbed nerve site. We do not, of course, condone the use of cortisone for systemic use (throughout the body), or for use in the traditionally applied manner to dampen the symptoms of pain. However, studies show that the form of cortisone described here acts only locally, thus is called "depot" for the fact that when "deposited" in one site it stays there, and only slowly dissipates without any of the dangerous conse- quences that normally accompany the traditional use of cortisone. (The mixture may be 1-1/2% procaine with a small amount of Depo-Steroid such as Triamcinolone Hexacetonide)

Pain in the joint will immediately disappear, even though the injection occurred remotely from the joint, and will stay gone so long as the body does not restore the cellular lesions that have occurred in the nerve centers treated. See Figure 7(a): "Right Hip (Posterior Aspect)" and 7(b): "Right Hand & Wrist (Posterior Aspect)".

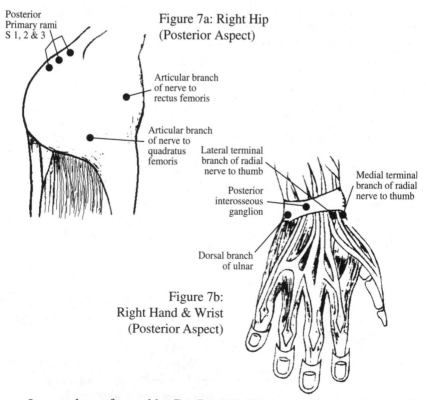

Posterior
Primary rami
S 1, 2 & 3

Figure 7a: Right Hip
(Posterior Aspect)

Articular branch
of nerve to
rectus femoris

Articular branch
of nerve to
quadratus
femoris

Lateral terminal
branch of radial
nerve to thumb

Posterior
interosseous
ganglion

Medial terminal
branch of radial
nerve to thumb

Dorsal branch
of ulnar

Figure 7b:
Right Hand & Wrist
(Posterior Aspect)

In a study performed by Dr. Paul K. Pybus, the average length of time that relief lasted in 393 pain points was 11.31 years, as shown in the following chart:

Patients Who were Followed Up by Dr. Paul K. Pybus[25]
Over a 4 year Period. Lost Patients are Unknown.

Type of Joint	Numbers	Numbers of Failures	Months of Relief	Average Relief of Joint Pain (Months)
Hips	37	3	385	10.4
Knees	124	7	1421	11.45
Ankles	44	5	491	11.15
Shoulders	44	1	716	16.27
Elbows	19	0	339	7.3
Hands	56	7	549	9.3
Sciatica	49	1	496	10.12
Neck	20	2	283	14.2
Totals	393	25	4740	11.31

The Case of Genevieve Watkerson

Genevieve Watkerson suffered from what she thought of as osteoarthritis in her right knee. Keith McElroy, M.D., Clinical Professor of Orthopaedic Surgery, College of Physicians & Surgeons, Columbia University, Columbia Presbyterian Medical Center & The New York Orthopaedic Hospital, described Genevieve "as a nice lady from Long Island with rather severe pain in her right leg, which she felt was primarily in her knee. An orthopaedist had recommended an operation on her knee. However, I could feel no tenderness in that knee, and all of the knee tests were completely negative. She did, however, walk with a limp favoring that leg." See Figure 8(a): (Right Knee (Medial Aspect): and Figure 8(b): "Right Knee (Anterior Aspect)".

Dr. McElroy examined Genevieve and   detected a very specific tenderness over a specific tendon   located in the buttock.

"I gave her an 'Injection Therapy' (Intraneural Injection) into that tender spot and, lo-and-behold, her knee pain completely vanished after injection of the local anesthetic into the buttock, a long way from the knee."

Dr. McElroy, who has independently developed Intraneural Injections, describes this phenomena of remotely located tender spots appearing painful elsewhere as "referred pain." He feels that this form of injection therapy is an important surgical alternative.

Intraneural Injections and Reconstructive Therapy cannot be performed on the patient at the same time, as the chemistry of the two therapies work in opposition to one another.[7, 27]

Chiropractic Manipulation

Concerned with the relationship of the musculoskeletal structures of the body and the spinal column to the nervous system, chiropractors usually adjust the spinal column to relieve pressure on nerves that can create pain or dysfunction in other parts of the body. This type of manipulation is called "subluxation," a method of increasing spinal motion.

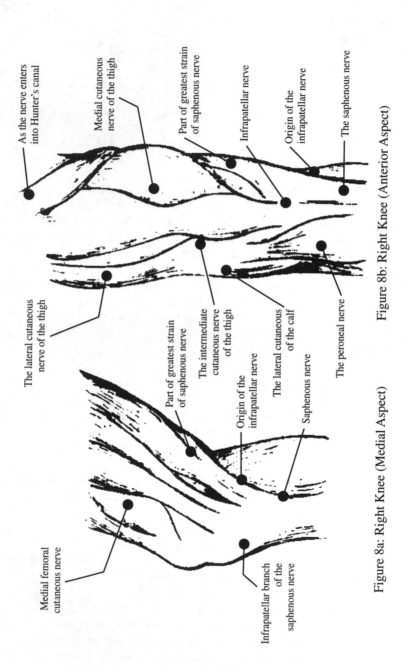

As the nerve enters into Hunter's canal

Medial cutaneous nerve of the thigh

Part of greatest strain of saphenous nerve

Infrapatellar nerve

Origin of the infrapatellar nerve

The saphenous nerve

The lateral cutaneous nerve of the thigh

Part of greatest strain of saphenous nerve

The intermediate cutaneous nerve of the thigh

Origin of the infrapatellar nerve

The lateral cutaneous of the calf

Saphenous nerve

The peroneal nerve

Medial femoral cutaneous nerve

Infrapatellar branch of the saphenous nerve

Figure 8b: Right Knee (Anterior Aspect)

Figure 8a: Right Knee (Medial Aspect)

When vertebral problems are corrected through subluxation, the overall health of the body can be improved, and such procedures can also act as a preventive measure.

Surprisingly, clusters of symptoms such as shortness of breath, heart palpitations, fatigue, depression and sharp pains radiating down the arm -- all traditionally accepted signals that heart and circulatory problems have begun -- may have started simply by mal-alignment of specific vertebrae associated with those regions, and, if this was the case, can easily be corrected by subluxation. The same traditional mis-diagnoses does and can occur on problems of inflammation of the tendons (tendinitis and synovitis), neck, back, hip, ankle and foot pain. So far as osteoarthritis is concerned, the major immediate relief is achieved for those problems that have an osteoarthritis-like appearance or have been mis-diagnosed to be osteoarthritis. Lower back pain is one of the most common complaints, with the lower lumbar region being a common source region for pain that stems along the buttock, down the leg, and may also be felt in the ankle. Left untreated, many of these problems can develop into observable osteoarthritis.

Sprains, injuries related to every joint in the body, various forms of arthritis and bursitis, and emotional problems are just a sample of where chiropractic subluxations may be useful.

Some studies have demonstrated that chiropractic combined with proper nutrition can reverse osteoarthritis. Nutrition is such an important component for the treatment of all bodily conditions, that many chiropractors have also become specialists in proper diet and supplements.

Chiropractors recognize that joints do not function independently of muscles, tendons, ligaments and other tissues, and therefore may also use treatment methods for improving blood flow , ridding the body's soft tissues of mineral deposits and tissue growths that inhibit movement.

One of us (Perry Chapdelaine, Sr.) can testify to the permanent relief of a long-standing (2 year) "tendinitis" ankle and foot pain that resulted from the 5th lumbar being displaced. Many other forms of traditional and alternative treatments were tried before trying chiropractic, which should have been tried first.

Osteopathic Manipulation

A doctor of osteopathy (D.O.) in the United States is able to combine the methods of both traditional and alternative medicine, and, like licensed medical doctors (M.D.s), can administer prescription medicines.

Osteopathic physicians use a very wide range of body manipulation techniques for soft-tissue problems, including soft-tissue arthritis (bursitis, fibromyalgia, etc.), as well as for both acute and chronic joint problems (osteoarthritis, tendenitis, etc.). Their methodology may range from gentle joint mobilization to specific thrust methods similar to those used by chiropractors.

As they are licensed to give injections, they may also provide when properly trained Reconstructive Therapy, Neural Injections, or Intraneural Injections.

They may also apply electrical stimulation and various other forms of mechanical therapy in order to trigger muscle relaxation, as do some chiropractors. These therapies may include gentle "muscle energy" techniques, and functional and positional techniques which are unique to osteopathic medicine.

Bodywork

There are many different forms of massage, deep tissue and movement awareness therapies that can be utilized to release pent-up energy, mobilize tissue flexibility, and to stimulate an increased flow of nutrients. Among these are Therapeutic Massage, The Alexander Method, The Feldenkrais Method, Rolfing, Hellerwork, The Aston-Patterning, The Trager Approach, Bonnie Prudden Myotherapy, Reflexology, Acupressure, Qigong (Oriental), Therapeutic Touch, and Polarity Therapy.

Which form of bodywork to use is often a matter of individual needs or preferences and of regional availability.

Two well known forms that have been useful for arthritics are Rolfing and Hellerwork. Both involve the strenuous manipulation of muscles, connective tissue, and joints in order to allow the body, muscles, and connective tissues to realign themselves.

Rolfing has been found useful for various forms of arthritis, including osteoarthritis and rheumatoid arthritis, particularly when the underlying disease mechanism is related to improper structural alignment and the failure of fascia -- the fibrous tissue that surrounds muscles -- to slide effortlessly because of fascial adhesions.

Pressure to fascial adhesions is applied with fingers, knuckles and elbows to release the adhesions, after which the muscles are free to operate throughout their proper range, and skeletal realignment naturally reoccurs.

In addition to body realignment, Hellerwork seeks to bring about a conscious awareness of the mind/body relationship, unlocking tension and unconscious holding patterns to achieve fuller and natural breathing, and later to learn to sit, stand, walk, or run in a manner that is natural to one's physical design.

To the extent that osteoarthritis stems, or may stem, from physical stress and poor posture, Hellerwork can provide relief. It is also useful for any sustained suffering or emotional stress, painful and stiff muscles, and injury.

Planned Exercise for Osteoarthritic Spurs

One of the most frequent consequences of age, imbalanced chemistry, or stretched or torn tendons and ligaments, is the production of compensating bone spurs, especially along the spine.

These bony spurs will often tend to close in the openings from which stem major nerve branches from the spinal column, and in so doing, they will also pinch the nerve, especially during movements, and cause pain elsewhere in the body or limbs.

Reconstructive Therapy can often assist in reducing the excess motion that causes the nerve pinch, but cannot dissolve the calcium spurs. Diet, supplements and enzyme therapy, joined with proper use of the Bruno Chikly Lymph Drainage Therapy and/or Vodder Lymph Therapy used in conjunction with the Light Beam Generator or Omega Ray, has been reported to help reduce the size of the spurs. According to Joel Wallach, D.V.M., N.D., author of *Rare Earths: Forbidden Cures*, "Bone spurs, heel spurs and calcium deposits can be reversed and eliminated by supplementing with significant amounts of chelated and colloidal calcium sources."[141] (See this chapter, "Energy Medicine.")

The use of permanent magnets of the correct polarity, properly placed, may also help, according to William Philpott, M.D. (See this chapter, "Magnetic Therapy.")

Exercise performed daily, in a properly planned manner, accompanied by appropriate traction has been reported to alleviate the pain, and apparently solve the calcium spur problem.

The Case of Harold R. Babcock

Ten years ago Harold Babcock,[97] 76 years-of-age, Colorado Springs, Colorado, found painful arthritic spurs stemming from his vertebrae. His chiropractor, D.L. Driscoll, Colorado Springs, Colorado, advised the use of a traction system.

Harold performed traction exercises as follows:

1. Gripping the seat in front, turn head as far as possible to the left, then to the right. Repeat for a count of 12.

2. Raise head as far back as possible, then bring chin to rest. Repeat for a count of 12.

3. Lean head as far as possible left shoulder, then right shoulder. Repeat for a count of 12.

These exercises were performed with approximate five minute gaps between each of the trials.

Another X-ray taken a few months later showed no spurs.

About fourteen years later Harold's right arm and hand started to go partially numb. After chiropractic manipulation, it did not improve, and so Harold was sent to an osteopath, who sent him to a hospital for a series of X-rays. Spurs were beginning to develop on the inside of Harold's neck vertebrae.

With the intent of eliminating the growth of arthritic spurs on the vertebrae, Harold developed the series of motions as follows:

1. *Facing forward*, rotate head in *clockwise* motion 12 times.

2. *Facing forward*, rotate head in a *counterclockwise* motion 12 times.

(Steps 1 and 2 act as a relaxer between the other steps.)

3. With face turned to the left, then the right, *inhale*, and raise head back as far as it will go. Repeat for a count of 12.

4. With face turned to the left, then the right, *exhale*, and bring chin to chest. Repeat for a count of 12.

5. Repeat step 1, then step 2.

6. Repeat step 3, then step 4.

7. Repeat step 1, then step 2.

8. *Gripping the seat in front of you*, turn head as far as possible to the left, then the right. Repeat for a count of 12.

9. Raise head as far as possible, then bring chin to chest. Repeat for a count of 12.

10. Lean head as far as possible toward left shoulder, then right shoulder Repeat for a count of 12. You need to go through all 10 steps three times.

Repeat these ten steps *twice* more.

Harold says, "As soon as you learn it, the routine can be accomplished in from ten to fifteen minutes. Thinking that my neck needed as much exercise as possible to put pressure on the developing spurs, I developed the series of motions as described. After one year of this, I started going through the routine only twice, and after six months have shown no ill effects. I still do it daily, and the results are still good. However, I would suggest going through it three times for the first year.

"I'm glad to report that my arms no longer have any numbness, and I have experienced no pain in my neck, although I've had no X-rays, as I haven't felt they were needed.

"I also take a 750 mg tablet of calcium per day (which should be balanced with the same amount of magnesium).

"I use 16 lbs. of weight on the traction, but I recommend that the weight be specified by a chiropractor or osteopath.

"I hope that people can make good use of what has done wonders for me. I'm sure that this routine can help a lot of people if they'll only go through it like they meant it and stay with it"

Homeopathy for Foot Bone Spurs and Soft Tissue Calcification

A common osteoarthritic problem is the growth of bone spurs and calcification of soft tissues.

Dr. Catherine Russell[98] of Guadalajara, Mexico, reports great success with the reduction of foot bone spurs and soft tissue calcification using 6C homeopathic remedies -- *Rhus tox* and *Calcarea carbonica*. "Usually in about 2 or 3 months, my patients are OK, but I've had patients who've had to take this remedy for as long as 6 months. The *Calcarea carbonica* normalizes the calcium metabolism, so that these spurs are reabsorbed.

"As the symptoms are frequently the same for calcium spurs in the cervical region, I have successfully used the same treatment.

"For painful calcium nodules in the foot or wrist area (soft tissue calcium deposits), I've successfully used homeopathic *Calcarea carbonica* or *Silicea*. Sometimes it's administered every 2 hours when the pain is present, and then every 4 hours later. This also works for bunions, which are such a serious deformation. People are very happy to be relieved of this horrible overgrowth, as this homeopathic remedy does help to shrink the bunion."

Other Treatments
Acupuncture
Background

The history of acupuncture, as briefly mentioned in "Energy Medicine," extends backward more than 4,500 years. Chinese knowledge was slowly acquired by scholarly study, intuition, experiments on war prisoners, and through trial and error during which there was much dispute. In 1029 A.D. Dr. Wang Wei-Yi forged the model of a human in brass that, like a road-map, clearly depicted and summarzied what was known about biological energy lines to that day. These energy lines were called "meridians," and this casting of a brass man served to consolidate knowledge of the flow of the body's "vital life energy" in a manner analogous to a suddenly revealed unifying, scientific principle, such as Newton's Law of Gravity, or Einstein's equation showing the relationship of energy to matter. Disagreements disappeared, and the developmental work of applying acupuncture for the good of society had begun.

Lacking modern concepts of electrical current flow and its associated magnetism, ancient Chinese explanatory models described a vital life energy which they called "qi," pronounced, "chi." Qi is present in all living organisms, and from some perspective, is in all things.

Qigong (pronounced "chi gong") is the Chinese science of working with qi energy within the body. Yang Jwing-Ming, Ph.D., physicist, master of qigong, and author of more than a dozen books on the subject -- defines "chi" in modern physics terms, as "bio-electrical energy." (See *Qigong for Arthritis*, Yang Jwing-Ming, Ph.D.)

In the human body, qi should flow smoothly and evenly, that is, it should be well-balanced so that its many tributaries, like a network of rivers, ebbs and flows, but never becomes so great that river banks overflow, or so little that rivers themselves cannot flow.

Continuing with the metaphor of a system of rivers for meridians, the rivers have overflow basins that capture and store excess water during periods of heavy rain. The Chinese discovered eight reservoirs which they believed should be full and strong for the body to regulate itself efficiently. These reservoirs were, in turn, connected to

12 channels, the meridians, which run vertically from the front of the head to the foot, returning to the head via the back. Whenever the river flow -- energy flow within the meridians -- is not normal, these reservoirs serve to regulate the qi flow and bring it back to normal.

Every organ and system in the body is visited by one or more of the meridians, the acupuncture points being analogous to control gates or pumping stations that can shut down or increase the flow. All meridians interconnect, so that every acupuncture point has a pathway to every other point. Additionally, there are a few isolated acupuncture points called "Extra" which have an affect on human organs which do not seem to be directly attached to meridians, although they would be indirectly connected through the affected organs themselves.

Each meridian has been given a name which represents its function, as viewed from a historical perspective that knew little of modern physiology. Keeping in mind that these are descriptions related to physiological function, and not necessarily physiological structure, they are described as Spleen-Pancreas (S), Stomach (ST), Gall Bladder (GB), Governor Vessel (GV), Conception Vessel (CV), Liver (L), Kidney (K), Bladder (B), Lung (LG), Large Intestine (LI), Master of the Heart (MH), Triple Warmer (TW), Heart (H), and Small Intestine (SI).

Each acupuncture point lying on each meridian is numbered, so that LI15 would refer to a position on the large intestine (colon) meridan located near the left or right shoulder, LI1 to a position on the large intestine (colon) meridian located on the first finger of the left or right hand, and so on.

As an example of how an imbalance of the flow of vital energy can occur between the meridians, and the qi reservoirs that should keep the meridians full, according to Dr. Jwing-Ming,[79] "when you experience a sudden shock the qi flow in the bladder will immediately regulate the qi in this channel so that you recover from the shock. However, if the reservoir qi in this channel is also deficient, or if the effect of the shock is too great and there is not enough time to regulate the qi, the bladder will suddenly contract, causing unavoidable urination."

Acupuncture points are connected together by the meridians, and although more than 2,000 acupuncture points have been discovered using modern energy sensing devices, such as Dr. Reinhold Voll's Dermatron described in the section on "Energy Medicine" about 1,000 are customarily used and when penetrated with a fine needle stimulate the flow of bio-electrical energy, or chi.

By selecting the proper acupuncture points pain can be alleviated -- even major surgery can be performed without anesthesia -- the immune system is enhanced, and there is accomplished a healing of many conditions, including colds and flus, and even allergies and addictions.

Although ancient Chinese wisdom had identified the functional concept of flow of chi energy, the reality of its structure was not verified until the scientific work of Korean Professor Kim Bong Han and his researchers in 1960, and later the French researcher Pierre de Vernejoul. Robert O. Becker, M.D. under a grant from the National Institutes of Health and Maria Reichmanis, a biophysicist, were able to prove that the electrical currents did flow along the ancient Chinese meridians, and that 25 percent of the acupuncture points exist structurally.

In a study reported in *Medical Tribune*, 29 patients with severe arthritis who were candidates for knee replacement surgery were treated by acupuncture in which needles were inserted at specific nerves near the surface of the skin to reduce pain. Half of the patients received standard pain killers, while half received the acupuncture twice a week for nine weeks. After nine weeks, those receiving acupuncture had significantly less pain and better function than those who were taking the pain killers, according to Hans-Henrik Bulow, M.D. of the University of Copenhagen. Seven patients responded so well that they did not need the surgery. Seventeen patients continued with acupuncture for a full year, once a month, and were able to maintain their improvement.[68]

Barbar Sage, through internet, shared her good experiences with the use of acupuncture. "I have degenerative joint disease (osteoarthritis) in my neck and upper back, accelerated from working at a computer all day.

"I tried physical therapy, exercises, chiropractic, and drugs. Nothing gave any lasting relief. Then I was referred to Peter Eckman, M.D., an acupuncturist in Palo Alto, CA. The very first visit I left with pain free neck -- the first time in two years. The stuff works rapidly. Through successive treatments, my back and neck pain is so much better."

The Typical Acupuncture Treatment

While all acupuncturists do not use a standardized patient diagnosis, there is a commonly used method that applies to all Chinese medicine. In addition to medical history and interviews which discovers current complaints, health history, family health history, patterns of sleep, appetite, weight, elimination, menses, stress and so on, the patient is studied to observe complexion, eyes, tongue, nails, hair, gait, stature, secretions and so on. The acupucturist also listens to sound of voice, breathing and identifies odor of breath, skin, secretions and so on. On touching the patient, the acupuncturist learns the texture, humidity, temperature and elasticity of skin, the strength and tone of muscles, the flexibility and range of motion of joints, radial pulse (12 of them), and so on.

After observations, fact collection, and diagnosis, an evaluation of treatment points is made, and needles are painlessly placed in any one of a thousand acupuncture locations. Normally no more than 10 or 12 are used per treatment. Modern acupuncturists use sterile disposable needles to avoid any possibility of transfer of infection. The needles are of various lengths and gauges, but usually they are hair-thin and made of stainless steel.

A substitute for needles has been found in the use of laser acupuncture which consists of a safe, cold light beam about the size of a penlight which is held at the acupuncture point for perhaps 30 to 40 seconds. Wherever the point to be reached is deeper than the light beam can penetrate, then needles must be used.

Treatments with the needles may last for forty-five minutes, or perhaps but a few seconds. Occasionally an ear needle is taped to an acupuncture point in the ear, and permitted to stay for a week. Twenty to thirty minutes seems to be the norm.

Acupressure, a substitute for either light or needles, can sometimes be used. This consists of applying finger tip pressure to an acupuncture point, or, as some health professionals have discovered, rubbing a painful point for a few minutes.

For maximum beneficial effect Chinese herbs in the form of teas, pills, and capsules may be given as a supplement. Changes in lifestyle, diet and physical activity may also be advised.

Acupuncture Treatment for Arthritis

Traditional Chinese medicine seeks to re-balance or restore the flow of qi along the meridians, and toward that end all acupuncture treatments are directed. Assuming an optimum flow of vital life energy, there will then be no cause for any kind of illness. The body can then heal itself.

Specific treatments have been designed to handle the problem of pain, or poor repair in, say, a knee or finger, and there are identified acupuncture points for each of these. Prior to an operation, for example, in lieu of anesthesia, specific acupuncture points will be utilized which permits the cutting of skin and organs without a sense of pain, and after the operation the flow of qi is restored by means of other selected points.

Also in Chinese acupuncture, arthritis is not divided into segments, such as osteoarthritis, rheumatoid arthritis, gouty arthritis, and so on. If there is a joint problem, it is treated as "arthritis."

During the acute stages of arthritis, the acupuncture treatment is used every day. In the chronic condition, acupuncture is used every other day. In each case the needles may be retained beneath the skin but 15-20 minutes, and the patient will also be asked to exercise to promote recovery, as well as advised on herbs, lifestyle changes and diet.

A rough measure of the number of treatments required is one month for each year the arthritis has existed.

According to the parts of the body in need of treatment, the following table lists the appropriate acupuncture points to be used:

Table of Acupuncture Points to be Used in the Treatment of Arthritis

Location of Arthritis	Meridian	Acupuncture Point	Approximate Position of Acupuncture Point
Upper Extremities	Colon	LI1	First finger left or right hand
		LI4	Base of thumb and first finger back of left or right hand
		LI15	Left or right shoulder
	Extra (Outside)	Extra28	In between webbing of back of all of the fingers and thumb, back of left or right hand
	Hypothalmus	SJ5	Back of forearm just above Left or right wrist
Lower Extremties	Gallbladder	GB30	Left or right outer hip
		GB34	Outer left or right lower leg, just below knee
		GB39	Outer left or right leg just above ankle
		GB40	Outer left or right ankle
	Stomach	ST35	Front of Left or right knee
		ST36	Just below front of left or right knee
		ST41	Front of left or right front ankle
	Extra (Outside)	Extra36	In between webbing of all of the toes, top of left or right foot
Pain in Vertebral Column	Governing Vessel	GV15	Upper neck
blade	Urinary Bladder	UB46	Below lower tip of shoulder blade
	Extra (Outside)	Extra21	Left or right of the vertebrae, at the particular point corresponding to pain
	Extra (Outside)	Extra36	In between webbing of all the toes, top of left or right foot
Pain in Mandibular Joint	Colon	LI4	Base of thumb and first finger, back of left or right hand
	Gall Bladder	GB2	In front of left or right ear
	Stomach	ST7	In front of left or right ear

(See Figure 9: "Front and Back Views of Partial Meridian Lines and Important Acupuncture Points for Treating Arthritics.")

In addition to decrease of pain and drug addiction, and restoration of freedom from allergic reactions to pollens and foods, acupuncture has been shown to be a complete system of healing by balancing the vital body energy, and strengthening the immune system, an important aspect for many forms of arthritis.[19]

Bee Sting Therapy

The American Apitherapy Society of Vermont, with 1600 members, estimates that as many as 10,000 Americans now practice bee sting therapy. A few arthritics receive "bee stings" -- apitherapy -- from a hypodermic in their physician's office, but most get the real thing. There are about 300 physicians who use bee venom on their patients. According to Dava Sobel and Arthur C. Klein,[91] authors of *Arthri-*

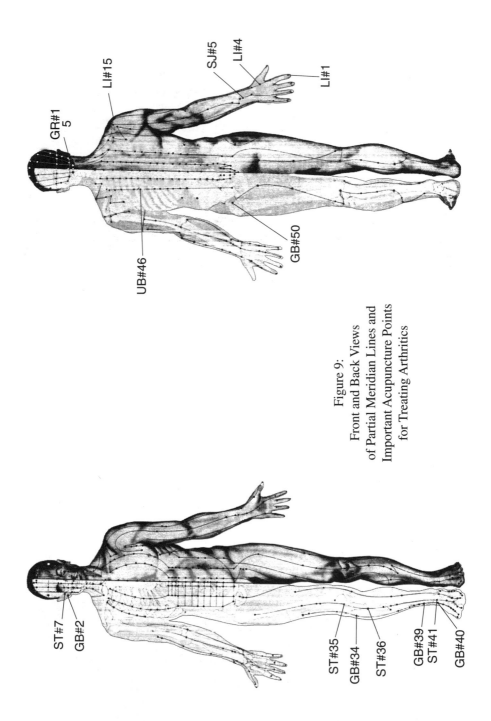

Figure 9:
Front and Back Views
of Partial Meridian Lines and
Important Acupuncture Points
for Treating Arthritics

tis: What Works, in a survey of 23 participants who tried bee venom for the pain of their arthritis, 48% (11) found it dramatically effective, 11 (48%) found it ineffective, and 1 (4%) felt it made arthritis worse.

Dangers are allergic reaction and anaphylactic shock. One participant wrote that "I had no idea of my allergy to insect venom until four years ago when I was stung by a yellow jacket and had to be rushed to the hospital emergency room for treatment."[91]

Prior to taking bee venom, an allergy examination should be made for possible allergic reaction to bee sting. Provided allergy from bee stings is not a problem, the arthritic can take as many stings each year as necessary. For example, Bradford S. Weeks, M.D., cofounder of the American Apitherapy Association,[91] reports that "patients with multiple sclerosis who use bee therapy take about 4000 stings a year, at the rate of 20-40 live bee stings per sitting, three times a week." An International Apitherapy Study (IAS) begun in 1983 gathers data on more than 12,000 bee-stung patients.

Christopher Kim, M.D. of the Monmouth Pain Institute in Red Bank, New Jersey, is a leader in the practice of apitherapy. During the past 10 years Dr. Kim has treated more than 2000 patients, using about 3 million injections.

"Bee venom can be injected into the skin of the patient either by hypodermic needle or by the direct contact of the honeybee." For direct contact by the honeybee, "the practitioner holds a live honey-bee in a pair of tweezers, places it in contact with a particular spot on the patient's body, and lets nature do the rest. Dosage is determined by how long you let the stinger remain in the skin; . . . , you can remove it instantly or let it remain for 5 minutes."[91]

According to information compiled by the International Apitherapy Study (IAS) osteoarthritis symptoms can be stung away in 2-6 weeks. "One case of severe osteoarthritis, a condition endured by a patient for 16 years, required 24 stings every second day for 8 months for full relief."

Bee venom contains anti-inflammatory substances, with the ability to reduce the swelling of inflamed tissue with an effect 100 times stronger than standard drugs, such as hydrocortisone. One needs 100 to 10,000 times less bee venom to get the same anti-inflammatory effects as from conventional anti-inflammatory drugs.

If you're not one of the 2% of the population allergic to the venom, there are no lasting unpleasant side-effects.

Yellow-jacket and wasp stings apparently do not provide the same benefits as the bee stings, and one can respond allergenically to these as well.

According to Bradford S. Weeks, M.D., and cofounder of the American Apitherapy Association, if you try honeybee sting therapy at home, you should first have an examination to see if you might be allergic to bee venom. Then, even if not, you should always have on hand allergy-antidoting medicines, such as epinephrine or antihistamine. Some folks can develop an allergy, and it would be "needlessly reckless," not to be prepared.

"It's natural for the arm to swell up, get red, and itch for a short period after a bee sting," says Dr. Weeks, "and this should not be confused with an allergic reaction."

You must also prepare your immune system by "nurturing" it ahead of time with megavitamins, a typical intake of vitamin C being at least 3 grams daily. It's also useful to take cold-pressed flax-seed oil (1 tablespoon daily) and magnesium (200 mg, 3 times daily). [See *Bee Pollen: The Perfect Food*, Anthony di Fabio, this Foundation. Recommended pollen: C.C. Pollen Co., 3627 E. Indian School, Road, Suite 209, Phoenix, AZ 85018-5126; (800) 950-0096]

Avoid alcohol, reduce or eliminate intake of refined foods, sugars, and dairy products, and start using bee pollen (1/2 teaspoon daily, minimum) and propolis (1/4 teaspoon daily, minimum). "People get great results intially from the bee stings but these results won't be sustained unless they support their immune system," Dr. Weeks explains.

The International Apitherapy Study begun in 1983, has gathered follow-up data on more than 12,000 bee stung patients. It may take up to 3-4 months of regular stings to change inflammatory conditions of rheumatoid arthritis.[204]

For More Information Contact American Apitherapy Society, Inc., PO Box 54, Hartland Four Corners, VT 05049; tel: 800-823-3460. For technical information on research studies, contact International Apitherapy Study (IAS), Bradford S. Weeks, M.D., PO Box 740, Clinton, WA 98236; tel: 360-341-2303. Fax: 360-341-2313. Dr. Weeks encourages readers to report their personal experiences with bee products to IAS.

Chelation Therapy

There are some health treatments that address themselves to such basic, underlying bodily functions that they apply to almost every condition. Among them, of course, is good nutrition and acupuncture. The following describes another which applies to such a wide range of conditions -- especially with physical aging -- that no one can afford to overlook its potential.

Pronounced "Key-lay-shun," chelation therapy is one of the most effective treatments for a wide spectrum of diseases or aging conditions, because, by it's use, 80% of peripheral -- hands, feet, arms, legs, heart, head -- problems of lowered circulation, hence insufficiency of cellular nutrients, are resolved. Cells that are healthy contribute to healthy organs, and healthy organs contribute to properly operating systems. Healthy systems contribute to overall health.[3,34]

At the same time the use of chelation therapy helps to clean up damaging molecules, called "free radicals," which bind to, and inhibit normal tissue from functioning properly. Other benefits of its use include removal of the subtle toxicities acquired through a life-time intake of many pollutants and metals, reduction of pain, and discomfort and disability from various degenerative diseases including osteoarthritis.

Intravenous chelation therapy uses an amino acid called "ethylene diamine tetracetic acid" (EDTA) which helps to remove fatty plaques that plug up   arteries. These deposits decrease or prevent blood from flowing freely, and, as it is the blood which must supply nutritional elements from our food intake and breathing, these nutrients are not received by individual cells in the abundance required for healthy tissues. By removing the plaque binding agent -- the calcium -- from the plaques that plug up arteries, the smaller plaques themselves disappear. Removal of even a small amount of arterial plaque increases blood flow a great deal. (In proportion to the third power of the increase in arterial diameter.)

With age the lining and the flexible arteries can began to have similar characteristics to an old bowl of jelly, or aged, cracked and stiffened rubber. After using a number of intravenous EDTA infusions, the inner lining begans to soften, becomes more flexible, and lowers blood pressure in a natural way.

When arteries become plugged too badly, traditional medicine recommends bypass surgery, where about one foot of thinner vein is used to replace the most occluded portion of the arteries, usually near the heart. EDTA therapy quite frequently makes this expensive, somewhat dubious procedure unnecessary. After all, replacing one foot of plugged up artery while ignoring the other nearly 528,000,000 feet of arterial occlusions brings about temporary relief, at best.

There 's hardly any disease or bodily condition that would not be benefited by opened arterial flow including osteoarthritis, as essential life elements are thence made more easily available to each cell. As each cell is better nourished, so are tissues, and therefore organs and bodily systems. Better opportunity for better nutrition at the cellular level also means enhanced capability of fighting off disease and of repairing damaged tissues.

Decomposed joint cartilage, as occurs in arthritis, contains free radicals -- chemicals with a high degree of undesirable attraction to other tissues. Chelation therapy assists in cleaning out these damaging molecules. More importantly, the cartilage itself -- with it's otherwise poor arterial blood supply relying essentially on expansion and squeezing action for nourishment -- is better fed and repaired with better arterial and capillary flow.

While intravenous chelation with EDTA   is efficient for improving blood circulation, it is not suitable for removal of damaging metals that contribute to various forms of disease such as mercury, iron, copper, arsenic, cobalt, chromium, cadmium and silver. When metal toxicity is suspected, physicians such as Mark Davidson, D.O., N.D. of North Carolina, usually first uses a different chemical called "di-mercaptopropane sulfonate (DMPS)" to remove these toxic metals, and then afterward uses the EDTA (ethylene diamine tetracetic acid) to improve arterial flow.[83]

Another substance used by health professionals for the same purpose is dimercaptosuccinic acid (DMSA). DMPS and DMSA are both effective in removal of arsenic, lead, mercury, and cadmium. DMPS has been reported by Chinese physicians to be effective in Wilson's disease, a condition of excessive copper, and is also useful for chelating copper sulphate.[140]

Many other metals besides those mentioned can also be chelated out with the use of of the three named: EDTA, DMPS, or DMSA. Deferoxamine may also be used for bivalent or trivalent metals.

More than half a million people have been safely treated with chelation therapy in the United States during the past 40 years. Following the treatment protocol recommended by the American College for Advancement of Medicine and the American Board of Chelation Therapists, more than 1,000 physicians routinely recommend it's use. In fact, it may be one of the rare examples of a therapy where the knowledgeable physician, impressed by its performance, routinely administers it to self and loved ones.

It's safety, as measured by standards applied to all drugs, shows that when used properly it is 3-1/2 times safer than the use of ordinary aspirin.[7]

In retrospective studies privately funded and performed by Cypher, Inc. of Ohio, founded by a group of interested scientists and physicians, 20,000 patient records were studied gathered over a 15 year period. Statistical evaluations on these records were performed by an independent agency free from all bias.[7]

Statistical analysis demonstrated beyond any possible doubt that 80% of peripheral circulation was improved, including impressive improvement in flow of blood to the brain through the carotid artery, intermittent claudication (cramping up of leg muscles) which affects many arthritics. And, in a 1% sample of the measure of bone density, conclusive proof was found that bones hardened by use of chelation therapy, thus reversing osteoporosis. Osteoporosis is a condition of weakened bone structure leading to fractures especially of the hip in the elderly where 1 in 4 women may suffer from weakened bone. Bone fractures from osteoporosis, a condition that often accompanies osteoarthritis, affects about one million three hundred thousand American woman annually.[7]

During the past 15 years, one of us has been chelated more than 200 times, while the other 100. In both cases laboratory examinations and physical signs and symptoms, such as stamina, cramping of muscles, heart/lung capacity, color of skin and so on, have obviously been favorable, or we would not continue.

How Chelation Therapy is Administered

Normally, unless a patient is already hospitalized, chelation therapy is administered on an out-patient basis, usually over about 3-1/2 hours of intravenous infusion. It is well known -- confirmed by our own experiences -- that 8 to 10 infusions, 2 to 3 times per week, are necessary before any changes at all can be noticed.

Most physicians use comfortable reclining chairs for their patients and are placed in a room with others who are also to be chelated. One can visit other patients, sharing experiences, watch television, or read.

Following a well-developed treatment protocol developed by the American College for Advancement of Medicine and the American Board of Chelation Therapy, the physician will often make tests before, during, and after treatment related to:

• Blood pressure and circulation
• Cholesterol and other components
• Kidney and organ function
• Tissue minerals, if indicated

For optimum benefits from this relatively inexpensive treatment, the patient is advised on the following:

• Smoking will cancel the benefits of chelation therapy, and therefore the patient is advised to halt this damaging habit.

• Whole foods as described in "Nutrition and Supplements," this chapter, is recommended, or specific diets and nutritional supplements are tailored to fit individual needs.

• Exercise is encouraged.

After receiving initial treatments a minimum of six treatments per year are recommended for maintenance of good circulation, particularly in the elderly.

When used properly, and in sufficient numbers, bypass surgery can be avoided. No other known traditional treatment, no amount of drug consumption to control symptoms, can bring about the improvements noted in the use of chelation therapy.

Chelation therapy should be considered by everyone with a disease related to circulation, such as a gangrenous leg or foot, thus most probably saving the leg from surgery.

Since most diseases that accompany aging have a strong component of inhibited circulation, virtually all elderly citizens should consider chelation therapy both as a preventive measure and as a healing treatment. (See *Chelation Therapy*, Anthony di Fabio, this Foundation.)

Environmental Medicine

Environmental factors can simulate, intensify or create arthritic symptoms. It is therefore important to explore the relationship of one's illness to these factors.

"Environmental medicine" refers to all those external factors that adversely influence health, such as dust, molds, chemicals and certain foods that cause allergic reactions, including asthma, hay fever, headaches, and depression.

Assuming no genetic defects, the human baby is born with a set of wholly functioning, self-repairing instructions, unless the mother has disturbed the ordinary course of pre-natal growth by poor nutrition, exposure to toxic chemicals, or by attempted or actual abortion. Newly born human organs and systems will operate efficiently until disturbed by an outside influence. The number of these environmental influences are accelerating as our society uses more and more pesticides, herbicides, organic fertilizers, fluoridated water, metal amalgams in teeth, prescription drugs, and so on.

The saddest part is that otherwise well-meaning practitioners of traditional medicine or dentistry for the most part either do not recognize these damaging influences; or, if they do, have been terribly slow in warning the general population of its dangers.

Theron G. Randolph, M.D., prominent allergy specialist and professor at four medical schools pioneered in the development of environmental medicine. He taught that "sensitivity reactions to commonly eaten foods can cause a range of symptoms in susceptible individuals, including headaches, eczema, fatigue, arthritis, depression, and a variety of gastrointestinal disorders."[5]

Later research added environmental chemicals to the list of items that can adversely affect sensitive individuals.

Harold Buttram, M.D., Quakertown, Pennsylvania, says that "Volatile organic compounds (VOCs) consist of a very large class of commercial chemicals which tend to evaporate into and contaminate indoor air of buildings. They enter the human system not only by inhalation but also through skin absorption. There are now about 70,000 chemicals used in commerce, of which several hundred are known to affect human nerve tissue, yet but 10% of these have had any testing. Ten of these chemicals were found in indoor air, drinking water, and exhaled breaths of 400 residents of New Jersey, North Carolina, and North Dakota." (See *Who Is Looking After Our Kids?* Harold Buttram, M.D.)

When New Hampshire passed a consumer protection act requiring produce retailers to post conspicuous signs on individual produce bins listing all ingredients in the waxed produce, signs revealed the presence of twelve fungicides.[107] The other 49 states did not require their produce retailers to make such a revelation, and even New Hampshire has since watered-down their pioneer law.

The inert ingredients in pesticides are not always inert. According to the Environmental Protective Agency (EPA), 40 of the ingredients that fall under the "inert" category are considered toxic, and can probably cause aching joints, cancer, brain/nervous system poisoning, and reproductive problems. Another 60 are potentially toxic because of their chemical similarities to known harmful compounds. Why consumers are not warned that certain "inert" ingredients are dangerous is a puzzle, but even more puzzling is why the EPA has not required disclosure on the labels.[108]

Metal amalgams in tooth dentures, surgical root canal work, fluoridation of water, and many more socially accepted toxic exposures go unknown by the general population and unknown or ignored by the professional who adminsters these.

Numerous books have been written covering only a fraction of the dangerous influences surrounding us from ordinary commerce, the above recital hardly doing justice to the total.

Furthermore all of the external influences that affect us adversely, once taken into the body, can, in turn, open the door to organisms-of-opportunity -- micro-organisms that set up residence in our bodies -- which then generate additional chemical toxins that create additional adverse effects.

Bio-detoxification

"Bio-detoxification" is simply the process or means for ridding the body of all undesireable, foreign pollutants, such as those described above. Environmental physicians and other health practitioners have designed methods for eliminating pesticides, herbicides, food preservatives, legal and illegal drugs, heavy metal toxicities, allergens, microorganisms and their toxins from the body. This is important, because these foreign elements interfere with enzymes, utilization of nutrients, cellular reproduction, restoration of healthy tissues and systems, and every other bodily component.

Virtually all of these methods also rely on proper nutrition and nutritional support, including appropriate vitamins, minerals and fatty acids. Among the important bio-detoxification vitamins and minerals of osteoarthritis are those described earlier in this chapter under "Nutrition," as anti-oxidants.

The process of bio-detoxification is basic to most natural health programs, and to achieving wellness from virtually every disease, but in particular for the eighty or so collagen tissue or so-called auto-immune diseases, including the various forms of arthritis. Treatments described here are useful for the condition of rheumatoid arthritis. They will not be repeated in that chapter. In like manner, bio-detoxification treatments such as colonics, the sauna sweat detox program, and others described in the chapter on rheumatoid arthritis will be wholly applicable to osteoarthritis, but not repeated in this chapter.

(See *Allergies and Biodetoxification for the Arthritic*, Warren Levin, M.D., Anthony di Fabio, this Foundation.)

The Dental Connection

According to Lee Cowden, M.D., Dallas, TX, "Osteoarthritis will always show up eventually in a joint associated with a bad tooth, a root canal tooth, or a place where infection has been left behind after an extraction."

Jerome S. Mittelman, D.D.S.,[105] Past President of the International Academy of Nutrition and Preventative Medicine, writes that "While dentists fill the root canal, there are still over three miles of inaccessible, untreated tubules from which these germs can pour toxins into your body. These poisons can affect your heart, kidneys, lungs, eyes, stomach, brain, and countless other body tissues."

Pat Connolly,[105] Executive Director of the Price-Pottenger Nutrition Foundation, writes, "After years of personal health problems -- severe sinus flareups, very painful headaches, chronic fatigue -- all disappeared with the extraction of an upper bicuspid and depriding the socket."

Even without root canal work, or tooth extraction, sometimes food that has lodged between a tooth and the gums can cause an infection at the base of the tooth.

Reinhold Voll, M.D. discovered that each tooth in the mouth relates to a specific acupuncture meridian, and that when a tooth became infected or diseased, organs found on the same meridian also were affected. Similarly, dysfunction in a particular organ could lead to a problem in the related tooth.

Osteoarthritis can also occur when older people have had teeth removed without removal of dental ligament and the dead bone has not been scraped out from beneath the dental ligament. One of Dr. Cowden's 50 year old patients was crippled with osteoarthritis so badly that he came into the office in a wheelchair. On questioning, Dr. Cowden says, "I found that he'd had some dental work. His gums went bad first, and then his teeth fell out. He never had dental extractions or the surgery to clear up the infection underneath the teeth."

When Dr. Cowden tested this patient with a device similar to Dr. Reinhold Voll's Dermatron described in "Energy Medicine," he found multiple infections in the jawbone. Dr. Cowden sent him to a dentist, called a "Biological Dentist," specially trained to treat the teeth, jaw, and related structures regarding how that treatment will affect the whole body. The hidden infection was scraped out of the jawbone, and the patient's arthritis disappeared.

According to George Meinig, D.D.S.,[106] founding member of the

American Association of Endodontists (root canal therapists), recipient of many awards, and also health columnist and book writer, "Since the discovery of penicillin and antibiotics, root canal specialists and some physicians have come to believe infections of teeth and tonsils no longer cause diseases in other parts of the body. They incorrectly claim focal infections are a thing of the past. Most disturbing is their failure to accept the existence of bacteria that become trapped inside the dentin tubules which make up 90 percent of the structure of the teeth. Added to that fact is the inability of antibiotics and other medicaments to be able to get at and kill these organisms." (See *Root Canal Coverup*, George Meinig, D.D.S.)

Another reason for retention of a foci of infection, according to Lida Mattman, Ph.D., Professor Emeritus, Department of Biology, Wayne State University, Detroit, Michigan, is that antibiotics strip off the cell wall of many bacteria, thereby preventing our immune systems from recognizing their presence, as their cell wall is the vehicle whereby our protective mechanisms know that a foreign microorganism is present. These cell wall deficient organisms can restructure themselves at a later time, and continue the pathogenic colony. (See *Cell Wall Deficient Forms: Stealth Pathogens*, Lida H. Mattman, Ph.D.)

Another reason relates to the environment surrounding the micro-organisms. Initially adapted for survival in an oxygen environment, after closure of root canal surgery oxygen is quickly depleted and then a number of original microorganisms produce off-spring that are adapted to an oxygen starved environment. These multiply and infect the 1,000 miles or so of dentin tubules, eventually also affecting remotely located organs either directly, or through bioelectrical influence and/or actual passage along acupuncture meridian lines.

Following the lead of Weston Price, D.D.S.who conducted extensive root canal research for 25 years, George E. Meinig, D.D.S., Ojai, California, investigated and reported on extensive research studies involving 5000 animals, clearly demonstrating how bacteria escape into the circulation of a tooth's surrounding bony socket, where these organisms are responsible for a high percentage of the chronic and degenerative diseases that are epidemic in America today.

Twenty-five percent of individuals who have root canal fillings are free from trouble for extended periods of time. "These are individuals who have excellent health and exceptionally good immune systems." Unfortunately, this group's freedom from side effects, such as arthritis, has led many root canal specialists to believe that their treatment of infected teeth has been successful, and will cause no harm.

Seventy-five percent of individuals whose immune systems have been compromised by illnesses, accidents, faulty nutrition, and so on, develop a variety of conditions which causes them to go from doctor to doctor in a desperate attempt to find the cause of their problems. A very high percentage of these cases are due to hidden root canal bacteria which, along with their toxins, enter the blood stream.

Many patients will remember that their problems began after root canal surgery, and when their infected teeth are removed -- or the infection actually cleaned up -- their illnesses disappear.

"To visualize what happens," Dr. Meinig reports, "picture the bacteria trapped in the dentin tubules; see them mutate and become more virulent and their toxins more toxic. In their escape into the blood circulation of the tooth's socket, these bacteria, like cancer cells, metastasize to other parts of the body. As they migrate, they infect the heart, kidneys, joints, nervous system, brain, eyes -- can endanger pregnant women and in fact may infect any organ, gland or other tissue."

Body Part Often Affected by Microorganisms
Left Behind After Root Canal Work
According to Lee Cowden, M.D.

Foci of Infection	Body Part Usually Affected
1st and second molars	Temporo-mandibular (jawbone), anterior (front) hip, knee and medial (middle) part of ankle
1st or second bicuspids or	Shoulder, elbow, hand (radial aspect), pre-molars foot and great toe
1st and 2nd incisors	Posterior (rear) knee, sacrococcygeal joint and posterior ankle
3rd tooth or wisdom tooth	Shoulder, elbow, ulna, part of hand, sacroilliac joint, foot and toes
Canine or cuspid	Posterior (rear) of knee, hip and the lateral ankle

"These foci of infection show up but 50% of the time on the best x-rays that most dentists do, so that means you have to use an electrodermal [or kinesiology] diagnostic technique to find the problems." [Dr. Voll's Dermatron as described in "Energy Medicine," is an electrodermal diagnostic device. Kinesiology is the testing of muscles to determine the state of organs and glands as determined by interpretation of muscle weaknesses and strengths.]

Dr. Cowden 's patient, a woman with multiple sclerosis and joint pains who had an inflammation in the cavity of the jaw-bone detectable by applied kinesthiology, was sent to her dentist and, after x-rays, the dentist said, "There's nothing there. I'm not going to do a surgical procedure on your jaw without evidence of it on x-ray.'"

The patient insisted on the surgery because of her faith in Dr. Cowden, so when the dentist agreed to make a very small puncture at the indicated place, he was surprised and dismayed to find a great deal of "gray goop start oozing out."

"I find that sometimes people have infections, chronic infections, elsewhere in their body and they'll have arthritis as a result . . . chronic appendicitis, or chronic diverticulitis (colon problem), or chronic tonsilitis. . . even after they've had the tonsils out, like an abscess near the base of where the tonsil used to be in the throat. Arthritis will improve if these infections are treated and cleared up . . . ."

These hidden infections bleed over into osteoarthritis, rheumatoid arthritis, scleroderma, Sjogren's disease, fibromyalgia, ankylosing spondilitis, systemic lupus erythematosus, and many other diseases.

A dental malocclusion can cause several different problems. If the tooth were to be capped or a filling placed in it, and the dentist didn't get it adjusted correctly, hitting the tooth too soon creates stress on the tooth which can cause the tooth to die and create an abcess at the base of the tooth.

This also throws off the muscles of the head and face which then translates into muscle spasm of the neck, which translates into muscle spasm of the back, which then causes problems with autonomic nervous system dysfunction, which then causes organ dysfunction, which then causes all kinds of other problems, including that of osteoarthritis.

According to George Meinig, D.D.S., "Even though infected teeth and tonsils are a frequent cause of arthritis tissue changes, the overzealous ordering of extractions was a leading factor in the cover-up of this important research.

"In spite of the fact of the many different causes of arthritis, too many doctors assumed oral infections were the cause. Dr. Weston Price, the dental research director of this 25 year research program, never made such claims.

"Whether or not oral infections are the direct cause of arthritis and other disease entities, the compromising effect of their presence on patients' immue systems is so severe that satisfactory treatment proves difficult and often impossible unless all oral focii are eliminated."[106]

Dental Fillings

Dental amalgams consist of mercury, tin, copper, silver, nickle, and sometimes zinc. Each of these metals when used as a so-called "permanent" filling or cap corrode or slowly disassociate into chemically active ions which are released into the body. These ions migrate from tooth to the root of the tooth, mouth, bone, connective tissues of the jaw, and finally into nerves, and into the central nervous system where the ions will attach themselves to organic tissue and disrupt the normal functions of the body. (See *It's All In Your Head*, Hall Huggins, D.D.s.)

While all of the above named materials can be toxic, the most toxic according to Joyal Taylor, D.D.S., Rancho Fe, California, are so-called "silver fillings," which are actually 50 percent mercury and only 25 percent silver.

Since the year 1500 A.D. mercury was known to be hazardous to human health . It was known to cause "mad hatter's disease" which

Hal Huggins, D.D.S. Urges Caution Prior to Potential Exposures!!

Fish

We've noted there is very little difference between highest and lowest concentrations of mercury in fish. Mercury is undisputedly dangerous, however, the methyl mercury form is considered more dangerous because it can cross the barriers of the body, including blood brain and placental. All the mercury in fish is in the methyl mercury form, whether salt water or fresh water. In fact some of the highest concentrations have been found in the high lakes of Colorado. So fish is out for the mercury affected person interested in his/her health.

Cosmetics

Cosmetics still contain high amounts of mercury, so read the labels. Thimerisol is the mercury compound most often found. Specifically, mascara is high in mercury, and close to the eye. The more "water resistant" the mascara, generally the more mercury present.

Over the Counter

Many over the counter medications contain mercury. Some are obvious like Merthiolate and Mercurichrome. Others don't have to list mercury because it is present in all drugs of that category. Contraceptive creams and jellies fall into that category. Mercury is the spermicide. I know of none that are mercury free.

Most skin "color lightening" creams have mercury as the active ingredient. Be sure to check labels on Fungicides. Acne preparations are not all mercury laden, but it would be well to check. Eye drops have cleared up their act substantially over the past 10 years. Drops for contact lenses (wetting solutions) are much better, but which ones? It's hard to read the label without your lenses in, I understand. Most of the drops used by eye doctors to "dilate" your eyes contain mercury.

Basically, eyes, ears, nose and throat preparations should be considered suspect until proven otherwise. Throat lozenges may have the code "mer" in their trade name. At the other end of the spectrum check out hemorrhoidal ointments and suppositories.

Occasionally hair tonic, scalp treatments and even bar soaps will include mercuric chloride. Veterinarian products are highly suspect, and household chemicals.

Paints

Many paints are touted to be mercury free, but upon testing have levels higher than allowable. After all, who is going to check? The kicker is that the coloring agent added may be a mercury compound -- especially shades of red.

Mildew resistant anything can use mercury as the active ingredient.

Gardening

Gardeners and especially farmers are exposed to multiple chemicals. Be careful of protectants, fungicides, and disinfectants.

Industrial Processes

It's surprising that in large industry one may find "vats" of mercury with no warning signs or protection cautions. In short, there are around 4000 commercial uses for mercury, and even experts in the field of mercury toxicity cannot name more than a few dozen. But no one is going to protect you. It is your responsibility to monitor exposures that might injure your health. One way to do this is to call (usually an 800 number) directly to the manufacturer about a product you suspect, and tell the person answering that you are highly "allergic" to mercury and want to make sure you don't become a liability to the company by using their product thinking that it was mercury free.

It's all in Your Head by Hal Huggins, D.D.S. is available through this foundation.

formed the basis to the Mad Hatter character in the "Mad Hatter's Teaparty" created by Lewis Carroll (Lewis Dodgson, 1865: *Alice in Wonderland*). Mercury was used for "sizing" or stiffening and shaping hats, the poisonous process eventually driving the hatter mad. Also in 1820 mercury began to be used for fillings in teeth.

Mercury is still being used for fillings today, although in 1988 the Environmental Protective Agency (EPA) declared dental scrap amalgam a hazardous waste. They state that there is no known lowest level that is safe for human consumption or exposure. So dangerous is mercury to the health of dentists and their assistants that governmental procedures have been developed to be followed by dentists who use mercury on their patients. No one, especially the influential American Dental Association trade association, has yet rationally explained how a substance can be so dangerous to dentists and their staff as to require special handling and disposal procedures, but when placed in the human mouth loses its danger.

Those who have not studied the matter of metal -- especially mercury -- toxicity, believe that once the metals are combined in an amalgam with other metals they are no longer free to form dangerous ions. This belief has been proven not to be true. By measuring the amount of mercury that remains in the amalgams of removed fillings, and comparing this amount to length of time that the filling has been in the mouth, it's quite clear that mercury decreases in direct proportion to length of time in the mouth in a linear relationship. The mercury must go somewhere. It combines with organic matter in the mouth and accumulates in the body, there to create serious health problems; and it also travels ionically, as would other postively charged materials, along body electrical paths that offer least resistance; and these ions end up somewhere in the body, often combined with organic cellular materials, particularly nerve ganglia.

Two different metals that make up an amalgam are saturated 24 hours daily by either an alkaline or an acid solution, the saliva and food mixtures that we drink and eat. Two different metals -- of which amalgams are composed -- in such a solution will form a small battery, creating an electric current affecting surrounding fluids and tissues. Each filled teeth, then, becomes a small battery which, when working together with other filled teeth, acts very much like two or more batteries connected together to strengthen the flow of current. Current flow also creates a magnetic field which influences release of certain hormones and neurotransmitters, chemicals that control the transmission of nerve impulses.

Also in each small "tooth battery" there is a constant disassociation of metalic ions that form the terminals of the battery. These ions combine with compounds in our tissues, migrate throughout the body, and accumulate. It is this accumulation of organic poisons that creates all of the different adverse health symptoms, among which can be found the symptoms of osteoarthritis in some patients.

Removing Mercury Fillings is a Growing Movement

Based on completed studies and clinical practices, Keith W. Sehnert, M.D., Gary Jacobson, D.D.S., and Kip Sullivan, J.D.[126] write that we often overlook the single most important source of auto-immune disorders -- the toxic mercury fillings in our teeth. "The use of mercury amalgams has been banned and are on a scheduled phaseout in Germany, Austria, Denmark and Sweden." Mercury toxicity leads to generalized morning stiffness, skin rashes, dry eyes and mouth, joint pain, immune dysfunction, and many other symptoms many of which are the same as can be found in one or more of the eighty auto-immune/ collagen tissue diseases.

The Case of Connie Anderson

Connie Anderson suffered miserably from muscle and joint aches, headaches, and overall, extreme lethargy, with repeated infections from yeast, colds and flu. After more than a year of ineffective antibiotics from various physicians, Connie read a book by Hal Huggins, D.D.S., *It's All in Your Head*.[107] She traveled 250 miles to Knoxville, Tennessee to consult with Biological Dentist Stephan Cobble, D.D.S., who began Connie on a planned program of mercury fillings replacement.

On completing her course of treatment, almost immediately Connie's immunological system recovered, and during the past five years Connie has not had her otherwise persistent muscle and joint aches, headaches or lethargy. She's seldom been sick since that moment forward.[107]

Treatment for Metal Toxicity

A Biological Dentist will understand the dental connection to osteoarthritis, including root canals and mercury toxicity. After testing by non-invasive diagnostic methods you'll know if underlying infection or mercury leakage is a possible cause of your joint pain, or other symptoms. Infection can be treated and mercury can be replaced with a safe substance.

The Biological Dentist will test each filling for current flow with an electrogalvanmeter, and, based on that flow, will make a decision as to which fillings should be removed and replaced with safe materials. Testing may also be by kinesiology, using certain indicator muscles to determine which are weak, thus indicating source of interference with the bio-electrical and musculature systems. The order in which the fillings are removed is quite important, as removal in the wrong order may increase the flow of current, thus increased mercury vaporization, per tooth.

Hal Huggins, D.D.S., then recommends a thorough detoxification, as simply removing the fillings does not remove the organic compounds that have accumulated over a long time. His detoxification regimen includes nutritional support, acupressure -- patterned pressure on spe-

ARTHRITIS: RHEUMATOID DISEASES CURED AT LAST WITH OSTEOARTHRITIS 121

cific acupuncture points -- massage treatment, chelating agents such as those mentioned in this chapter -- Ethylene Diamine Tetracetic Acid (EDTA) and Di-Mercaptopropane Sulfonate (DMPS) -- and both oral and intravenous vitamin C.

Rushing to a dentist to have your filings removed, in the absence of proper training and equipment by that dentist, can result in worsening your condition, or producing an added problem, such as chronic fatigue as a result of further spreading of mercury contamination. You must have a Biological Dentist.

Fluoridation

Fluoride is another of the governmentally approved poisons that over long periods of consumption can lead to a variety of osteoarthitic aches and pains, osteoporosis and dozens of other symptoms, many of which are based upon creation of an excess of free-radicals, chemicals that are actively seeking to join with otherwise healthy tissues, inhibiting their normal functions. (See *Fluoridation: Governmentally Approved Poison*, Anthony di Fabio, this Foundation.)

Fluoride is found in drinking water, mouth washes and tooth pastes. Over 121 million Americans have been wrongly told that artificial fluoride -- a toxic waste product of the aluminum ore industry -- will prevent tooth decay.

In 1930 Dr. Trendley Dean established the theory that fluoridation was safe and would protect teeth from cavities. In 1945 he established trials of fluoridation in the water supply of Grand Rapids, Michigan. These trials appeared to prove his theory. In 1950 the Public Health System recommended placing artificial fluoridation into public water systems to fight tooth decay. Since that time there have been an increasing number of health problems wherever fluoride has been added to municipal waters, tooth pastes and to dental treatments -- with no decrease in tooth decay!

And since the time of Dr. Dean's theory and trials, he has twice testified in court that statistics from his early studies were invalid.

Numerous independent scientific studies have established that Dean's theory is untrue and, in fact, that fluoride is a dangerous poison whose consistent use -- and especially overuse -- can lead to mottling, pitting, and crumbling of teeth, overgrowth and weakening of bone, hip fractures, adverse effects on red blood cells, cancer, neurotoxic effects, and arthritic pains.

Pennsylvania Supreme Court Judge John P. Flaherty, after extensive and meticulous study of the scientific data presented before him, wrote an opinion saying, "I entered an injunction against the fluoridation of the public water supply for a large portion of Allegheny County. . . . In my view, the evidence is quite convincing that the addition of sodium fluoride to the public water supply at one part per million is extremely deleterious to the human body, and a review of the evidence will disclose that there was no convincing evidence to the contrary."[45]

In a manner reminiscent of the American Dental Association's intransigent attitude toward removal of metal fillings from their industry, the Public Health System encourages the use of fluoride throughout the nation as though it were a beneficial treatment for all to partake of in drinking waters. However, after reviewing the scientific evidence for and against fluoride, it has now been banned in Austria, Denmark, France, Greece, Italy, Luxembourg, the Netherlands, Norway and Spain.

Since there is little control over individual consumption of fluoride taken by means of municipal water supplies, soft drinks, foods, tooth pastes and dental fluoridation, all consumers, particularly children, are in danger of obtaining more toxic fluoride than the body can handle safely. Levels that become excessive will first give rise to chalky-white, irregularly distributed patches on the tooth surface enamel, then become infiltrated with yellow or brown stains giving rise to the mottled appearance called dental fluorosis. Severe dental fluorosis weakens the enamel resulting in pitting.

Meanwhile, equivalent chemical changes occur in the bones that make up our skeletons. Prolonged intake of fluorides -- say around 20 years -- even at low levels -- brings about serious changes that weaken the bone leading to fractures, bone spurs, joint pains, and curvature of the spine called "skeletal fluorosis."

According to nutritionist and author Rex E. Newnham, D.O., N.D., Ph.D., North Yorkshire, England, who first discovered the importance of boron for human health, and especially for arthritis, skeletal fluorosis is the bone's counterpart to dental fluorosis. He relates that in some parts of India and Africa, where from two to five parts per million (ppm) fluoride is found in the drinking water, there is a serious development of skeletal fluorosis which affects many people. "They cannot work normally and can barely stand up; they cannot stand up straight since their backs are nearly parallel with the ground."[9,12]

At least ten percent of fluoride consumed by adults is deposited in bones, and studies have shown a positive correlation between decreased bone mass and strength. According to John R. Lee, M.D., Sebastapol, California, bones become weaker, increasing the risk of hip fracture.[5]

Richard A. Kunin, M.D., San Francisco, California, an orthomolecular physician, one who seeks to administer the right foods, vitamins, minerals, and other supplemental support for restoring health, writes, "I've seen spinal arthritis cases that have responded to removing fluoridated water. I've been amazed to find that some arthritis and osteoporosis patients are still being treated with fluoride therapy, at doses of 12 to 50 mg per day of sodium fluoride, 3 to 10 times the tolerance level recognized by the Environmental Protection agency -- and naturally they get worse: more back pain and less range of motion."[108]

As mercury has historically formed the backbone for many chemicals used as pesticides, fluoride has been used for generations as a most potent insecticide. While insects and rodents are not composed of human tissue, there is sufficient commonality of tissue structure in all to signal danger to us, also.

True Causes of Declining Dental Caries

According to John R. Lee, M.D., "If one were to argue that swallowing fluoridated water leads eventually to higher fluoride levels in dental enamel, one would then have to explain away the fact that dental enamel fluoride concentration in children from fluoridated communities in the U.S. is no different than the fluoride concentration in teeth of children from non-fluoridated communities."[109]

More than likely, the true causes for decrease in dental caries are the following factors, given by Dr. John R. Lee, M.D.

• Better nutrition
• Less sugar intake (e.g., use of artificial sweetners in kids' diets).
• Better dental hygiene (tooth brushing)
• Rising immunity to *Strepococcus mutans*, the plaque germ responsible for the conversion of simple dietary starches into acids that dissolve enamel
• General use of antibiotics that kill or hold in check the germ *Strepococcus mutans*.
• Use of fluoridated toothpaste. This latter factor does not vindicate water fluoridation or tooth treatment with fluoride. The concentration in toothpaste (which is applied directly to dental enamel) is 1000-1500 ppm whereas drinking water (which passes the teeth into the gut and then is excreted in urine) contains only 1 ppm fluoride [but can be considerably higher in some communities]. The higher concentration in toothpaste is sufficient to kill or seriously impair the enzyme processes of *Strepococcus mutans* plaque germs, whereas the low concentration in drinking water is simply ineffective.[19]

More than likely safer substitutes are available for the same teeth brushing purpose, that will serve to kill *Strepococcus mutans*.

Dangers of Using Fluoride

Gerard P. Judd, Ph.D.[109] summarizes the actual and indicated dangers from forceful feeding of fluoride as follows:

• Slightly poorer teeth (more decay, missing teeth, fillings), with egg-shell white fluorosis and brittleness.

According to Professor Cornelius Steelink, Department of Chemistry at the University of Arizona, who headed up a subcommittee for study of addition of fluoride to the Tucson, AZ water supply, their study showed that ". . . the more fluoride a child drank, the more cavities appeared in the teeth."[21]

• More brittle bones in the aged;

• Destruction of at least 60 out of 63 enzymes, including cyto-chrome C, cholinesterase and others handling oxygen. Enzymes are necessary for all of our life processes of digestion, absorption of essential nutrients, and tens of thousands of other vital functions;
• Genetic change, both in the sperm and other cells;
• Dramatic heart death increase in Antiogo, Wisconsin, where a long-term study was made;
• Down's syndrome increase of 250%;
• Probably a major cause of sudden infant death sydrome (SIDS) and chronic fatigue syndrome (CFS), since allergic (toxic) symptoms the same;
• Infant mortality increase: for Washington, D.C. African-Americans 4 times, for Caucasians 3 times (48 years of fluoridation) and for the average U.S. population 1.4 times;
• Infant birth defects increased 3 times in Chile during its experiment with fluoridation;
• 39% increase in cancers overall, with 80% for rectal cancer in the U.S. after 33 years;
• Fluoride accumulates about 50% daily in the bones and soft tissue;
• Miscarriages and spontaneous abortions increase;
• Possibly Alzheimers, multiple sclerosis (MS) and other viral disease are made worse due to antibody destruction.
• Fifty other side effects among which is arthritis.

How to Avoid the Consequences of Fluoride

Of course, the safest way to avoid the consequences of fluoride is to become politically active, forcing those who have less knowledge of its effects than you to confront truth, and to prove or supply adequate proof of erroneous claims -- and to get the fluoride out of your family's drinking water.

The second most effective way is to purchase only non-fluoride toothpaste, or to mix bicarbonate and salt together for your brushing.

Faced with the problem of an immovable, ill-educated, emotional-stimulus-response public works bureaucracy, most knowledgeable physicians will recommend   for all of their patients the purchase and installation of a reverse osmosis filter, along with an activated charcoal filter for your house or apartment water system. The reverse osmosis filter will remove the fluoride and chlorine, whereas the activated charcoal filter will remove other undesireable pollutants. Cost savings for you and your family's health will be well-worth the additional capital outlay, and can have a direct effect on one kind or another of the various arthritic diseases.

Treatment for Excessive Fluoride and the Ideal Clinic

Rex Newnham, N.D., D.O., Ph.D., North Yorkshire, England, Dr. Catherine Russell, Guadalajara, Mexico, and other physicians use homeopathic remedies to help the body counteract and discharge fluoride, others will employ whole-body detoxification procedures. One such is described by Mark Davidson, D.O, N.D.,[83] who described an ideal clinic that would address the whole person and their lifestyle training, not just components that make up the person.

Dr. Davidson says that "So many people say they've got the cure, they've got the whole picture. I tend to see little parts of a puzzle. You get a better picture when you get more viewpoints. . . . We look at the patient's physical, emotional, electromagnetic, biochemical and spiritual being, using a team of experienced practitioners, each contributing their health expertise in a particular area but applying it in such a manner that the whole individual is treated."

The following is a brief description of Dr. Davidson's recommended treatments:

• The patient is placed in an environment conducive to peace and serenity surrounded by woods and forests with pure water, fresh air, biodynamic gardens, and a spring-fed, solar-heated swimming pool.

• Dr. Davidson, and the other health-care professionals, believe that how a person thinks influences their emotions and physical conditions. "In treating degenerative problems, our emphasis is on our modern way of life. Change of habits and patterns that get to the core of things. If you can advise people on how to handle stress factors in their life, relationship factors, communication skills, work problems, you're looking at a multi-factorial approach in dealing with stress." If a person's beliefs, thoughts and emotions are chaotic, scattered, or confused, they will have a difficult time healing. "The physical problem is the end-stage of unresolved, strong emotions." Staff members help clients confront the issues that they need to address.

• As most people with chronic illness have major toxicity problems, usually stemming from the bowels, Dr. Davidson believes that cleansing of the bowels is of primary importance. This is done by means of fiber, herbs, enzymes and nutrients, plus ozone colonic irrigation. Dr. Davidson says that "Usually toxicities found in the gallbladder, liver and kidneys are cleared only through proper bowel cleansing."

Ozonated colonics and other forms of cleansing will also rid the burden of parasites, of which there are many forms. This is an important factor, as getting rid of the lining of the small bowel, because behind the lining you'll usually find a lot of parasites: worms, amoeba, flukes and so forth.

Dr. Davison's team would also flushe out the liver and gallbladder with the use of herbs, nutrients, acupressure, acupuncture, shiatsu (Japanese "finger pressure"), Swedish massage, and by stimulating the lymph system. People who finally deal with their unresolved anger may have a spontaneous detoxification of their liver and gallbladder.

Body tissues are cleansed by using steam cabinets, Turkish baths, herbs that cause sweating, ozonated baths, all of which help toxins to come through the skin. Homeopathic remedies and herbs help to speed up the metabolism and therefore also help detoxification.

• After the bowel and organs are detoxified, Dr. Davidson starts giving the right nutrients, preventing additional toxicity from entering into tissues, liver and gallbladder from poor food choices."We also educate people. We teach them about water purity, air pollutants and how to find foods low in or free of toxins, so that when they return home, they can continue their process of detoxification."

• As many people develop clogged lymph systems, preventing toxins from being removed from the body, we use lymphatic massage therapy accompanied by a device that combines magnetic therapy with soft laser principles. This is a gentle massage, and it breaks up congealed lymph, permitting the free flow of lymph drainage again. Dry skin brushing is taught, or bouncing regularly on a trampoline-rebounder, as these will also help lymph to drain. (See this chapter, "Energy Medicine.")

• "Most chronically ill people have toxin-producing infections," Dr. Davidson believes. "This stems from root canal teeth or previous tooth extractions. As these infections are tied in with acupuncture meridians which pass through internal organs, these organs are also affected. Therefore it's important to clean out pockets of dental infection and 'dead' teeth."

• Uneven bites or malocclusions -- where teeth do not match up perfectly -- can also affect health.

As mercury amalgam is one of the primary sources of accumulated toxicity and immune suppression, these fillings should be considered for replacement.

A Biological Dentist would be provided to assess and to solve these otherwise hidden problems.

Although not necessarily related to teeth, Dr. Davidson feels that geo-magnetic fields (geo-pathic lines) can also influence a persons health, and education is important to avoid certain electromagnetic stress.

• Once there is sufficient metal removed from the teeth, intravenous chelation therapy is used as described in this chapter under "Chelation Therapy."

• Dr. Davidson says that "These approaches must be combined with changes in the person's diet, lifestyle, and nutrient supplementation. One of our prime goals would be for people to come to our clinic, learn the techniques, and take them back home to use and to show others. We're not interested in treating diseases, but in building health." Health Restoration Systems, Inc. under guidance of Lee Cowden, M.D., conducts a similar educational program. For more information contact them at 1202 West Executive Drive, 75081, Richardson, TX 75083;

(972) 480-8909; Fax (972) 480-8807.
Homeopathy
Homeopathy is a natural approach to medicine that works without side effects, stimulating the body's curative responses so that the body heals itself. In addition to healing, homeopathy, properly used, strengthens the immune system.[94]

Where conventional medicine defines health as the absence of symptoms, homeopathy defines health as lack of disease. For example, if your nose is runny, and you are rid of the runny nose by means of a decongestant, does that mean that you're well? Of course not, because while the decongestant dried up the runny nose, it didn't solve the physical problem that caused the runny nose.

Homeopathy would solve the physical problem -- that is, your body would learn to solve it -- and the runny nose would clear up as a consequence.

Background
Dr. Samuel Christian Hahneman, one of Napoleon Bonaparte's physicians, founded and defined the basic outlines of homeopathy. On Napoleon's route to conquer most of Europe, Napoleon used Dr. Hahneman to keep his troops free of typhoid fever. Hahneman created a new concept of medicine, which he called 'homeopathy,' derived from the Greek words, 'homeos,' which means 'similar,' and, 'pathos' or 'disease'.

Hahneman's basic law was, "Let's cure a disease with the disease itself, or, like cures like."

Many success stories, with every form of disease, have been reported through the use of homeopathy. Used by hundreds of millions worldwide, homeopathy is two hundred years old, and was once a widely practiced healing discipline in the United States until the dominance of "allopathic" medicine.

The practice of allopathic medicine, or "allopathy," is that method which seeks to cure disease by the production of a condition of the system either different from or opposite to the condition produced by the disease. For example, if one has a joint pain, then the allopathic solution is to provide a drug that will decrease or suppress the joint pain -- the opposite sensation from the pain. As all know -- or should know -- who suffer from any form of arthritis, although halting the pain provides a short measure of comfort the disease continues onward.

"Homeopathy," the granddaddy of vaccination theory, is the opposite of allopathy. Homeopathy is a theory or system of curing diseases with very minute doses of medicine which in a healthy person and in large doses would produce a condition like that of the disease treated. The basic principle is that symptoms of a "disease" are a natural part of the healing process. As such, they must be allowed to occur, even augmented, rather than be suppressed. For example, if a particular substance would normally create a joint pain when given in large doses, the dosage of the substance is diluted drastically -- to the point of disappearance -- and provided to the arthritic. Substances, therefore, are diluted to such an extreme dilution that scoffing allopathic physicians will describe the resulting mixture as being "the essence of residual vibrations of a ghostly spirit passing through the room quickly one time."

Initial substances chosen for dilution are   products of diseased tissues or bodily secretions, protoplasm of animal cells, various components of plant tissue, or from chemical compounds. If the initial substance is the product of disease tissue or bodily secretions, it is called a "nosode." If the initial substance is from the protoplasm of animal cells, it is called a "sarcode."

Sterilized nosodes and sarcodes, are both used to prepare a "mother" by dissolving them in either water or alcohol in usually a 1 to 9 ratio, and this mother is the actual fluid used to create the homeopathic remedies. These carefully selected substances are sequentially diluted (and struck, vigorously shaken, or tapped; i.e., "succussion") to concentrations such as 0.9×9^{-61}. The more dilute the homeopathic remedy, the more "powerful" its effect -- a phenomenon which stretches normal imagination beyond training of allopathic physicians as it is unlikely that any one vial of any substance diluted 1 to 99 in successive manner 18 times will   contain even one molecule of the orginal substance.

Hahnemann originally published the results of his trials of various homeopathic remedies in a book titled *Materia Medica* where was listed under each remedy the symptoms that the remedy produced in healthy people. Later work by others has increased the number of substances used as remedies to three thousand, although not all of these have been tested with the same thoroughness as Hahnemann's original investigations.

To become entered in the *Materia Medica* one had to "prove," the homeopathic solutions. Proving is done by applying the possible homeopathic remedy to a healthy person, and, over a given time period, carefully observing symptoms. This same experiment is performed with a number of healthy people until confidence assures that a given dilution of a given substance in fact produces given symptoms. Such observations are complicated by the fact that people vary in their response to a given remedy, some developing severe symptoms, some mild, and others inbetween.

Later researchers have developed remedy finders or *Reperotires*, classifying sections with a series of headings concerned with parts or systems of the body, such as mental, vertigo, head, eyes, nose, and so on down to toes. Under each heading there is a list of symptoms, such as pain, redness, or swelling. Alongside each symptom are printed all the remedies known to produce that symptom, together with any factors that might affect it. Symptoms are graded, with the most well proven in bold type, the second in italics, and the third in plain roman type.

Basic Laws of Homeopathy

Based on Hahnemann's early observation and research, the doctor who established homeopathy in the United States, Dr. Constantine Hering, was able to isolate out healing rules that apply universally to those who receive homeopathic remedies. These are:

• Cure takes place from the top of the body downward, and from the inside to the outside, and from the most important organs to the least important; and

• Cure takes place in reverse order to the onset of symptoms.

For example, an ill person will start to feel better emotionally before physical symptoms disappear, and a long-standing problem will take longer to disappear than a recent one. Many physicians such as Louis J. Marx, M.D.,[112] Ventura, California describe this phenomena to their patients as "Like unpeeling layers from an onion. One unpeels layer by layer, and, when various symptoms disappear at last one reaches the core, and total healing has taken place."

Other homeopathic laws that apply are these:

• Small stimuli (very dilute) encourage living systems, medium stimuli impede them, and strong stimuli (as with drugs) tend to stop living systems. The greater the dilution, the better the response, the less the dilution, the poorer the response.

• The quantity of action necessary to effect a change in nature is the least possible, the decisive amount is always the minimum, perhaps even an infintesimal amount.

• Life forces produce functional changes in exact proportion to the degree of physical disturbance, and these functional changes always preceed structural changes. For example, pains in joints inhibit motion of the joint, which is its function. The joint is used less and less, until at last structural changes occur, which might be calcification of joints, weakened muscles, poorer blood flow, and so on, until at last the joint is rigid and unable to move properly, a structural change.

Homeopathic Research

While it is true that modern medicine has a difficult time reconciling healing with a dilution so tiny that no molecule of the original substance can possibly remain in a given vial, there are efforts to develop hypotheses to explain the mystery. According to Trevor Cook, Ph.D., DI Hom., President of the United Kingdom Homeopathic Medical Association, explanation for the successful activity of homeopathic preparations seems to lie in the domain of quantum physics and energy medicine. In a study using nuclear magnetic resonance (NMR) imaging distinctive readings showed subatomic activity in 23 homeopathic remedies.

130 ANTHONY DI FABIO, M.A. & GUS J. PROSCH, JR., M.D

Several clinical experiments have stood up to scrutiny, including increase in growth of wheat seedlings, diastase hydrolysis (enzyme reactions) of starch and growth rate of lymphoblast, a cell that gives rise to a white blood cell called a lymphocyte.

To the great chagrin and consternation of traditional allopathic practitioners, *The British Medical Journal* (Feb. 9, 1991) published a groundbreaking survey of clinical research on homeopathic medicine. Three experts on clinical research analyzed 107 controlled clinical studies which were published between 1966 and 1990. They noted that 81 trials -- a scientifically significant finding --indicated positive results.[96]

In a 1992 patent received by Robert A. Collins, Waukon, Iowa, *Method of Producing Remedies and Products of the Method* (Patent Number 5,102,669), deadly bacteria were killed and injected into the cistern of a cow (above each of four teats) prior to calving. The cow has the ability, as does any mammal, to prepare small molecules called "complement" that will protect the calf from dangerous, invasive organisms.

Colostrum, the cow's first milk after birth, was prepared in three homeopathic dilutions as was the later milk. Deadly bacteria were injected in groups of four mice each. In each of two studies completed, homeopathic remedies made from the milk or the colostrum, in the greatest dilution, achieved the highest survival of the mice.

Illustrating another of the homeopathic laws, when the dosage itself was cut from 1 cc to 0.5 cc and 0.25 cc, the greatest survival was achieved with the smaller dosages, the greatest survival rate being the 0.25 cc.

Described in the same patent, a sick herd of cows was isolated from which a mixture of various disease-causing organisms were obtained. These micro-organisms were killed, and were used to form a mother from which a homeopathic remedy was made. The homeopathic remedy was distributed in the feed of the cows and measures of the various disease-producing organisms made. The cattle receiving the homeopathic remedies showed a remarkable drop in their degree of infection as compared to the non-treated cows.

How Is Homeopathic Medicine Practiced?
Preventive role

Where allopathic medicine seeks a drastic benefit quickly, and often ignores a preventive role for medicine, the preventive role of homeopathy seeks to nudge the white cell populations, stabilize emotional states and attempts to bring the whole body to a state where it will be responsive and ready to ward off disease and further prevent disease from setting up shop, so to speak. When a homeopathic physician administers a prescription, he is prescribing for both the present ailment as well as for tendencies that have not yet come into being as a recognizable ailment.

Fetuses in the womb can be safely treated homeopathically through the mother. Infants and childhood ailments respond well to homeopathic remedies. In adults, immediate attention to minor illnesses can prevent serious complaints later on in life.

Choosing the Correct Remedy

Traditional medical practices -- allopathic medicine -- provides each arthritic with an analgesic or anti-inflammatory drug, usually of size to fit body weight, recognizing only pain as pain; that is, pain is evaluated in but one way. This drug, of course, merely suppresses the symptom of pain and does nothing to halt the progress of a diseased condition that set up the pain.

Homeopathic practices recognize many kinds of pain: pain that comes on suddenly, pain that disappears as suddenly as it comes on, pain that comes on and wears off gradually, biting pain, boring, penetrating pain, and so on, perhaps more than 30 in number. Within each of these categories are recommended homeopathic remedies, more than 200 in number.

Most ill people suffer not just the symptoms that are easily noted, but also a mal-functioning that is unique to them. Another way of stating this is that for a given symptom, such as a headache, or joint ache, there can be many different causes. In orthodox medicine these unique causes are unimportant, as only the symptom -- the pain -- is being treated. In homeopathic medicine, these unique causes assume primary importance to determine the correct remedy. This is why different patients may receive different remedies for the same disease state, or set of symptoms.

It's clear from the foregoing that, while it is simple to purchase a particular homeopathic remedy over the counter, without keen observation and classification of symptoms and the experience and background developed by a practicing homeopathic physician, and especially without a book of provings such as the *Materia Medica*, a chance selection of the proper remedy over the counter is remote. Still many do make such low probability choices of over-the-counter homeopathic remedies and find relief. Homeopathic remedies are generally recognized as safe, and can be purchased throughout the United States without prescription.

To evaluate a patient's needs, three aspects should be considered: (1) consitution: whether robust and strong, weak and sensitive, and so on; (2) mental: restless, easily excited, pain, and conditions under which pain occurs, dazed or stupid, and so on; (3) physical symptoms: sensitivity to light, thirst, coated tongue, pulse rate, nature of stools, and so on.

The example below describes only the symptoms of pain and conditions under which they occur.

A patient who suffers from arthritis will more than likely have a mixture of problems. For example, a patient may have a stiff, painful joint that occurs at the start of movement, but then disappears as the movement is continued. This same pain may be aggravated by damp weather, cold, and rest, but is improved by changing positions and in warm, dry weather. From the overall collection of symptoms, the homeopathic physician may decide that the fibrous connective tissue surrounding a joint needs assistance and will therefore prescribe Rhus tox *(Rhus toxicodendron)*, a derivative of poison ivy, 9 C from two to four times daily. This will be a remedy in solution or tablet form that has been successively diluted in a 1 to 9 ratio 9 times.

However if the joint pain is aggravated by rest and improved immediately by movement, the physician may decide that the tendons and the membrane covering the bones (periosteum) need assistance, and so prescribe Ruta *(Ruta graveolens)*, a derivative of herb-of-grace, 5C, 7C, or 9C, two to four times daily.

When symptoms in the lumbo-sacral region and knees are aggravated at night, by prolonged rest, and are improved by movement and heat, and if the patient has a feeling of joint weakness, as if the joints were about to give way, *Radium bromatum* is prescribed in the same manner as is Ruta, above.

As arthritic disorders may alternate with, or accompany digestive disorders such as diarrhea, when the joint pain is caused or aggravated by cold, damp weather, and also worsens with rest and improves with movement, then Dulcamara is used, often with Thuja *(Thuja accidentalis)*, and *Natrum sulphuricum*.

The patient whose joint synovial tissue causes irritation and effusion with joints that are red and hot, frequently swollen and sensitive to the slightest touch, with throbbing pain, aggravated by the slightest movement and improved by absolute immobility, prescribed may be 7C or 9C Bryonia *(Bryonia alba)*, two to four times daily.

Constitution, emotional state, and physical symptoms are all necessary patterns for choosing the correct homeopathic remedy.

Homeopathic Remedies Used as Traditional Medicines

Traditional medical practitioners may use homeopathic medicines, but not homeopathically. For example, *Cis platinum*, can be used homeopathically or as a drug. *Cis platinum* used traditionally -- that is, non-homeopathically -- is cancer-inducing, just as the allopathic use for rheumatoid arthritis of methotrexate and other cyto-toxic drugs are cancer-inducing.

Similarly use of quinine, digitalis and emetine -- although the basis to homeopathic remedies -- are used by traditional allopathic practitioners as drugs in greatly increased strengths. Many traditional remedies used for lumbago or sleeplessness may give some results -- but they are not used homeopathically, and they're given to all without regard to the cause of the symptoms. Also with some success, dilutions of allergens -- small allergy inducing proteins such as pollens -- are also used in varying dilution strengths (not homeopathically) to treat allergies by injecting them into the patient. These same allergens can be used homeopathically to produce safe and effective results.

Combination Remedies

Although the initial intent of classical homeopathic practitioners is to use but one remedy at a time, many today use combination formulas that contain remedies that may cover a broad spectrum of symptoms. For example, for an arthritic the symptoms of joint pain, stiffness on arising in the morning, muscle weakness, calcium deposits, depression and lethargy may all be treated at the same time, with combinations of remedies that will fit each problem. The view is that the body will shed off those remedies that have no effect, but will learn from those that do.

One such homeopathic combination is Zeel T, a commercial ointment to be applied to the skin over joint pain, and which consists of *Toxicondendron quercifolium, Arnica montana, Solanum dulcamara, Symphytum, and Sanguinaria canadensis,* homeopathic attenuations of the mineral substances sulfur, acidum siliccum, homeopathic preparations of organ extracts, *Cartilago suis, Funiculus umbilicalis suis, Embryo suis, and Placenta suis,* and also homeopathic preparations of the bio-catalysts nicotinamide-adenindinucleotide, coenzyme A, acidum alpha-liponicum, and sodium diethyloxalaceticum these latter being "capable of activating cell and tissue functions in homeopathic concentrations."

Zeel T was used in a study on 498 arthritics in 7 medical centers ranging from 28 to 200 patients per center. Arthritic conditions involved those suffering from pain in a single joint, many joints, backbone, and other degenerative disorders related to osteoarthritis.

According to the report of Professor R.E. Woodick, M.D., Specialist for Sports Medicine, K. Steininger, M.D., and Stefan Zenner, M.D. published in *Biological Therapy*[113], "Throughout the course of therapy, the patients experienced rapid and definite relief from such complaints as pain experienced during the night, pain upon onset of motion, and pain during articular movement.

"Participating physicians assessed overall results of therapy as either very good or good for 75.1% of the patients."

Traditional Diagnosis Can Determine the Correct Homeopathic Treatment

Joint pain, including rheumatoid arthritis, may start in the tonsils and throat, according to Dr. Catherine Russell,[233] Guadalajara, Mexico. Dr. Russell runs laboratory tests for the anti-streptococcus lyosome, parts of the microorganism's inner digestive system. If it is high, she'll administer the homeopathic remedy Streptococcus 200 X (diluted successively 1 to 9, 200 times), 1 per week. She reports that "Streptococcus usually starts in the tonsils, then after becoming chronic in the throat area, starts infiltrating in the joints. On starting treatment there is usually an aggravation in the joints, and the tonsils become inflammed again. The worse thing that can be done at this point is to give antibiotics which suppresses the removal of the bacteria. (Also see *Root Canal Coverup*, George Meinig, D.D.S.)

"One must give supportive treatment to get through this throat crises. After that, the joint pain decreases, the throat crises is resolved.

"Usually 8 or 12 doses of this medicine will see the patient through the crisis. Patients definitely start getting better.

"I also use the streptococcus nosodes for patients with rheumatic fever."

In addition to homeopathic remedies and herbals for some forms of arthritis, including rheumatoid arthritis, Dr. Russell may also use traditional anti-microorganism drugs [described in Chapter II, Rheumatoid Disease, "The Professor Roger Wyburn-Mason, M.D., Ph.D. Treatment for Rheumatoid Arthritis,"] starting with tinidizole (Tinidex® or Fasigyn®), which is easily available in Mexico over the counter. She reports that she always sees a herxheimer reaction, or "flu-like symptoms" also called the "die-off effect." (See Chapter II, Rheumatoid Arthritis, "The Herxheimer Effect.")

According to Dan Clark, M.D.,[112] Melbourne, Florida, chief executive officer of Sports, Health, and Fitness which offers safe alternatives to steroids for sports, and Bio Active Nutritional which supplies herbals, homeopathic remedies, and nutritional supplements, the chief beneficial function of homeopathic remedies for arthritics is with their ability to boost immune system, detoxify connective tissue cells, and for special purposes, such as stimulating the intake of calcium, where calcium is not being utilized efficiently, thus leading to conditions such as arthritis.

Dr. Clark says that, "seldom will homeopathic remedies reverse or cure arthritis, but is intended to be a supplement to other necessary treatments." Bio Active Nutritional and Sports, Health, and Fitness may both be reached at 1803 North Wickham Rd., Suite 6, Melbourne, Florida 32935; (800-311-5265).

Non-Traditional Diagnosis Can Determine
the Correct Homeopathic Treatment

***Dermatron*™**: Developed by Reinhold Voll, M.D., the Dermatron measures electrical resistance at acupuncture points. He discovered that other than normal readings -- higher or lower -- at specific acupuncture points meant a problem with a corresponding organ. A higher reading generally meant irritation or inflammation and a lower meant fatigue or degneration of the organ. There are more than 2000 control points that can be measured and assessed. A skilled Dermatron operator can quickly assess which organs need help. When the patient holds a sample of known disease substances, such as bacteria, viruses, or diseased tissue, the readings return to normal.

The reason is the homepathic principle that "like cures like." The body perceives the substance as "good medicine."

More than this, however, testing in the same way with various herbs, vitamins, minerals, or homeopathic remedies immediately tells the Dermatron operator which substances will effect a beneficial change in the condition.

The Vega™ is another electroacupuncture feedback device similar to the Dermatron. Computerized systems are now employed to speed up the process, and also to build a patient data base. Some of these newer systems have codified within the computer memory a vast array of electromagnetic "signatures" of microorganisms (antigens), and allergens. Simply by placing a particular acupuncture point along a desired meridian into circuit with the specialized computer, a reading is obtained that not only tells of a problem, but also identifies the name of the organism or allergen -- all done accurately without using invasive techniques. BIOSOURCE, Inc., 1388 West Center Street, Orem, UT 84057; (801) 226-1117, manufactures one such device.

Kinesiology: Kinesiology practitioners determine health imbalances in organs and glands by identifying specific muscles which show weakness. By stimulating or relaxing these key muscles, diagnoses and resolution of a variety of health problems occurs.

Similar to the Dermatron, when a patient holds a substance with negative influence on him or her, muscle testing will reveal this, and also vice versa. For example, if a patient is allergic to a substance, while simultaneously holding that substance and being tested with kinesiology the patient's muscles will respond with immediate weakness, and also vice versa. An easy test is this: have a friend or relative hold one arm at right angles to their body, and direct them to resist your downward push. In the other hand alternate a small container of sugar and salt. The sugar will produce weakness in efforts to resist your push. Your friend's or relative's body is telling him that sugar is not good for him!

Where is Homeopathy Practiced?

The Food and Drug Administration recognizes homeopathic remedies as official drugs and regulates manufacturing, labeling, and dispensing. The *Homeopathic Pharmacopoeia of the United States* published in 1897, is an official compendium.

While homeopathy is not licensed in all states, about three thousand medical doctors and licensed health care professionals practice it. Homeopathy has been available in many European countries for 200 years, where thousands use and practice homeopathy. Certain present-day royalty and other governmental leaders would not have any other kind. And, while John D. Rockefeller (the original) is said to have promoted allopathy in many American medical schools -- as drugs increased his oil-related profits -- he, himself, would not permit any other kind of physician than one who practiced homeopathy.

In the United States practitioners of homeopathy may be licensed as Medical Doctors (M.D.s), Doctors of Osteopathy (D.O.s), Chiropractors (D.C.), Naturopathic Physician (N.D.s), Doctors of Oriental Medicine (O.M.D.s). Dentists (D.D.S.s), Podiatrists (D.P.M.s) , and Nurses (R.N.s). The last three are often considered lay practitioners and, in some states, may be treading on the borderline of practicing medicine without a license.

For information on qualified practitioners of homeopathy, contact The Arthritis Trust of America/The Rheumatoid Disease Foundation, 5106 Old Harding Road, Franklin, TN 37064; International Foundation for Homeopathy, 2366 Eastlake Drive East, Seattle, Washington 98102; and National Center for Homeopathy, 801 N. Fairfax # 306; Alexandria, VA 22314.

Hormonal Replacement Therapy

A hormone is a chemical substance that originates in a gland, or body part, or tissue, which is conveyed through the blood to another part of the body where it stimulates by chemical action an increase in activity and increased secretions.

Hormones have many generalized functions, such as turning on the flight or fight mechanism during emergencies, control of growth, regulation of sexual characteristics and functions, regulation of bone density, sleep, immunological system -- to ward of invasive organisms -- and other functions.

Production of hormones may be too much, or too little, each resulting in   characteristic symptoms.

Although there are a wide range of hormones used in both traditional and alternative medical treatments, those that apply to osteoarthritis in particular are cortico-steroids (cortisone), estrogen, progesterone, testosterone,   dehydroepiandrosterone (DHEA), and thyroid.

Cortico-Steroids

The most commonly administered hormone for arthritis is corticosteroid or "cortisone" -- a product of the adrenal glands which must be used in increasingly greater dosages to alleviate pain symptoms, as the body constantly reduces its own production as more and more cortisone is injected or taken orally. Although cortisone is probably the fastest means for damping pain, and is widely used for this purpose by traditional medical practitioners, it has never cured any arthritic disease and, in fact, permits the disease to continue -- often faster -- as the symptoms of the disease are suppressed. Eventually with some arthritics, their adrenal glands quit manufacturing a sufficient amount of this chemical, and a dependency results on external cortisone sources for life itself. Except for use of a form of cortisone that does not act systemically -- "depot medrol" as described in this chapter, "Structure" -- we do not recommend the use of cortisone. If an arthritic is using it, we recommend a gradual decrease in dosage under a physician's care while alternative therapies are employed.

Sex Hormones

Since more woman after menopause suffer from osteoarthritis and osteoporosis (weakening of bones that lead to bone fractures with aging) than men, it is frequently assumed that an insufficiency of specific hormones are part of the basis to osteoarthritis as well as osteoporosis. Key hormones for the treatment of osteoporosis, according to Alan Gaby, M.D., Seattle, Washington, and Johnathan V. Wright, M.D., Kent, Washington, are estrogen, progesterone, dehydroepiandrosterone (DHEA), and testosterone.

Louis J. Marx, M.D., Ventura, California, will frequently treat osteoarthritis and osteoporosis in a similar manner.

For osteoarthritics, therefore, the object would be to replace important female or male hormones.

Dehydroepiandrosterone (DHEA) is produced by the adrenal glands and is a precursor to many other hormones. It decreases steadily as age increases in both sexes. It is one of the most reliable indicators of aging, and, according to Julian Whitaker, M.D., editor of *Health & Healing*, by age 80 is only 5% of what it was at its peak at age 20. Restoring to a normal level of DHEA will decrease blood platelet stickiness to help prevent heart attacks and strokes, lower blood pressure, assist in cases of cancer, Alzheimer's disease, multiple sclerosis, memory loss, chronic fatigue syndrome, Parkinson's disease and lower blood cholesterol levels. It's use will increase the level of the sex hormone estrogen in women and the sex hormone testosterone in men to levels found in younger men and women, and, according to Dr. Whitaker, may be a safer supplement in older men and women than the traditional prescriptions for estrogen and testosterone.

Traditional medical practices provide estrogen replacement for aging women at risk for bone fractures. According to Johnathan V. Wright, M.D. and Alan R. Gaby, M.D., editors of *Nutrition & Healing*, such replacement reduces the number of fractures by about 50%, but may also increase the risk of cancer. They recommend the use of a product called "estriol," which is a compound of three naturally occurring forms of estrogen in the body that are non-carcinogenic. "In fact some studies indicate that estriol actually prevents breast cancer."[110] Developed by Jonathan V. Wright, M.D., estriol is a combination of 80% estriol, 10% estrone, and 10% estradiol. This combination is called "triple estrogen," and can be obtained with a prescription through a compounding pharmacist.

Progesterone is traditionally prescribed in the form of "progestogens" (such as Provera®) to prevent uterine-cancer-promoting effects of estrogen. According to Dr. Gaby, "progestogens are not the same as

the natural progesterone manufactured by the ovary. Natural progesterone is not only much safer than progestogens but apparently more
effective against osteoporosis." Since reduction in the same hormones
as we age accompanies both osteoporosis and osteoarthritis, natural
progesterone would be advised for osteoarthritis also.

John Lee, M.D., a pioneer in natural progesterone therapy discovered that administering the substance directly to the skin as a cream
"invariably increased bone mass and prevented fractures in women
with osteoporosis.[110]

Dr. Gaby also advises switching over from progestogen to natural progesterone under a trained physician's care.

Testosterone and dehydroepiandrosterone (DHEA) are both customarily considered male hormones, but they are both produced in
substantial amounts by the ovaries. Both are bone builders, both stimulating the growth of new bone.

In both men and women, blood level tests of these hormones
should be made prior to their replacement therapy, as is true for the use
of the other hormones described. Dehydroepiandrosterone (DHEA)
should be measured as DHEA-sulfate.

One of us (Perry A. Chapdelaine, Sr.) has found that a skin application of a combined gel consisting of the proper ratios of testosterone
and DHEA to be extremely effective. Widely used in Europe, this process can only be obtained in the United States through a compounding
pharmacist under prescription. After the two hormones are measured
in the blood, the information along with prescription is mailed to a
compounding pharmacist who is knowledgeable in "percutaneous" (skin
applied) mixtures. On return of the gel -- usually enough to last 4 to 5
weeks -- 1 cc per side is applied across the skin on each side of the
body each day. The skin acts as a reservoir throughout the day, absorbing whatever is needed for hormonal replacement throughout the next
24 hours.

Similar mixtures are available for women, using their appropriate substances as described above.

Thyroid

A most important hormone to be considered in the treatment of
virtually all diseases, including osteoarthritis, is that of thyroid produced by a small gland normally weighing only one ounce found at the
base of the Adam's apple. The thyroid, like other glands, can produce
too much or too little hormone. A deficiency of thyroid is usually assumed from symptoms and is called "hypothyroidism," as blood and
laboratory measures do not normally reflect a deficiency unless glands
responsible for thyroid production are defective. The reason for this
paradox will be described.

Common symptoms include sluggish circulation, especially in
the hands and feet (always feeling cold), poor digestion, lack of men-

struation, dry skin, long-term nervousness, heart palpitations, loss of appetite, inability for the obese individual to lose weight or for the thin person to gain weight, emotional imbalance, chronic fatigue syndrome, and many other symptoms. The condition of hypothyroidism contributes to or causes more than 60 different disease symptoms, among which is also found various forms of arthritis. This cluster of disease symptoms is called "Wilson's Syndrome," or "Multiple Enzyme Deficiency."

There are several traditional laboratory tests for determining the sufficiency of thyroid production from the gland, itself, but none of them are good indicators for measuring hypothyroidism. While the thyroid gland may be functioning perfectly, the hormone secreted by the thyroid must be converted by cells to a form that turns on cellular metabolism, our heat engine. There are no blood tests that can measure how well our cells turn on their metabolism, or heat engine. Therefore, no matter how normal blood and laboratory tests may appear, none [until recently] are capable of measuring thyroid utilization by the cells. Unfortunately, many physicians are unaware of this fact.

Broda Barnes, M.D., who discovered how to determine thyroid deficiency by taking temperature before arising in the morning, E. Denis Wilson, M.D.,[113] Orlando, Florida, who discovered a means of reversing thyroid deficiency when all the glands were producing normally, one of us (Gus J. Prosch, Jr., M.D.), and many other alternative care physicians have learned that an underactive thyroid -- even marginally so -- is a common denominator for much of the Western world's illnesses, including that of osteoarthritis and rheumatoid arthritis.

How can a person's thyroid gland be operating normally, but the person still suffer from an under-thyroid condition?

The answer has to do with enzymes, those small molecules in the body described in the section on "Nutrition and Supplements," which are involved with every chemical reaction in the human body of which there are hundreds of thousands.

The section on "Nutrition and Supplements" has emphasized the importance of enzymes, but what if the enzymes cannot operate properly?

Of course, if enzymes are unable to operate properly, or are deficient, the body will behave as though there is a lack of proper enzymes or that there is a supply of defective enzymes, both cases causing disturbance in chemical processes throughout the body, thus resulting in the sixty or so hypothyroid deficiency symptoms, including that of arthritis.

How do enzymes become deficient?

What's supposed to occur is as follows, according to E. Denis Wilson, M.D.: The hypothalmus gland at the base of the brain releases a chemical called "thyrotropin releasing hormone" (TRH) which stimulates the pituitary gland located inside the human skull to produce a chemical called "thyroid stimulating hormone" (TSH), which signals the thyroid gland to produce its own hormone called "thyroxine" (T_4).

When the hormone thyroxine (T_4) is received by the body's cells, it's supposed to be changed to another chemical called "triidothyronine" (T_3). This last chemical -- triidothyronine (T_3) -- is supposed to fit into each cell at sites especially designed to interlock like a key to a lock, called "receptor sites," and there the thyroid hormone (T_3) signals the cell to increase metabolism, thus turning on the cellular heat engine, thus the heat of the whole body.

Enzymes are complex molecules that depend on just the right temperature for proper functioning. Like a coiled spring, they will stretch or compress depending upon their temperature. If too long or too short, they won't work. They, too, must fit into various receptor sites or chemical reactions throughout the body. When the temperature of the cells is between 98.4^0-98.6^0 Fahrehnheit, the enzymes function most efficiently, fitting properly where they belong, and entering into chemical reactions the way they were designed to do.

Dr. Wilson explains that in a hypothyroid condition there is an emergency state which we've inherited from our body's long evolutionary years that kicks in to conserve our energy. This occurs whenever we've experienced long periods of emotional or physical stress, or have fasted for a long period, have been ill for a long time, or have been subjected to cortisol (cortisone) and some other drugs.

To conserve energy, our body dampens down the heat cycle by substituting at the cellular level an imitation of the thyroid hormone, actually a chemical reverse image called "reverse liothyronine" (RT_3). This reverse image thyroid (RT_3) fits exactly in the cellular receptor sites just as does the proper heat-engine thyroid (T_3), and it is constructed identically the same, with the same chemicals in the same structure -- except for its reverse image -- like the right hand is the reverse image of the left hand. However, this reverse image thyroid has absolutely no ability to turn on the heat engine of the cells, thus conserving energy during our state of emergency.

When the emergency is over, we should stop producing this reverse image thyroid, but some of us get stuck with it, and the proper chemical -- the correctly structured thyroid -- is not produced in sufficient quantity to stoke up to normal the cellular heat engine.

The hypothalmus and pituitary properly send their chemical signals to the thyroid, which also performs properly, sending its hormone to the cells.

The cells improperly convert a large proportion of this thyroid to a reverse image thyroid, which takes up a large proportion of the receptor sites in the cells, and we do not heat up the cellular metabolism as well.

When above or below 98.4^0-98.6^0 Fahrehnheit -- in this case below -- the enzymes fail to function properly, and therefore the chemistry of the body cannot function properly. The result will be the sixty hypothyroid disease symptoms, including arthritis, now called Wilson's syndrome, or Multiple Enzyme Deficiency.

E. Denis Wilson, M.D. says that a new balance has been established between the properly formed thyroid and its reverse image so that many of us that suffer from hypothyroid symptoms continue to do so year after year.

Traditional thyroid therapy -- treatments for hypothyroidism caused by glandular insufficiency -- will be to supply a form of thyroid that is produced by the thyroid gland as a replacement hormone. Under the condition of insufficient production of thyroid, traditional therapy may be appropriate and beneficial.

When traditional thyroid therapy is used to stoke up the cellular heat when the thyroid gland is producing properly, even over years of treatment the hypothyroid conditions will not be resolved. Why? Because the cells are using this chemical to produce the reverse image thyroid, and that is where the problem lies -- at the cellular level -- not in the production or supply of glandular thyroid, itself. One of us (Gus J. Prosch, Jr., M.D.) estimates that 20% of Americans suffer from Wilson's syndrome.

Jonathan V. Wright, M.D., Kent, Washington, a consultant for Meridian Valley Clinical Laboratory and also president of the National Health Federation, writes, "For years, I've been bugging Meridian Labs to put out an accurate, inexpensive thyroid panel including thyroid stimulating hormone (TSH), thyroxine (T_4), liothyronine (T_3), and reverse liothyronine (RT_3). They've finally done it, and for [only] $85!"

Insufficient thyroid utilization may not be reflected by normal thyroid glandular tests. One of the problems that was faced by those who use the E. Denis Wilson, M.D. program to help patients in an attempt to reverse their thyroid utilization (hypothyroidism) was the lack of any definitive reverse liothyronine (RT_3) blood test. And so an extensive series of accurate temperature measurements was required by the patient for implementation of Wilson's recommended treatment.

This new laboratory test when used properly may prove to be a major clinical indicator, as the amount of reverse liothyronine (RT_3) produced by our cells determines our temperature (metabolism), and our bodily temperature determines how well tens of thousands of essential enzymes function, and those enzymes determine the health of our cells, organs, systems, and overall bodily processes.

Before asking your doctor to obtain this new test, they should read *Wilson's Syndrome*. The book is available through this foundation for a tax-exempt donation of $25.

Meridian Valley Clinical Laboratory requests that your doctor "draw blood in a Serum Separator Tube (SST) and allow it to clot for 20 minutes, then centrifuge it for at least 10 minutes. The serum should then be poured into a transfer tube. A minimum of 3.0 ml of serum is required. It should be frozen and shipped via Overnight Mail in a pre-paid kit. Monday through Thursday delivery only," they advise.

Meridian Valley Clinical Laboratory can be contacted at 515 W. Harrison Street, Ste. #9, Kent, Wa 98032; (800) 234-6825; fax (206) 859-1135.

The Case of Elizabeth Wendell, Ed.D., R.N.

Eilizabeth Wendell suffered a cluster of symptomatic complaints that neither she nor her doctors could understand, among which was debilitating osteoarthritic joint pain in feet, ankles and finger joints, dry itchy skin, general fatigue and depression, dyspepsia, flatus, night sweats, brittle hair and nails, constipation, frequent respiratory infec-tions, frequent and severe migraine type headaches, a tender abdomen, easy bruising, irritability, and difficulty with memory.

A pyschologist told her that, except for mild depression due to stress, she was very healthy.

Elizabeth's job was quite stressful, and when her mother was di-agnosed with terminal cancer, her stress increased until she had to give up her job.

A puzzled and concerned Elizabeth visited E. Denis Wilson, M.D., as she knew she was not physically normal. Dr. Wilson placed her on a program to measure her temperature three times daily, take the aver-age, and to report back in three weeks. Her oral temperature averaged about 1 degree Farhenheit below the normal of 98.4^0-98.6^0. This fact told Dr. Wilson that his patient was marginally hypothyroid, a condi-tion that most physicians would have ignored as being close enough to normal not to be a physical problem. Or, had they considered it impor-tant, they would have supplied Elizabeth with thyroid supplements for the rest of her life.

After four months of treatment using the right kind of replace-ment thyroid administered in just the right way, Elizabeth's tempera-ture stabilized at an average of 98.4^0-98.6^0. During that period she found that her osteoarthritis pain symptoms disappeared completely, as did fatigue and depression. Nails and hair grew normally, and nails be-came stronger.

Elizabeth reported that "My quality of life has improved a 100 percent and my husband and I have even started playing golf and other recreational activities together that we have not done in years. How I wish that 20 years ago this had been diagnosed. Even 5 years ago would have been a blessing."

Reversing Hypothyroidism

E. Denis Wilson, M.D.[113] says, "Of all *chronic* medical problems, I believe that Wilson's Sydrome is *the* most common and has *the* greatest impact and is *the* easiest to address and is *the* most likely to be remedied and is *the* most rapidly responding and is *the* most inherent or non-foreign of treatments." For these reasons Wilson's Syndrome should be the first of impairments to be considered in the treatment of patients rather than the last."[175]

You can determine whether or not you're a candidate for thyroid treatment -- which has the promise of reversing the hypothyroid condition provided your glands are otherwise operating properly.

First, calibrate a thermometer, usually by means of comparing the thermometer against others. A glass thermometer is best, as many of the digital thermometers are not sufficiently accurate. Be sure to shake down the thermometer before each reading.

Measure your temperature three times daily about four hours apart, each time at the same time, but the first temperature should be checked 3 hours or more after arising for the day. Record these temperatures for three weeks. Average each series of three daily readings, and record them for a daily average.

A review of the three week averages should give you information as to whether or not you are habitually below the 98.4^0-98.6^0 Fahrehnheit optimum for efficiently functioning enzymes. If so, you are a candidate for E. Denis Wilson's multiple enzyme deficiency treatment program, and you should seek assistance from a knowledgeable physician.

If you and your doctor decide that you're a candidate for reversal of hypothyroidism, then you'll be given   a small amount of thyroid called "sustained released triiodothyronine" (T_3SR) to take orally each day; and you will continue recording daily average temperature, unless your doctor chooses to use the new measures available through the aforementioned Meridian Valley Clinical Laboratories.

Caution: the triiodothyronine (T_3 SR) must be made up special under prescription by a compounding pharmacist, called T_3SR, (T_3 compounded with a sustain release agent to be taken every 12 hours).

The thyroid triiodothyronine (T_3) on the commercial market, packaged for non-compounding pharmacists, is not used because a sustained release substance triiodothyronine(T_3SR) must be used that is compounded in the correct dosage increments. One of us (Gus J. Prosch, Jr., M.D.) has 13 different doses of the sustained release thyroid (T_3SR), compounded for patient use: 7.5 mcg, 15.0 mcg, 22.5 mcg, 30.0 mcg, 37.5 mcg, 45.0 mcg, 52.5 mcg, 52.5 mcg, 60.0 mcg, 67.5 mcg, 75.0 mcg, 82.5 mcg, 90.0 mcg.

The amount of thyroid triiodothyronine (T_3SR) will be increased incrementally each day; and you will continue recording three temperatures a day, three hours apart, and determining average daily temperature.

If at any time from the first dosage forward, your symptoms resolve

-- temperature reaches between 98.4 ^{0} and 98.6^0 Farenheit -- then the medication is maintained at that dosage for three weeks, after which it is slowly discontinued by decreasing it incrementally, twice as slow as it was increased incrementally, and you will continue recording daily temperatures three times a day, three hours apart and averaging them..

Although somewhat simplified, if all has worked well, the body's thyroid balance should be reversed. One should be able to discontinue the medicine -- you will be down to zero dosage by then -- and one's multiple enzyme dysfunctioning should be solved, along with a disappearance of any one, or all, of some 60 different symptoms, including arthritic symptoms that are based on enzyme deficiencies.

There are some who have to repeat through this total cycle several times before their body gets the message, inhibiting an over-production of reverse thyroid liothyronine (RT$_3$), and increasing one's own thyroid triidothyronine (T$_3$) production.

Good results are seen in about 70 to 80 percent of the people that follow this program. One must take care to do everything just right, and it's a lot of precision work keeping track of temperatures and dosages on time.

One patient, the worst case seen, had to go through 14 cycles before her body reset, but this is unusual.

E. Denis Wilson, M.D., a dedicated pioneer, has given up his practice to spread the good news. He's picked out 200 doctors to teach. The book, *Wilson's Syndrome*, and the publication, *How to Quickly and Easily Obtain Proper Treatment for Wilson's Syndrome* is available from the Wilson's Syndrome Foundation, PO Box 916206, Longwood, Florida 32791-6206; (800) 621-7006. This patients' guide helps you to find treatment in your area, discussing each of the three easy ways you can obtain treatment for Wilson's Syndrome. The book *Wilson's Syndrome* is also available through The Arthritis Trust of America, 5106 Old Harding Road, Franklin, TN 37064 for a tax-exempt donation.

Thyroid-Stimulating Foods

Lita Lee, Ph.D.[114] uses a 24-hour urinanalysis developed by Howard Loomis, Jr., D.C., Forsyth, Missouri, which will determine the following:

Acidity/alkalinity (pH), specific gravity, too little or too much volume, chloride, calcium, food intolerances and nutritional deficiencies, indican (determines need for colon cleansing and other conditions), sediment (determines need for multiple enzymes), and abnormal solutes.

According to Lita Lee, Ph.D., Eugene, Oregon, fruits or fruit juices, which provide magnesium that works with thyroid to moderate stress, also helps modulate blood sugar and calm down adrenal glands. Fruit juices can also help to stimulate increased production of triiodothyronine (T$_3$).

Raymond F. Peat, Ph.D., Eugene, Oregon, recommends a salad recipe consisting of grated carrots, vinegar, coconut oil and salt. Fatty acids in the coconut oil are thyroid-stimulating. Carrot fiber tones the bowel and binds toxins.

Salt mobilizes glucose and calms adrenal glands, according to Peat.

Coconut oil has several thyroid-promoting effects. It contains butyric acid which helps thyroid hormone move into the brain [triiodothyronine (T_3) uptake into glial cells]. It opposes anti-thyroid unsaturated oils. It contains short and medium chain fatty acids which help modulate blood sugar, are anti-allergic, and protect mitochondria -- the cellular power unit, source of protein synthesis, and lipid metabolism -- against stress injuries.[195]

Of course, while useful, unless production of reverse triiodothyronine (RT_3) has been minimized at the cellular level, these nutritional assists will be of lessened value.

Once thyroid utilization has been normalized, determination of actual enzyme deficiencies can be important for treatment of all health conditions, including arthritis.

Enzyme supplementation can be obtained through licensed health care providers available from Howard Loomis, D.C., 21st Century Nutrition, 6421 Enterprise Lane, Madison, Wisconsin 53719; (800) 614-4400; or Nutritional Enzyme Support System, 2903 NW Platte Rd., Riverside, Missouri 64150; (800) NESS-893.

Hydrotherapy

Hydrotherapy uses water, ice, steam and either hot or cold temperatures to assist in maintaining or restoring health. Treatment procedures may include full body immersion, steam baths, saunas, sitz baths (pelvis immersed), colonic irrigation, and the application of hot, and/ or cold compresses.

As part of home care, as well as through professional assistance, hydrotherapy can be utilized for a wide range of conditions, including osteoarthritis.

The rule is that heat relaxes, while cold stimulates.

Douglas Lewis, N.D.,[5] Chairperson of Physical Medicine at Bastyr College Natural Health Clinic, Seattle, Washington, says, "Hot water produces a response that stimulates the immune system and causes white cells to migrate out of the blood vessels and into the tissue where they clean up toxins and assist the body in eliminating wastes.

"Cold water discourages inflammation by means of vasoconstriction (constricting blood vessels), and by reducing the inflammatory agents by making the blood vessels less permeable. Cold water also tones muscular weakness and may be useful in cases of incontinence.

It is the opinion based on clinical experience of one of us (Gus J. Prosch, Jr., M.D.) that bathing in heated swimming pools or Jacuzzi will help to spread the distribution of infectious microorganisms that cause rheumatoid arthritis including those who suffer osteoarthritis as a secondary consequence of rheumatoid arthritis, about one out of ten osteoarthritis patients. For that reason it is recommended that heated pools be avoided for the arthritic until the arthritis itself has been solved, or at least in the case of osteoarthritis that one is reasonably sure it is not a secondary condition of an infectious organism. It has been shown that some organisms -- the main offending ones -- grow rapidly in warm water, or spread more rapidly throughout the body.

Hyperthermia

Hyperthermia is any method that induces a fever in the patient who is unable to produce a natural fever response against disease-causing organisms. Although fever is often thought to be undesirable by traditional medical practitioners, it is actually nature's means for ridding the body of invasive microorganisms, and, unless the fever reaches a dangerous level around 104^0 to 106^0 Fahrenheit, should be permitted unabated.

Fever signals the immune system to produce antibodies and a group of proteins that are released by white blood cells to combat viruses.

To solve the drug addiction problem during the 1960s, known as the "hippie" or drug era, philosopher, mind/emotion researcher, and writer L. Ron Hubbard, also creator of the philosophy of the Church of Scientology, developed a successful method of sauna hyperthermia as a means of ridding the body of fat-stored drugs and other chemicals such as pesticides and herbicides. This program was successfully tested by funding from the Environmental Protective Agency by David W. Schnare, and Megan Shields, M.D.,[115] Los Angeles, California. Their study showed that PCBs and PBBs and chlorinated pesticides were reduced considerably through use of Hubbard's regimen. Later studies verified this finding, and extended the range of detoxified elements possible by Hubbard's method to include many otherwise intransigents, so-called recreational drugs and prescription medicines that have similar effects on the body and appear to be very difficult to shed by other means.

According to the Environmental Protective Agency, by 1980 over 400 chemicals had been detected in human tissue; 48 were found in adipose (fat) tissue, 40 in breast milk, 73 in liver, and over 250 in blood.

The National Academy of Sciences reports that an average American today ingests about 40 mg of pesticides each day as DDT, and carries approximately 1/10th of a gram permanently stored in body fat. "Human accumulation of such compounds as DDT, PCP (phencyclindine -- angel dust), PCB (polychlorinated biphenyl), THC, and dioxin (agent orange ingredient), reflect biologically persistent chemicals which are partitioned within the body from water into lipids (fatty parts of cells). . . . Chemicals stored in the body pose a serious threat to both physiological and psychological health. . . . the human body has no previous experience with these chemicals and there is no natural machinery in the body to break them down, much less eliminate them."[114]

When Zane Gard, M.D. and his wife and daughter suffered from agent orange poisoning, Hubbard's method, called, *Purification Rundown*™, turned their lives about, and Dr. Gard started a San Diego, California medical clinic very successfully using the Hubbardian procedure. While Dr. Gard was not the only physician to utilize Hubbard's techniques, he was the first to write up for general publication literally dozens of case histories demonstrating that as the sauna progressed, laboratory measured toxins reduced, and symptoms lessened or disappeared simultaneously.

The Chilocco Indian Tribe of Cholocco, Oklahoma, in cooperation with the Church of Scientology, established a one thousand bed facility called the Chilocco Biodetoxification Center for the purpose of treating alcoholism and drug addiction, and for training others in the Hubbardian procedure. This program has the lowest recidivism rate of any known drug program, being 33%, or 67% success rate!

Despite scientific proof of success of Hubbard's *Purification Rundown*, the continuing successes at the Chilocco Biodetoxification Center in Chilocco, Oklahoma, and Dr. Gard's successes in San Diego, California, California, and other physicians' clinical successes, authorities withdrew Dr. Gard's license to practice medicine. However, the treatment is available at every Church of Scientology outlet in the world, regardless of church affiliation, as the church makes no medical claims regarding this "spiritual" experience.

A medical certificate based on a physical examination by a licensed medical doctor is a pre-requisite for undergoing detoxification via Hubbard's *Purification Rundown*.

Whirlpool Baths

Support for joint rehabilitation for the arthritic, or for otherwise injured muscles and joints, can be obtained through the use of whirlpools which are usually available through hospital physical therapy departments, private clinics, physiotherapists, or the office of some private health professionals. Whirlpools improve blood circulation, and alleviate the stress and strains of life.

Neutral Baths

Water at a body temperature of 92^0-98^0 Fahrenheit -- close to normal body temperature -- sooths the nervous system and calms emotions, mental disturbances, and assists with insomnia.

Studies have shown that neutral baths are beneficial for swollen and painful joints.

Alternative Heat and Cold Packs

The symptoms of any acute inflammation can be improved by

148   ANTHONY DI FABIO, M.A. & GUS J. PROSCH, JR., M.D

alternating hot and cold packs.

For acute inflammation, an ice pack is applied for twenty minutes every hour for the first 24 to 36 hours.

For chronic inflammation, use a hot pack for 3 minutes, then cold for 30 to 60 seconds. Repeat 3 times in one sitting, finishing with the cold. Do the same cycle 3 times per day, depending on severity of symptoms.

<u>Hot Pack for Joints</u>

Agatha Thrash, M.D. and Calvin Thrash, M.D.[116] describe a method for giving hydrotherapy, using a heating pad to apply heat to a joint: "Wring out a large towel from tap water, and wrap it around the affected joint. Cover the towel completely with two layers of plastic wrap. A large plastic bag can be used, and for an extremity, both ends of the sac can be opened and the bag used as a sleeve over the wet towel, the excess being folded over and taped with scotch or masking tape.

Next, place a heating pad over the plastic cover and attach in place, turning the control to low or medium.

Apply this once a day for one to two hours at a time.

A radio placed at the bedside, using the same electrical outlet as the heating pad, will crackle with static as a warning if the heating pad is getting wet and beginning to short. Tune the radio to a blank place on the dial and set the volume loud enough to attract attention. (Caution: A heating pad may produce undesireable magnetic disturbances. See "Magnetic Therapy," this chapter.)

<u>Colon Detoxification[117]</u>

The health of the colon is vital in support of our ability to absorb nutrients, and to eliminate wastes that are generated by each of our body's cells. Toxins produced by invasive microorganisms, and also accompanying air, water and food intake, are also eliminated to some large degree by a healthy colon, along with elimination channels such as the skin, kidneys and lungs.

A colon that is sluggish, or operating inefficiently, can contribute to a wide range of diseases, including various forms of arthritis. While we may find it socially unacceptable to think in such terms, the human anus is just as important as the mouth. What we put into our mouth determines our state of health; what we pass through our anus, and how frequently, also determines the state of our health.

Colon detoxification is the irrigation of the large bowel with water or other solution (ozonated water, coffee, etc.) for the purpose of improving colon microflora, creating a healthy mucosa, toning up contractive muscles, improving timely evacuation, ridding of colon toxemia -- a burdening of accumulated waste material -- and lowering the opportunity for foreign substances to provoke immune reactions. As this subject can assume large importance for all diseases such as osteoarthritis, but also including rheumatoid arthritis, it is discussed in more detail in Chapter II, Rheumatoid Arthritis. (See *Tissue Cleansing Through Bowel Management*, Bernard Jensen, D.C.; *Guess What Came to Dinner*, Louise Gittleman.)

Qigong for Arthritis
What is Qi ("Chi")?

Pronounced "chi gong," chinese energy work, or "qigong" (also referred to as *chi-kung*) has exploded into Western awareness during the past twenty years.

According to physicist and master of qigong, Jwing-Ming Yang, Ph.D.,[79] Jamaica Plain, Massachusetts, lecturer and author of several dozen books explaining and translating ancient Chinese knowledge into Western terms -- including some methods that have remained secret until the 1970s -- qi is the body's bioelectricity whose strength is subject to "balance, harmony and interactive influence." This bioelectric field can be measured by modern scientific instruments, and strengthened and balanced through qigong exercises, spiritual contemplation, emotional rebalancing, and thought.

There is also a glimmer of hope that modern technology can enhance the electromagnetic field effects of one's own bioelectric activity. (See this chapter, "Energy Medicine.")

Sometimes referred to as "vital life force," Dr. Jwing-Ming Yang's description of qi is "the energy or natural force which fills the universe," of which there are three general types: heavenly qi, the forces which heavenly bodies exert on the earth, Earth qi, which absorbs the Heaven qi, and human qi which is influenced by the other two. The pervasive theme within and between all three is "balance, harmony and interactive influence."

Until the exceptional journey of Marco Polo in the thirteenth century, Europeans viewed scientific, religious, medical, and philosophical ideas in a limited manner, perceiving themselves as the known world's, if not the universe's center.

Marco Polo brought to Western consciousness but a tiny fraction of long accumulated Chinese wisdom, including knowledge of the invention of gunpowder, printing press, rocketry, and, of course, the shocking details of a hugh civilization already thousands of years old.

Had thirteenth century Western thought-leaders been sufficiently open to new ideas, Marco Polo could have prepared us for a workable medical system based on the Chinese concept of primary energy, a subtle bio-electrical force pervading our every cell, common to us all, and capable of preventing illness, healing when ill, and extending life and it's quality.

Perhaps one reason why ancient Chinese healing lore has taken so long to penetrate Western civilizations is that, historically, Chinese medical emphasis was not upon solving a specific disease problem, but rather on restoring the balancing energy of vital life forces -- the qi forces -- from which all health then flows. The result is that disease states disappear when the life force is strengthened and rebalanced. Similar to other basic fundamentals of good health such as the control and mastering of stress, nutrition and supplements, acupuncture, and chelation therapy, the qigong form of energy therapy underlies all that we are and do.

Roger Jahnke, O.M.D.,[118] Santa Barbarba, California, Doctor of Acupuncture and Oriental Medicine, author of books and tapes on qigong, has had dozens of patients with arthritis. "We feel that arthritis is an overall degenerative disorder that is not really a muscle/joint disease, . . . that the symptoms are not the cause.

"We found through regular massage, acupuncture and qigong, that most cases will improve very dramatically."

With the guidance of men such as Drs. Jwing-Ming Yang , and Roger Jahnke, we may learn simple exercises which condition our tissues and permit us to increase the flow of blood, thus oxygen and other nourishment, to those parts of the body in need.

More importantly, we're taught to "lead" our qi forces ourselves, so that we can direct the flow of this primary subtle energy. According to Dr. Yang, "In order to use qigong to maintain and improve your health you must (1) know that there is qi in your body, and you must (2) understand how it circulates and (3) what you can do to insure that the circulation is smooth and strong."

While the more than 4,000 year history of shrewd Chinese observations resulted in many beneficial methods for preventing illness, or achieving wellness, none is more basic to the arthritic than the practices of qigong. (See *Qigong for Arthritis*, Jwing-Ming Yang, Ph.D.)

Master Jwing-Ming Yang

Jwing-Ming Yang,[39] who has written a series of books clearly explaining this ancient Chinese knowledge, was born in Taiwan, Republic of China in 1946. He started his Gongfu/Wushu (Kung Fu/Wushu) training at age of fifteen under a Shaolin White Crane master Cheng Ging Gsao. He later studied Yang Style Taijiquan (or Tai Chi Chuan) under Master Kao Tao for three years. From Master Kao Tao, Dr. Yang learned the barehand Yang style form, Taiji breathing, and Qi (Chi) exercises.

When Jwing-Ming Yang was eighteen-years-of-age he entered Tamkang College in Taipei Hsien to study physics, and while there he studied Shaolin Long Fist (Chang Quan) with Master Li Mao-Ching, and advanced his Taiji training with Master Li. Later he practiced and studied together with a classmate, Mr. Wilson Chen "who was learning Taijiquan with one of the most famous masters in Taipei, Master Zhang Xiang-San."[39]

Dr. Yang completed his master's degree in physics at the National

Taiwan University, served in the Chinese Air Force, returned to Tamkang College to teach physics, and to continue his study under Master Li Mao-Ching. In 1974 Dr. Yang studied mechanical engineering at Purdue University (United States) where he founded a Chinese Kung Fu Research club and also taught accredited courses in Taijiquan, also to be awarded his Ph.D. in 1978.

In Houston, TX, while working for Texas Instruments, Dr. Yang founded Yang's Shaolin Kung Fu Academy.

In Boston, where he moved, Dr. Yang founded Yang's Martial Arts Academy (YMAA), later giving up his engineering career to research, write and teach in Boston.

Besides extensive travel to lecture and teach in many foreign countries, Dr. Yang has written twenty-four books and published twenty-one videotapes on qigong and martial arts. There is little doubt that Dr. Yang can authoritatively blend western thinking with health/martial arts discoveries that are far, far older than Western civilization itself.

<u>Master Jwing-Ming Yang Historical Background of Qigong</u>

The Chinese way of healing and prevention began more than 4,000 years ago, with a remarkable interweaving of the healing arts, physical combat, and spiritual search. During its vast historical development it also absorbed philosophies and techniques from many adjacents cultures. One book -- certainly not a section in a chapter -- can hardly do justice to the necessary interweaving of important principles found in Chinese methods of prevention and healing, martial arts, philosophy, and religion, when explaining qigong. It is nonetheless helpful to look at a brief history of the discovery and development of qigong.

Dr. Jing-Ming Yang divides the history of Chinese Qigong into four periods:

• 2690 B.C. to 1154 B.C.: While acupuncture was not mentioned in Chinese writings dating back to 1766-1154 B.C., the *Oracle-Bone Scripture* (*Jia Gu Wen*), there is evidence that "stone probes" (Bian Shi) were used during the reign of the Yellow emperor from 2690-2590 B.C., and that these probes were being used to adjust qi circulation.

• Before 1122 B.C. to Han Dynasty 206 B.C.: *Book of Changes* (*Yi Jing*) was introduced before 1122 B.C., lasting until Buddhism and its meditation methods were imported from India, bringing qigong practice and meditation into the second period, the religious qigong era.

• 1122 B.C. to 934 B.C.: Breathing techniques were mentioned in Lao Zi's (Li Er) Classic on the *Virtue of the Dao* (*Tao Te Ching*), stressing the way to obtain health was to "concentrate on qi and achieve softness."

• 770 B.C. to 221 B.C.: *Historical Record* (*Shi Ji*) described more complete methods of breath training.

• 300 B.C. (approximately) Zhuang Zi, Daoist philosopher, described the relationship between health and the breath in *Nan Hua Jing*. "The men of old breathed clear down to their heels. . . ."

• 206 B.C. to 502-557 A.D.: Discovery that Qigong could be used for martial purposes. Thousands-of-years-old Buddhism imported to China from India. Buddhism became popular through emperor's influence. Since much of the training was aimed at obtaining Buddhahood, the principles were kept secret. Zhang Dao-Ling combined traditional Daoist principles with Buddhism, creating a religion called Dao Jiao, combining Daoism with Buddhism.

Tibetian training systems and methods were also imported, and absorbed. "Contemporary documents and Qigong styles show clearly that religious practitioners trained their qi to a much deeper level, working with many internal functions of the body, and strove to obtain control of their bodies, minds, and spirits with the goal of escaping from the cyle of reincarnation."

During the 3rd century, Hua Tuo, a famous physician, used acupuncture for anesthesia in surgery.

Daoist Jun Qian used the movements of animals to create the *Five Animal Sports* (*Wu Qin Xi*), "teaching people how to increase their qi circulation through specific movements."

Physician Ge Hong used his mind "to lead and increase qi."

During the period of 420 to 581 A.D. Tao Hong-Jing complied *Records of Nourishing the Body and Extending Life* (*Yang Shen Yan Ming Lu*) which showed many qigong techniques.

From 220 B.C. to 220 A.D. there are written references to (1) breathing to increase qi circulation by Bian Que in *Classic on Disorders* (*Nan Jing*); (2) the use of qi and accupuncture to maintain good qi flow by Zhang Zhong-Jing in *Prescriptions from the Golden Chamber* (*Jing Kui Yao Lue*); (3) the relationship of nature's forces and Qi by Wei Bo-Yang in *A Comparative Study of the Zhou* [dynasty] *Book of Changes* (*Zhou Yi Can Tong Qi*).

• 502-557 A.D. to 1911: Martial qigong styles were created based upon Buddhist and Daoist qigong. A Buddhist monk, Da Mo, former Indian prince, was invited to China to preach Buddhism. As the emperor did not like the monk, Dao Mo withdrew into a Shaolin Temple where he found the priests were weak and sickly. After nine years of seclusion, and consideration of the problem, he wrote two classics: *Muscle/Tendon Changing Classic* (*Yi Jin Jing)* and *Marrow/Brain Washing Classic* (*Xi Sui Jing*).

According to Dr. Yang, "the *Muscle/Tendon Changing Classic* taught the priests how to gain health and change their physical bodies from weak to strong. "The *Marrow/Brain Washing Classic* taught the priests how to use qi to clean the bone marrow and strengthen the blood and immune system, as well as how to energize the brain and attain enlightenment."

The *Marrow/Brain Washing Classic* training was held in secret, passed only to a few disciples each generation, because it was harder to understand and practice.

After the priests used the muscle/tendon changing exercises, they found that not only did they improve their health, but they also greatly increased their strength. When this training was integrated into the martial arts forms, it increased the effectiveness of their techniques.

Shaolin priests also created five animal styles of Gonfu (Kung Fu) which imitated the way different animals fight. The animals imitated were the tiger, leopard, dragon, snake, and crane.

• 581 A.D. to 907 A.D.: Chao Yuan-Fang compiled the *Thesis on the Origins and Symptoms of Various Diseases* (*Zhu Bing Yuan Hou Lun*) listing 260 different ways to increase the flow of qi.

Sun Si-Mao described the method of "leading" qi -- directing qi to specific body parts -- in *Thousand Gold Prescriptions* (*Qian Jin Fang*) and also described Six Sounds to regulate qi internal organs, the Six Sounds having already been in use by Buddhists and Daoists.

Sun Si-Mao introduced his Lao Zi's Massage Techniques in *The Extra Important Secret* (*Wai Tai Mi Yao*) which discussed use of breathing and herbal therapies for disorders of qi circulation.

• 960 A.D. to 1279 A.D.: "Chang San-Feng is believed to have created "great ultimate fist," Taijiquan (or Tai Chi Chuan). Taiji followed a different approach in its use of qigong than did Shaolin. While Shaolin emphasized "External Elixir" (Wai Dan) qigong exercises, Taiji emphasized "Internal Elixir" (Nei Dan) qigong training. External, here, means the limbs, as opposed to the torso which includes all vital organs. Internal means in the body instead of in the limbs. After thousands of years of searching for elixer, a hypothetical life-prolonging substance, elixer was found inside the body. "In other words, if you want to prolong your life, you must find the elixer in your body, and then learn to protect and nourish it."

In 1026 A.D. the famous brass man of acupuncture was designed and built by Dr. Wang Wei-Yi. Before that time there was much disagreement about acupuncture theory, principles and techniques. Dr. Wang Wei-Yi also wrote *Illustration of the Brass Man Acupuncture and Moxibustion* (*Tong Ren Yu Xue Zhen Jiu Tu*).

Dr. Wang Wei-Yi explained for the first time the relationship of the 12 organs and the 12 qi channels, also systematically organizing acupuncture theory and principles. As the success of acupuncture spread, Dr. Wang also dissected the bodies of prisoners and added more information to the advance of qigong and Chinese medicine, describing the circulation of qi in the body.

From 1127-1279 A.D. Marshal Yue Fei created several internal qigong exercises and martial arts. It is believed that he created the set of exercises applicable to medicine known as the "Eight Pieces of Brocade," to improve the health of soldiers. Marshal Yue Fei "is also known as the creator of the internal martial style Xing Yi.

Eagle style martial artists also claim that Yue Fei was the creator of their style.

• 960 A.D. to 1368 A.D.: Zhang An-Dao wrote *Life Nourishing Secrets* (*Yang Shen Jue*) discussing several qigong practices.

Zhang Zi-He wrote *The Confucian Point of View* (*Ru Men Shi Shi*) describing "the use of qigong to cure external injuries such as cuts and bruises."

In *Secret Library of the Orchid Room* (*Lan Shi Mi Cang*), Li Guo describes qigong and herbal remedies for internal disorders.

A Further Thesis of Complete Study (*Ge Zhi Yu Lun*), written by Zhu Dan-Xi, provides a theoretical explanation for the use of qigong in curing disease.

From 1279 A.D. until 1911 A.D. many other qigong styles were founded, and many documents related to qigong were published.

• 1911 onward: Chinese qigong training was mixed with qigong practices from India, Japan, and many other countries. Qigong practice entered a new era, as China became known by the remainder of the world. What had been taught secretly either by martial artists, or by religious organizations, found its way into the stream of the world's consciousness, and also people were able to compare Chinese qigong to similar developments in India, Japan, Korea and the Middle East.

Categories of Qigong

Many people think that qigong is a difficult subject to understand. No matter how difficult theory and practice of a particular recommended exercise, called a "style," may seem, all qigong theory and principles are very simple, and remain that way for all recommended styles. All qigong practices aim at rebalancing qi bioelectrical energy, maintaining its strong flow, maintaining health, healing when necessary, for spiritual enlightenment, and for fighting, which are also the categories of qigong.

Theory of Qigong

During the past twenty years, western medicine has gradually begun to accept the existence of qi and its circulation in the human body. It is also a growing trend to accept that disease is an imbalance in the electrical flow of the body, such a concept corresponding rather well with the concept of qi as developed several thousand years ago. If all disease states are an imbalance of the bioelectrical flow of the body, then all disease states including arthritis can be conquered, or changed, by changing the flow of bioelectrical energy.[79]

According to Roger Jahnke, O.M.D., "Qi, in China, is not thought of as an energy the way we relate to it. The best definition that I've come up with is 'naturally occurring internal self-healing resource.' By this definition you're including physical as well as electromagnetic as well as chemicals, as well as whatever performs the functions."[118]

According to Dr. Yang,[79] "In order to use qigong to maintain and improve your health you must (1) know that there is qi in your body, and you must (2) understand how it circulates and (3) know what you can do to insure that the circulation is smooth and strong."

The Flow and Storage of Qi

Factors necessary for proper creation and conduction of bioelectrical energy are (1) natural energy received by interaction with electromagnetic fields; (2) food and air; (3) the way we think, as thought creates the electromagnetic force that leads to Qi to energize emotion which energizes appropriate muscles to action; and (4) exercise. The mind and movements are two major sources of electromotive force.

There are two divisions of qi: Managing Qi (Ying Qi), sometimes called "Nutritive Qi," and Guardian Qi (Wei Qi). Managing (or "Nutritive") Qi is energy that has been sent to the organs so that you can function. Guardian Qi has been sent to the surface of the body to protect you from negative influences such as the cold. To keep yourself healthy, you must learn to manage these two types of qi.

Corresponding to the now well-known acupuncture meridians, the human body has twelve major channels through which qi circulates. There are also eight vessels that store qi. The twelve channels are like twelve electric lines, with capacitors for excess electrical storage located throughout the body; or like 12 rivers that each interconnect, and having common storage basins, a total of eight in all. When the qi in the eight reservoirs is full and strong, the qi in the rivers is strong and will be regulated efficiently. When stagnation occurs in any of these twelve channels or rivers, the qi which flows to the body's extremities and to the internal organs will be abnormal, and illness may develop.

The function of the reservoirs are to replenish the flow in the twelve major channels that interconnect all bodily organs whenever qi becomes low in various bodily parts. (See this chapter "Other Treatments" Acupuncture.)

The Treasures of Life

According to Dr. Yang, "Before you start your qigong training, you must first understand the three treasures of life -- essence (Jing), internal energy (Qi), and spirit (Shen) -- as well as their relationship. If you lack this understanding, you are missing the root of qigong training, as well as the basic idea of qigong theory. The main goals of qigong training are to learn how to retain your essence (Jing), strengthen and smooth your internal energy (Qi) flow, and enlighten your spirit (Shen), as well as their interrelationship. To reach these goals you must learn how to regulate the body (Tiao Shen), regulate the mind (Tiao Xin), regulate the breathing (Tiao Xi), regulate the internal energy (Tiao Qi), and regulate the spirit (Tiao Shen)."

Regulation of Qi

Regulating the body includes understanding how to find and build the root of the body, as well as the root of the individual forms you are practicing. To build a firm root, you must know how to keep your center, how to balance your body, and most important of all, how to relax so that the qi can flow.

Regulating the mind involves learning how to keep your mind calm, peaceful, and centered, so that you can judge situations objectively and lead qi to the desired places. The mind is the main key to success in qigong practice.

To regulate your breathing, you must learn how to breathe so that your breathing and your mind mutually correspond and cooperate. When you breathe this way, your mind will be able to attain peace more quickly, and therefore concentrate more easily on leading the qi.

Regulating the qi is one of the ultimate goals of qigong practice. In order to regulate your qi effectively you must first have regulated your body, mind, and breathing. Only then will your mind be clear enough to sense how the qi is distributed in your body, and understand how to adjust it.

How Qigong Works[5]

Qigong practices vary from simple calisthenic-type exercises combined with breath coordination to complex exercises coupled with measures of brain wave frequencies, heart rate, and other organs, to techniques which use biofeedback that assists in learning to modify each of these.

The result of regular practice combining movement, deep relaxation, and breathing can improve strength and flexibility, reverse damage caused by previous injuries and disease, and promote relaxation, awareness, and healing.

According to Roger Jahnke, O.M.D., qigong practices stimulates and nourishes the body's internal organs by circulating qi, breaks down energy blocks and facilitates the free flow of energy throughout the body, promotes blood and lymph flow and the flow of nerve impulses all necessary for maintenance of proper health.

Illustrating how electrical charge freely flows throughout the body using a simple exercise, Dr. Jahnke describes breathing regulation and deep relaxation while lifting the arms and rising upward on the toes. This combination can "help prevent tension headaches, constipation, insomnia, and other disorders by improving circulation of the cardiovascular and lymphatic systems, as well as modulating brain chemistry."[5]

Dr. Jahnke has summarized research reports showing that through the regular use of qigong there are many benefits, including that of decreasing heart and blood pressure, dilating blood capillaries, optimizing delivery of oxygen to tissues, moderating pain, depression, and addictive cravings, as well as strengthening and optimizing immune capability, increasing rate and flow of lymphatic fluid and accelerating elimination of toxic substances from tissues, organs, and glands through lymphatic system, increasing circulation of oxygen and nutrient rich blood to brain, organs and tissues, promoting deeper sleep, reduced anxiety, and mental clarity, and optimizing the body's self-regulating mechanisms by decreasing activity of the sympathetic nervous system.

Conditions Benefited by Qigong

According to Roger Jahnke, O.M.D., in addition to active physical exercise, qigong can be practiced by those who cannot move at all, those who are bedridden, those who have limited mobility, sitting or walking. Meditation is an example of one form of qigong that can be accomplished by anyone who is conscious.

Accordingly, just as acupuncture, proper nutrition, energy therapy, and chelation therapy are treatments that apply to virtually all disease states, including all forms of arthritis, those helped have had every bodily condition, including digestive problems, asthma, insomnia, pain, depression, anxiety, cancer, coronary heart disease, and many other human medical problems.

Stephan Chang, M.D., author of *The Complete System of Self-Healing*, cites one study where 2,873 terminal cancer patients practiced qigong for 6 months, and 12 percent of the patients were cured and 47 improved significantly.[5]

Qigong is virtually a way of life in many hospitals in China, and has often been found to be more effective than traditional Western medical practices in a host of diseases.

Dr. Jahnke cites a group of arthritis patients who've participated regularly in qigong classes, reporting that, "After approximately six months, several patients remarked that the stiffness and pain in their hands had diminished and the deformed knuckles characteristic of arthritis had begun to return to normal. The most incredible thing about qigong practice is that people actually can feel the operation of the physiological mechanisms of healing in their body. The increase of blood and lymph flow, and a shift in neurotransmitters creates an actual sensation that is clearly perceptible to the individual. The Chinese call this 'qi sensation'."

Qigong Practices

For those beginning qigong, Dr. Jahnke has prepared advice and a series of exercises that can be performed by almost anyone, regardless of health, age, or physical condition.

- Take it easy, and don't rush.
- Dedication can mobilize healing forces.
- Results come over time.
- When performed correctly, qigong is safe to practice as often as you wish.

- You can make up your own routines.
- Relax, direct your mind toward quiet indifference.
- Regulate your breathing so that both inhaling and exhaling are slow and deep, but not urgent or exaggerated.

Circulating Vital Life Energy by Tracing Acupuncture Meridians

1. Rub your hands together to increase qi. The hands will become warmer when you are relaxed and the environment is comfortable.

2. Stroke palms upward as if washing your face -- across the cheeks, eyes, and forehead, continuing over top and side of head, down the back of neck, and along the shoulders to the shoulder joint, then under arms and down sides to the rib cage. At rib cage's lower edge move palms around to back, across buttocks, down the back and sides of legs and out sides of feet, then trace up inside the feet and the inner surface of legs, up front side of torso and onto face again, beginning a second round to 1 above.

Directing Vital Life Energy to Internal Organs

1. Rub your hands together.

2. Place right hand over liver at lower right edge of rib cage. Visualize the liver receiving and benefiting from qi.

3. Place left hand over spleen and pancreas at lower left side of ribs. Move hand circularly continuing to create heat, and breathing full breaths, and relaxing. Feel heat passing through skin and penetrating organs.

4. Hold hands over organs continuing to feel heat penetrate. On exhaling, visualize qi circulating from center of body out the arms, into hands, and penetrating from hands into organs.

5. Cover naval and breastbone with hands. Visualize qi pouring into navel, heart, and thymus.

6. Cover lower back with palms. Rub these areas. Visualize kidneys and adrenals receiving qi and becoming better able to eliminate waste products and produce more energy while activating healing throughout body.

Massaging Acupuncture Points

1. Press your thumbs vigorously against all areas of the palms and soles of feet. Concentrate pressure on any sore points discovered, and do this several times.

2. Press along each segment of fingers and toes, including tips, lateral sides of the base, near the fingernail or toenail. Roll the finger or toe between pressure of the thumb and forefinger. Return to those points that are particularly tender. Massage both ears with thumb and forefinger simultaneously, beginning with moderate pressure and work over entire ear on both sides until they begin feeling hot. Rub vigorously any areas that feel tender.

Breathing to Build Up Vital Energy

1. In a sitting or standing position, close eyes loosely, or just

slightly open. Focus attention inward. Relax shoulders with head resting directly on top of shoulders and spine. Hold hands palm facing upward with fingertips pointing toward each other about two inches below navel.

2. Bring hands slowly upward to lower edge of breastbone while also slowly inhaling. Take in three short puffs of breath to fill lungs, raising the hands a bit with each puff. Hold for a moment, then slowly turn palms face downward while also slowly lowering hands to the navel.

3. Exhale three additional puffs while lowering hands to beginning location. Hold for a moment, then repeat from 2, above.

Relaxing and Contracting With Breathing

1. While sitting or standing, bring hands to heart and breastbone. Exhale, pressing hands forward as if pushing something heavy. Contract as many muscles as possible. Grip floor or ground with toes, and, while hands slowly push forward, contract the muscles located on pelvic floor between genital and anal area.

2. Completely exhale when hands are extended and muscles contracted. Release tension from muscles and float hands back toward heart, with deep inhalation. Release toes, and other muscles.

3. Repeat same cycle, pressing hands upward as high as possible, as if lifting great weight, exhale and contract.

4. Relax completely, inhale slowly, return hands to position before heart.

5. Repeat same cycle, pushing hands out to side, then pressing downward, then continue forward, then up, then to sides, and finally downward.

Twisting the Waist

1. Seated or standing, with feet at shoulder width, rotate torso. Upper body movement should come from moving waist. Shoulders follow waist and arms follow shoulders, they just dangle and swing. Turn head completely as far as comfortable.

2. Breathe fully, noting relationship between action and relaxation. Relax with the movement as much as possible. Arms and hands hit the body, which can be purposeful when aimed at kidneys, spleen, liver and lower torso.

Spontaneous Movement

Rather than follow a set of orchestrated movements, you can move or not move at all according to your inner feelings, or intuition.

Meditation

One can practice meditating in any posture. If severely ill, it can mobilize resources, but if healthy, it can help maintain health, coordinate the body, mind and spirit.

(For a more complete description of qigong routines, see *Qigong for Arthritis*, Yang, Jwing-Ming, Ph.D., this foundation. Also see books by Roger Jahnke, O.M.D., *Qigong: Awakening and Mastering the Medicine Within, The Self Applied Health Enhancement Methods; The Most Profound Medicine;* tape, *Deeper Relaxation for Self Healing,* Health Action Publishing, 243 Pebble Beach, Santa Barbara, CA 93117.)

<u>The Chinese Approach to Arthritis</u>

Chinese physicians evalute the imbalances of qi (or "bioelectricity") by noting the actual physical symptoms. According to ancient Chinese lore, qi becomes unbalanced before a disease or sickness appears. If the unbalance is not corrected, then physical damage results, because every cell in the body requires qi to survive, and without its normal abundance, the cell functions improperly, or dies.

Chinese physicians, and their patients, try to correct the imbalance before it results in destruction to the cells, joints, and systems.

Chinese medicine does not differentiate between different forms of arthritis, as does the West, because they are all caused by an imbalance in the body's bioelectrical energy, which, in any case, must be corrected for the body to repair itself as far as it can do so after damage has resulted. Consider, for example, the case of Crystal Starburger who suffered from fibromyalgia. Had she suffered from any other form of arthritis, including osteoarthritis or rheumatoid arthritis, her qigong therapy component would have been the same.

The Case of Crystal Starburger

Crystal had a very severe case of fibromyalgia, a condition of fatigue, muscle and tissue inflammation and weakness, pain and local tenderness with stiff joints and muscles, joint swelling and redness, and other symptoms. She had gone off work using workman's compensation. She was "stagnating in her house and dissatisfied with numerous doctors who had given her a whole array of medications, all of which did nothing."

Dr. Jahnke reports that, "Our strategy was to help her understand fibromyalgia, that it is caused and then perpetuated by the person's choices -- their personal choices.

"In this case it seemed acupuncture was somewhat helpful, but the shift in life style and practice of qigong was the most important parts of Crystal's wellness, because she discontinued the acupuncture treatments and kept improving. What I believe she found most important was that she learned to meditate into gentle body movement types of exercises, which is what qigong is."

Crystal began having steady improvement to the extent that she returned to work, basically completely cured. Most people seen by Dr. Jahnke who've had arthritis work too hard, they don't rest efficiently, and they build up a deficiency in stimulating the body's ability to eliminate toxic substances. They build up toxicity.

"We see that when people began to meditate, chew their food more slowly, do gentle exercise on a regular basis -- and that means never doing aggressive exercise -- and when they do gentle massage of the hand, foot, and ear, and do deep breathing exercises -- this contributes to producing less metabolic byproducts that are toxic, and to removing more toxic materials."[55]

Restricting negative enviromental exposures as well as proper diet are considered important in Chinese medicine, although the latter is often enhanced with a vast store of data related to the use of herbs.

Chinese Ways of Treating Arthritis

Dr. Jwing-Ming Yang[79] lists these ways as means for treating arthritis, preventing arthritis from happening, or from getting worse:

• Massage, when properly done, can improve qi circulation in the joint area.

• Acupuncture can temporarily halt pain and also increase qi circulation. (Western physicians have also shown that it can strengthen the immune system.)

• Herbal remedies are used to alleviate pain, increase qi circulation, help healing of injuries, and speed up healing.

• Use Cavity Press (Dian Xue), a "method of using the fingertips (especially the thumb tip) to press acupuncture cavities and certain other points (pressure points) on the body in order to manipulate the qi circulation."

While it may take years to learn to use acupuncture properly, according to Dr. Jwing-Ming Yang, Cavity Press can be learned quickly and requires no equipment.

"In Cavity Press, stagnant qi deep in the joint is led to the surface. This improves the qi circulation in the joint area, and considerably reduces the pain. The use of cavity press to speed up the healing of injured joints is very common in the Chinese martial arts." (See *Qigong for Arthritis*, Jwing-Ming Yang, Ph.D.)

Summary of Benefits

Qigong exercises for arthritis have the main purpose of rebuilding the strength of the joint by improving qi circulation. As long as there is a proper supply of qi at the joints, they can be repaired and, in some cases, even be rebuilt.

Practicing qigong can not only heal arthritis or joint injury and rebuild the joint, it is also known to be very effective in strengthening the internal organs. Many illnesses, including some forms of arthritis, stem from abnormally functioning internal organs.

According to Roger Jahnke, O.M.D.,[118] qigong accelerates oxygen distribution in the body at a time when your muscles are not rapidly using it as they would be in aerobics or running. This enables cells to begin their repair work.

Second, there is a tremendous benefit to the immune system. Qigong shifts the body into a state where the autonomic nervous system moves toward the parasympathetic-sympathetic balance, which then supports and enhances the activities of the immune system.

Third, qigong helps to turn on the body's 'garbage disposal system' known as the lymph system, thereby eliminating toxins, metabolites, and pathogenic factors from the tissues. (See this Chapter, "Energy Medicine.")

With a healthy flow of qi circulation, internal organs will be healthy, the immune system will be strengthened, and the spirit will be at peace.

Stress

The Importance of Stress

A person's overall nutritional intake is the most important single factor for preventing sickness and achieving wellness, and it is fundamental to every disease condition. Good dietary habits are a most necessary condition for reversing or controlling all disease states, but may not, in themselves, be a sufficient condition.

Absence of stress, like a good nutritional status, is also a necessary condition for preventing and achieving wellness, and, like good dietary habits, may also not be sufficient.

There is such a strong interplay between many basic factors   that none can be overlooked when seeking wellness. For example, one of the causes of stress can be poor nutritional habits, while poor nutritional habits can also lead to physical and emotional stress. Both fasting and long-term or chronically stressful lifestyles can lead to hormonal unbalances which lead to many different disease states.

Aside from the interactive, underlying and pervasive nature of good nutrition, however, stress becomes the most important single factor in virtually every disease state. It's also a subject that physicians tend to ignore, and patients wish to avoid.

Just as physicians are generally not taught nutrition, so they are not taught the skills of stress management in medical school. Most of their education is heavily oriented toward drug treatments. Even those who later specialize in mental, emotional and psychic disciplines are not provided with techniques that work effectively; and so, having at best a failed technology, psychiatrists resort to the use of damaging, mood-altering drugs.

The best that drugs can do for a distraught mental/emotional state is to temporarily occlude painful effects, and delay the individual's need to confront "real-world" stimuli. A continual drugging of sensitive mental/emotional problems continually delays solutions to the problems. Meanwhile, the physical aspect of the problem -- which, like two faces of a coin, is the obverse side of the mental/emotional state -- continues to seek resolution, that is, restoration to the normal state. Failing this, a "disease" process is established, and whatever we are genetically susceptible to kicks in.

L. Ron Hubbard,[119] creator and developer of the philosophy of Scientology®, early in his researches discovered that hypnotism, while appearing to be effective in allaying physical or mental problems, was deceptively dangerous. He was able to demonstrate that the act of suppressing an unwanted emotional response via hypnotic command actually turned on a corresponding physical ailment; and vice versa, the act of suppressing a physical ailment by hypnotic command turned on a corresponding mental/emotional problem. After this research, he abandoned the use of any kind of hypnotic commands or positive suggestions on patients in favor of a technology that would permit and teach each individual to confront his or her innermost emotional pain, and to resolve the pain so that it's founding memory-experience was confrontable, and comfortable thereafter. By doing so, he learned that, as a byproduct, people became free of their recorded trauma, sickness and stress, and also became better human beings.[119]

Some physicians who do recognize the importance of stress reduction in bringing about the disease-free state have learned to use techniques that will hopefully reduce their patient's stress. Among techniques used are bio-feedback training, visualizations or guided imageries, aroma therapy, light and sound therapies, meditation, Yoga, qigong, Alcoholics Anyonymous, religion, and so on. All of these can be important, if they satisfy the patient, and if they work. C. Norman Shealy, M.D., Ph.D.[142] writing in *Miracles Do Happen: A Physician's Experience with Alternative Medicine*, says, "Nothing is more important or powerful in stress management than physical exercise."

It is no deep, complex psychological mystery that our greatest source of stress is from personal relationships and from our work. These, after all, thrust at the very heart of survival.

The impact of stress on our bodies was neatly demonstrated by Hans Selye, who described the bio-physical details of the "flight or fight" syndrome, and the exhaustion of adrenaline and its affect on our systems.

In simplified form, what happens is that a threat to survival triggers production of cortisol, a substance from the adrenal gland (cortex) very much like cortisone. Cortisol activates the body to produce quick energy, which we need during our emergency state. We are programmed to convert certain T-cells -- microorganism protecting cells found in the blood stream that are also part of our immunological system -- into a form of quick energy. While this T-cell conversion is excellent for a real emergency, like running away from a saber-toothed tiger or an automobile that is bearing down on us, the tragic effect of a sustained emergency state soon becomes evident.

If we continue to unbalance our immunological system by converting some of its defense factors (specialized T-cells) into quick energy, we also permit organisms-of-opportunity to utilize their new opportunity, and infection -- a cold or other pathogenically "derived disease" -- hits us[5].

There are also other effects, such as those which stem from an unbalanced hormonal system, and perhaps even other effects not yet categorized.

In any case, a continuous emergency state -- threat to survival, flight or fight syndrome -- is a continuing stress, and continuing stress is damaging mentally, emotionally and physically.

How the Body Adapts to Stress to Create Arthritis

Canadian physiologist Hans Selye described a generally accepted physical model of the effects of prolonged stress at different stages on the human body, called the general adaptation syndrome (GAS). There are three stages (1) Alarm Stage; (2) Resistance Stage; and (3) Exhaustion Stage.

Alarm Stage of Stress

A young person filled with vitality and health will often overwork muscles and come home with "aches and pains" that soon disappear, as the ability to bring nourishment to individual cells, to dispose of excess cellular wastes, and to repair tissue proceeds rapidly. An older person, however, may take considerably longer and, if the muscles are continually overworked or subjected to additional strain from other stress factors, the body will began to adapt in other mechanical and biochemical ways. One example of such adaptation has been described by Carl Reich, M.D., Ottawa, Canada, who has shown through his research and clinical practices that biological stress from persistent lack of vitamin D_3, calcium, and sunshine causes the body to adapt to any of dozens of different disease states including various forms of arthritis. Rex E. Newnham, N.D., D.O., Ph.D., England, has shown a similar result when the body lacks boron. (See Chapter 2, Rheumatoid Arthritis, "Nutrition and Supplements.")

Repetitive stress factors beyond the individual's ability to swiftly compensate leads to the second stage, or resistance stage in the general adaptation syndrome (GAS).

Resistance Stage

The middle aged man or woman who works two jobs and who also leads a very stressful life at home because of the absolute need to take care of small children during periods when rest, peace and recovery are demanded of the mind, emotions and body may think that, though often fatigued, s/he is coping rather well. Years may go by with such super-stress at home and work as the body slowly uses up resources and also functions with less efficiency due to aging. Circulation decreases minutely year by year, as does the secretion of hormones from aging glands. The heart, kidneys, liver and pancreas function with less efficiency -- meanwhile the body like a very good soldier continues to attempt to repair itself from daily stress.

Additional stress may be acquired in the form of nutritional deficiencies; emotional trauma such as loved ones who've died; toxicity from traditional drug therapy that treats symptoms and not the causes, thus providing the illusion that with the drug one is coping; surgeries that interrupt the natural flow of energy --qi -- along meridian lines, or incapacitate organs by destroying or deleting them; and other forms of stress -- all take their toll.

Soon minor symptoms are acquired and small complaints begin: "I feel tired all the time." "My skin has broken out, and nothing I use clears it up." "When I get up in the morning, my joints ache and I feel stiff all over, but I'm OK after I've moved around a bit." "I get head-aches at work, and my back and wrist hurt all the time." -- and so on!

When treated by means that simply hide symptoms -- which is a way of saying "left untreated and hidden" -- a persistently overworked muscle manifests pain, stiffness, and often inflammation, becoming less and less elastic and more fibrous. Additional stress is placed on tendon and ligament attachments to bones and muscles, which creates additional pain and structural mal-adaptations.

Left untreated with appropriate rest and nourishment, muscles and joint structures finally reach the exhaustion stage of the general adaptation syndrome.

Exhaustion Stage

Joints are not just places where bones move in well-oiled sacs. Joints consist of interacting bones, muscles, skin, nerve tissue, fluids and so on. All components must be healthy and working well with one another.

When certain peripheral nerves leading to joints become bio-chemically unstable, they can fire impulses that signal both as a spi-nal reflex action back to the joint and also to the brain and back to the same joint as a pain signal. This can create a condition in the joint of insufficiency of nourishment which factor, in turn, leads to cartilage degeneration, free radical chemical damage, and finally inflammation, swelling, and permanent joint damage. (See this chapter, "Intraneural Injections.")

Muscular imbalances that derive from tendon and ligament im-balances lead to further structural stress. Although we're not aware of the fact -- as we have no internal sensing mechanisms to tell us -- our body's attempt to compensate creates calcium spurs and further joint damage.

Two adverse factors also become evident at this stage, viewed especially in rheumatoid arthritis, but also seen in some osteoarthritis: (1) various forms of microorganisms gain entrance to bodily tissues. The resulting tissue sensitivity to the toxins or protein products of the microorganisms sets up an internal "allergy" reaction, an antigen/anti-body response. If the protein substances have a DNA structure -- a genetic sequencing of basic protein molecules -- similar to the tissues infected, the body's immunological system apparently attacks both the

foreign agents and its own joint   tissues; (2) "external" immuno-complexes, substances formed from other forms of antigen/antibody combinations, usually from food allergies, also lodge in joint tissues creating additional irritating foreign substances that lead to pain, inflammation, swelling and general cartilage (that is, joint) destruction.

By this time the lymph system (designed to sweep out   impuri-
ties) is often overloaded and backed up, like a clogged house drain,
and the concentrated toxicity problem simply cascades, looming ever
larger.

Pain, swelling, and joint destruction, of course, lead to more stress.
Thus is established a well-known poistive feed-back loop, where stress
has initiated a physiological/emotional/mental sequence which creates
more stress.

The Many Faces of Stress
Stress Has an Infinite Number of Faces

No one knows how many life forms have inhabited our planet,
Earth. There must be trillions, if not an order of magnitude or so more.
Life has adapted to deserts and oceans; to extreme cold and excessive
humidities; to the depths of long-buried oil pools and sulphur-bearing
rocks; it is found amidst scalding heat and caustic chemicals spewed
up by hydrothermal vents; life is found far beneath the earth in solid
rock; it is present in oxygen deficient environments, algae   live out
their complete existence in the swiftly vanishing, fleecy white clouds
above us -- life is everywhere on earth, and, for all we know, may be a
fundamental characteristic of the universe itself.

The powerful engine that drives life into every niche and cranny
is stress: biochemical, mechanical, nutritional, mental and emotional,
environmental, electromagnetic, radioactive, and so on. A supreme
beingness has devised a small DNA molecule that through various
mechanisms can adapt or change successive progeny so that survivors
can live comfortably, indeed, demand, the particular factors that previously represented serious stress factors for their parents.

This powerful engine -- stress -- is a wonderful force for species'
development and evolution, but an extremely   costly one for individuals within the species. Billions of individual bacterium must die before
one microbial form is produced that can survive the onslaught of a
new antibiotic. This individual then propagates a whole new genus
from which springs certain individuals that can only live in the presence of the formerly deadly antibiotic.

As each species' adapts in response to radically changing environments, eventually a totally new species is born, one that cannot
cross-breed with the original, and so life spreads, filling every possible
niche and cranny.

From the preceding perspective it's easy to visualize that now,
today, all of us are undergoing tremendous stress factors that may be

producing a human species that can live in an oxygen deficient environment surrounded by deadly automobile fumes, pesticides, fluorides and herbicides, nourished by foods without enzyme content, vitamins or minerals or essential fatty acids: eggless eggs, fatless fats, creamless ice cream, and so on being the norm of the diet for those who survive all the deadly present-day stress factors.

But, oh, at what a cost to each of us as individuals. . . !

Advice for the Arthritic

Although there's no known special set of stress factors that apply to other forms of disease-states that do not also apply to the arthritic, there are some important mental and emotional problems that should be understood and ways to confront these problems that are appropriate for the arthritic.

The only difference between stress-relieving principles that apply to the osteoarthritic as compared to those that apply to the rheumatoid arthritic may be a much higher incidence of infectious microorganism in the rheumatoid victim.

Seven physicians   (Jack M. Blount, M.D., Ronald Davis, M.D., Paul Jaconello, M.D., Warren Levin, M.D., Rex E. Newnham, D.O., N.D., Ph.D., Gus J. Prosch, Jr., M.D. , John Parks Trowbridge, M.D.) were asked to review the subject of stress, and reduce advice for the arthritic to its most elemental form. Here is their consensus:

Physician-Approved Advice for Reducing Stress

Not only can controlling the stress in your life help prevent contracting arthritis but if you get the disease, controlling stress can help lessen the pain and its impact on the body.

Be conscious of stress in your life and use the following guidelines to reduce stress:

• Develop a positive attitude about everything you do; associate with "positive attitude" people,
• Learn to relax,
• Learn proper breathing exercises,
• Cultivate a good sense of humor,
• Listen to relaxing music,
• Visit with friends and do things that you enjoy,
• Exercise, get outside in the sunlight, take really brisk walks,
• Permit yourself to yawn when required, and to stretch from time to time,
• Take enjoyable vacations, at least get away from humdrum routine,
• Always get proper rest,
• Learn about your inner spirit, pray according to your conscience and beliefs. Stay in control, don't just become a drug user, as happens to many patients.

Drugs -- any kind of drugs -- contain a hidden danger that lay unknown until recently, with the work of biochemist Hermona Soreq of Hebrew University, and Alan Friedman,[149] physician at Soroka Hospital in Beersheva, Israel.

Fatty tissues surround the blood vessels that nourish the brain. These specialized layers prevent infectious agents and large chemical molecules from passing through what is called the "blood-brain barrier," adversely affecting brain cells, our health, and behavior. Medical scientists have assumed that most drugs taken by mouth do not pass through this protective barrier. Indeed, few, if any, drugs are tested with patients under stressful conditions. Now, it's clear from the work of Soreq and Friedman that under stress the fatty sheath around brain vessels is affected, and various drugs can pass through blood vessels, affecting brain cells, health, and behavior. It follows, therefore, that all of the carefully reported listing of possible adverse affects described in required FDA "counter-indications," is incomplete and may, in fact, be vastly understating the dangers of both common and uncommon drugs, especially whenever stress -- a common life factor -- is experienced simultaneously with drug usage.

Biofeedback Training[5]

Biofeedback training is a means of learning how to control nerve impulses and muscles that we would normally not be conscious of controlling. Usually, safe electronic mechanisms are used that help bring to our conscious awareness what our thought and muscle patterns are doing under a given stimulus.

Although biofeedback training is useful in eliminating headaches, controlling asthmatic attacks, reconditioning injured muscles, and relieving pain, it can be particularly useful for relieving stress, and emotions behind the stress.

Before the 1960s it was a commonly accepted Western belief that autonomic functions, such as the heart rate and pulse, digestion, blood pressure, brain waves, and muscle behavior were beyond our awareness control." They just happened." Now it is well known that many of these functions can be placed under conscious control, or modified if desired, to the benefit of the body's health. Of course, a few seekers after spiritual mysteries, some Yoga practitioners (an ancient healing discipline using breathing exercises, physical postures, and meditation), some who follow the spiritual path of Qigong teachings, and others have been able to control their autonomic nervous system in centuries past, but it was only the few who placed themselves under intense, long, usually life-time study, who obtained the ability. Modern instrumentation makes this chore relatively easy, often pleasant, and swift.

For example, once the physical attribute -- heart rate, pulse, skin electrical conductivity, etc. -- is chosen, a training signal is wired into the desired attribute -- such as a bell, moving needle, light, or other feedback stimuli -- and these signals will change according to changes in the chosen physical attribute. The individual will observe the training signal, and through practice, an individual soon learns to "think" or otherwise change internal signals so that the formerly autonomic function can now be consciously controlled.

One way that biofeedback might help the arthritic is in reducing the sensation of pain by reducing one's emotional response to the pain.

Biofeedback can also be used with visual imagery to reduce stress and also to reduce levels of destructive chemicals in the blood stream.

Exercise for the Relief of Stress

Exercise is absolutely essential for optimum bodily functioning. Physical exercise places demands on all of the body's systems, pumping blood faster, bringing nutrients to the cells, disposing of cellular wastes, breaking down and repairing tissues, and so on. When the metabolism operates efficiently throughout, suppressed emotions and other stress factors dissipate.

Arthritics are often pain-filled, and what is "moderate" exercise to such a person may be "excessive" exercise to another. Although the goal may be to exercise for the purpose of stimulating the overall metabolism, the over-production of undisposed cellular waste products and the tearing down of more tissue than is rebuilt can place the arthritic in a position where the arthritis and its accompanying pain is increased, rather than decreased.

An additional factor must be considered in the event that arthritis is actually a by-product of sensitivity to microorganisms (as is surely the case with many of those suffering from rheumatoid arthritis, other rheumatoid diseases, and may possibly be the case for about 1 out of 10 of those suffering from osteoarthritis). One of us (Gus J. Prosch, Jr., M.D.) therefore, would caution that exercising without first eliminating these potential organisms may serve to spread the disease faster, as increased blood flow enhances the rate, hence scope, of microorganism distribution.

Aside from the possibility of an infectious organism, however, exercise is a must for all individuals, even if it is no more than twisting and bending fingers and hands.

Although many health professionals will advise the employment of "moderate" exercise, the definition of what constitutes "moderate," may be between you and your health professional in consideration of your present health circumstances.

The arthritic's best goal is to slowly, safely increase physical exercise without also creating further damage to joints, and more lasting pain. Although pain will inevitably be present before joints have completely healed, there should be continued improvement for every kind of exercise employed. Start with a pad and pencil and record your ability to exercise by, say, counting the number of finger bends, or wrist twists, or even the number of attempts to stretch and touch your toes. From this information:

1. Set yourself a first safe goal.

2. Tomorrow, equal or exceed the goal, but not by so much that you create more suffering.

3. The third day, equal or exceed the goal of the second day. If you can't, don't be disappointed, as everyone's body has ebbs and flows in efficiency. Simply go back to day one, equalling or exceeding your accomplishment, if possible.

4. Continue as above, always recording your accomplishment -- or even graphing it against the number of days of trial. Your graph will wiggle up and down, which is natural, but overall it will rise, giving the appearance of a jagged outcropping reaching toward the clouds.

5. When you're satisfied with what you've done with one set of exercises, choose another, but don't forget the first. Now record both of them.

6. Continue expanding your abilities as above, adding number of movements, or attempts, and new exercises as your body permits.

Many arthritics are advised to exercise in water, because the water holds off the toll of gravity, allowing more movements for a given energy exertion and with lessened weight on joints.

If you're one of the fortunate ones, you'll want to take up a more active form of exercise: trampolining (which moves lymph faster); walking fast, or even running, dancing, swimming, etc.

Taking individual differences into account, then, John Hibbs, N.D. of Bastyr College, Seattle, Washington, recommends what he calls tissue aerobic exercise: relaxing exercise that allows blood flow to continue to the tissues. "The heart rate should increase and you should wind up sweating, but many doctors are switching over to a lower heart rate now. You don't need to go up to 140."

Don't pick an exercise that you despise, or even dislike, pick an exercise you enjoy, but try never to overdo, never over-achieve. Pamper your body, pet it, be nice to it -- and it'll one day return the favor with improved health, lessened suppressed emotion, and certainly lowered stress.

Guided Imagery for Stress Relief[5]

After a stressful day at work, filled with withering emotions, it is sometimes difficult to fall immediately to sleep, no matter the urgency of sleep. Many have learned that they can invent a scenario inside their mind somewhat more complex than counting sheep, but rather including something quite pleasant they'd like to do. Placing all of one's attention on the play-acting inside the mind quickly dissipates the wrought-up energies, and often one will fall asleep before finishing the scenario.

L. Ron Hubbard, founder of the philosophy of the Church of

Scientology, and author of many publications covering 40,000,000 words on how to truly know one's self, in 1950 published the first book, *Dianetics: The Modern Science of Mental Health*,[118] wherein was described the method of guided imagery. This book has stayed on the best-seller list since 1950, and has been translated to most of the major languages of the world, so it's not suprising that many of its concepts are now advocated by many health professionals.

Hubbard's first method for relieving illness, including arthritis and aberrant behavior patterns, involved a technology of assisted self-confrontation, where stored, but "unconscious," moments of pain and emotion could be wholly alleviated, thus resulting in disappearance of either the illness or its counterpart, the compulsory behavior pattern. The result was more freedom to choose, and less subjection to undesirable stimulus-response mechanisms.

In the process of uncovering deep pain and emotion, and even after its complete discharge, there was often undesirable, residual "restimulation," produced by associated recall of similar events. To ease these moments, Hubbard invented a technique of guided imagery. The one who does the guiding is called an "auditor," one who sits and listens.

After a session where emotion and pain memories have been reduced or "erased" so that they no longer create psychosomatic illnesses or aberrant behavior patterns, the auditor would say, "Remember a pleasant moment."

The subjects would then bring to their mind an earlier memory from his or her life when relaxation and pleasure ruled. They would describe what they were doing, what they saw, who was present, pleasant things said and heard, delightful odors, beautiful colors, laughing children, thoughts, feelings, and so on, focusing entirely on an image which they chose, and which they described in however much detail they could.

The result of this little exercise was that the subject lost any possible residual restimulation from associated memories containing similarities to those painful memories confronted and alleviated, and the session was ended.

While nowhere nearly as beneficial as that   obtained when releasing huge stores of undesirable, pent-up pain and emotion, the use of guided imagery by itself has been sufficiently positive to attract many health professionals.

Guided imagery relies on a natural function discovered to be common to all people from childhood upward: the ability to focus thoughts, and to either recall or imagine a specific time when the the body and emotions were at ease.

Meditation for the Relief of Stress[5]

The art of meditation is perhaps as old as modern man, for it is the tribal shamans (healers) and primitive tribesmen who learned its value for many purposes, including that of healing.

According to Joan Borysenko, Ph.D., pioneer in the field of mind/body medicine, meditation is defined as any activity which keeps the person's attention anchored in present time without being influenced by past memories, nor preoccupied with future considerations.

Another way of describing such meditation is that we learn to "key out," all currently functioning stimulus-response mechanisms of the body, whether these are triggered by past, recorded memories, or were conditioned under painful and emotional experiences.

There are many systems for achieving appropriate meditation which are beyond the scope of this book. Some will advise sitting quietly while concentrating on the breath, image, or a sound, while others advise becoming aware of our sensory impressions, such as feelings, images, sounds, thoughts, odors, and so on, without becoming involved with them.

Many stimulus-response mechanisms -- or as some have phrased it, "automatic circuits" -- operate daily to cause us to move our hands, head, and other body parts in almost random, meaningless behavior patterns (such as the desire -- sometimes overriding desire -- to scratch a particular place on the face, or behind the neck). To some extent we've all identified our personality, our beingness, our awareness-of-being-aware unit with these patterns, and if asked why we scratched, we'd answer that "I itched there," which is more of a justification after the fact than a statement of cause.

One of the easily observed phenomena when attempting meditation is the number of these overwhelming distractions that must be ignored in order to be in present time without computing conclusions about past events, or analytically predicting future actions or probabilities.

At the point where all these distractions disappear -- and they will -- one has usually achieved a meditative state.

There are physiological, psychological, and spiritual benefits from the daily practice of meditation.

Meditation lowers the body's core temperature, which is one of two factors that have been shown to extend life, the other being restriction of calorie intake.

Stress is more easily confronted, or handled, when we permit ourselves to simply "be," the distinguishing outcome of meditation. Of course, with stress under control, all disease states -- including arthritis -- are better handled, including pain and the emotional components of pain.

Jom Kabat-Zinn, Ph.D., founder and director of the Stress Reduction Clinic at the University of Massachusetts Medical Center, has taught meditation and Yoga to thousands of patients, mostly referred to him by other physicians. "In one study overseen by Dr. Kabat-Zinn, 72 percent of the patients with chronic pain conditions achieved at least a 33 percent reduction after participating in an eight-week period of mindful meditation, while 61 percent of the pain patients achieved at least a 50 percent reduction."[5] Additionally these patients improved their self-esteem and held more positive views about their bodies.

Meditative practices are quite easy to learn, and once the discipline takes hold, with frequency and time, the more benefits are received.

Meditation is not a substitute for medical or stress-related physical disorders. Although people can easily practice meditation by themself, physical problems should be attended to by those best trained in the art of healing.

Stress in Personal Relationships
The Suppressive Personality

According to the research of L. Ron Hubbard,[119,120] often there is one or more persons in the close work or home environment who are suppressive to the one who is sick, such suppression expressing itself in a way that constantly invalidates the sick person's actions, thoughts or emotions. It is a negative stimulus that depresses our beingness, our will to want to engage in friendly exchange of ideas or activities. Hubbard called these people "antisocial personalities." He estimated that about 15-20% of all humans have characteristics that can be called antisocial. An individual's intelligence, educational level or manner of earning a wage has no relationship to whether or not he or she is antisocial. Judges, administrators, physicians, ditch-diggers, taxi-drivers, editors, homemakers, teachers, any nationality, any race, any creed, any or all walks of life may fall into the 15-20% category.

A person who is so affected by another will often suppress his or her emotions and behavior in ways that express outwardly in the form of hormonal changes and accompanying clinical sicknesses.

The medical terminology is "psychosomatic," indicating that the person's state of mind governs his emotions and bodily condition. This is true to the extent that a person permits suppressive conditions and "suppressive" people to influence his or her mind and body.

As few physicians have training in recognizing the causative patterns, and would probably be resisted by their patients if they mentioned them, interpersonal stress sources are often ignored in treatment, although they may be the largest component of all diseases, acute or chronic.[7, 20]

Hubbard identified "antisocial" and "social personality," characteristics, the social personality being the opposite of those assigned to the anti-social personality. Those who would learn more will find the information easily available through many publications of this applied religious philosophy through any outlet of the Church of Scientology.

(Change in religious convictions not at all required.)

Yoga for Stress[5]

Yoga, one of the oldest known systems for health, is the practice of physical postures, breathing exercises, and meditation. Its practice in modern times has demonstrated the lowering of stress and blood pressure, regulation of heart rate, and even retardation of the aging process.

Yoga teaches an integration of the mind and body. The mind and body are one and the same, and should be written with a new symbol, as mind/body. The modern view of psychosomatic medicine may have stemmed from this ancient art, where whatever affects the body, also affects the mind, and vice-versa. Spelling out such a cause effect relationship is, in itself, inaccurate, as the true Yoga practitioner would view physical disease of the body, or aberrated behavior patterns, as being symptomatic of our forgetting the unity known as mind/body.

The thyroid gland, and its hormonal production, is basic to the stoking up of our cellular metabolic engines, which in turn is basic to the efficient utilization of enzymes, which is fundamental to good health for all disease states, including the arthritic. Indeed, many arthritic symptoms do stem from insufficiency of thyroid hormone, or in its conversion to a form that slows down the metabolic heat engine. The practice of Yoga has been shown to normalize the production of thyroid hormone.

As the thyroid is the master regulator of all the other glands (with the pituitary being the master gland over all, including the thyroid), and as the glands are intimately tied in with stress and emotion, the ability to increase or decrease thyroid activity without taking drugs can be an important self-help process.

There have been more than a thousand well-designed studies (since the 1970s) of meditation and Yoga. These studies have demonstrated that Yoga can bring about stress and anxiety alleviation, blood and heart rate reduction, improved memory and intelligence, pain alleviation, improved motor skills, relief from addiction, heightened visual and auditory perceptions, enhanced metabolic and respiratory functions, and many other benefits.[5]

In *The 1983-1984 Yoga Biomedical Trust* survey, 90% or 530 out of 589 people with either arthritis or rheumatism (a cluster of symptoms resembling several different kinds of arthritis) reported improvement with the use of Yoga practices involving physical postures, breathing exercises, and meditation.[5]

Yoga can be ideally suited to the personal health maintenance program of all arthritics. To learn more, you can obtain numerous books at any book store.

References

1. Personal conversation with Gus J. Prosch, Jr. 1990.

2. Anthony di Fabio, *Prevention and Treatment of Osteoarthritis*, The Art of Getting Well, The Arthritis Fund/The Rheumatoid Disease Foundation, 1990.

3. *Textbook of Internal Medicine,* J.B. Lippincott Company, 1989.

4. *The Merck Manual of Diagnosis and Therapy*, 16th Edition, Merck, Sharp & Dohme Research Laboratories, Division of Merck & Co., Inc., 1992.

5. Burton Goldberg Group, *Alternative Medicine: The Definitive Guide*, Future Medicine Publishing Co., 1994.

6. Anthony di Fabio, *Rheumatoid Diseases Cured at Last*, The Arthritis Fund/ The Rheumatoid Disease Foundation, 1985.

7. Anthony di Fabio, *The Art of Getting Well*, The Arthritis Fund/The Rheumatoid Disease Foundation, 1988.

8. Anthony di Fabio, *Treatment and Prevention of Osteoarthritis*, Part I, The Arthritis Fund/The Rheumatoid Disease Foundation, 1989. Also in *Townsend Letter for Doctors*, January 1990, #78; also Anthony di Fabio, *Arthritis*, The Rheumatoid Disease Foundation.

9. Anthony di Fabio, *Treatment and Prevention of Osteoarthritis*, Part II, The Arthritis Fund/The Rheumatoid Disease Foundation, 1989. Also in *Townsend Letter for Doctors*, February/March 1990, #79/80; also Anthony di Fabio, *Arthritis*, The Arthritis Fund/The Rheumatoid Disease Foundation.

10. Hector E. Solorzano del Rio, M.D., D.Sc, Ph.D, *Systemic Enzyme Therapy*, The Arthritis Fund/The Rheumatoid Disease Foundation , 1994.

11. Personal Communication with Gus J. Prosch, Jr., M.D.

12. Rex E. Newnham, D.O., N.D., Ph.D., *Boron and Arthritis,* The Arthritis Fund/ The Rheumatoid Disease Foundation, 1994; also Rex E. Newham, D.O., N.D., Ph.D., *Away With Arthritis*, Vantage Press, Inc., 1994; also personal correspondence.

13. William Kaufman, Ph.D., M.D.,"The Use of Vitamin Therapy to Reverse Certain Concomitants of Aging," *Journal of the American Geriatrics Society*, Vol. III, No. 11, Nov. 1955, William Kaufman, Ph.D., M.D. "Niacinamide: A Most Neglected Vitamin," *Journal of the International Academy of Preventive Medicine*, Vol. VIII, No. 1, Winter, 1983; William Kaufman, Ph.D., M.D. *The Common Form of Joint Dysfunction*, E.L. Hildreth & Co., 1949.

14. Pizzorno & Murray, *Textbook of Natural Medicine*, Rheumatoid Arthritis, VI: RA-5, John Bastyr College Publications, 1991.

15. Linus Pauling, Ph.D., *How To Live Longer and Feel Better*, Avon Books, 1986.

16. Louis J. Marx, M.D., *Healing Dimensions of Herbal Medicine*, Neo-Paradigm Publishers,.

17. Pizzorno & Murray, *A Textbook of Natural Medicine*, Rheumatoid Arthritis VI: RA-4, John Bastyr College Publications, 1991.

18. Pizzorno & Murray, *Textbook of Natural Medicine*, Rheumatoid Arthritis VI: RA-5, John Bastyr College Publications, 1991.

19. Luc De Schepper, M.D., Ph.D., C.A., *Peak Immunity*, 1989.

20. L. Ron Hubbard, *Dianetics: The Modern Science of Mental Health*, Bridge Publications, Inc.

21. Raymond F. Peat, Ph.D., "Hormone Balancing: Natural Treatment," The Journal of the Rheumatoid Disease Medical Association, volume 1, Number 1, Robert Bingham, M.D., Ed.: now available at The Arthritis Fund/The Rheumatoid Disease Foundation.

22. Anthony di Fabio, *The Master Regulator*, The Rheumatoid Disease Foundation, 1989; also Broda O. Barnes, M.D., Lawrence Galton, *Hypothyroidism: The Unsuspected Illness*, Harper & Row, New York, 1976.

23. Julian Whitaker, M.D., *Health & Healing*, Vol. 2, No. 6, June 1992.

24. Robert Bingham, M.D., *Fight Back Against Arthritis,* Desert Arthritis Medical Clinic, 1993.

25. Paul Pybus, *Intraneural Injections for Rheumatoid Arthritis and Osteoarthritis and The Control of Pain in Arthritis of the Knee,* 1989.

26. Arabinda Das, M.D. "A Doctor's Case: What Happens When a Physician Becomes a Rheumatoid Arthritis Patient?" *The Townsend Letter for Doctors,*"July 1992.

27. William J. Faber, D.O. and Morton Walker, D.P.M., *Pain, Pain Go Away,* Milwaukee Pain Clinic & Metabolic Research Center, 1990.

28. James Carlson, D.O. personal visit.

29. William J. Faber, D.O. and Morton Walker, D.P.M., *Instant Pain Relief,* Milwaukee Pain Clinic & Metabolic Research Center, 1990.

30. Peter Dosch, M.D., *Manual of Neural Therapy According to Huneke,* Eleventh Edition, Haug Publishers, 1984.

31. Personal Communication with Thomas Gervais.

32. Personal visit to James Carlson, D.O.

33. Ida P. Rolf, Ph.D., *Rolfing the Integration of Human Structures,* Harper & Row Publishers, 1977.

34. Anthony di Fabio, *Chelation Therapy,* The Arthritis Fund/The Rheumatoid Disease Foundation, 1993.

35. From personal knowledge of patient.

36. William H. Philpott, M.D., *Magnetic Resonance Bio-Oxidative Therapy for Rheumatoid and Other Degenerative Diseases,* Supplement to The Art of getting Well, The Arthritis Fund/The Rheumatoid Disease Foundation, 1994.

37. Buryl Payne, Ph.D., *The Body Magnetic,* 4264 Topsail Ct., Soquel, CA 95073, from "Book Notices," *Townsend Letter for Doctors,* April 1993.

38. William H. Philpott, M.D., *Magnetic Research Protocols,* Philpott Medical Services, Choctaw, OK 73020.

39. Thomas Gervais, Courtland Reeves, Anthony di Fabio, *Lymphatic Detoxification,* The Arthritis Fund/The Rheumatoid Disease Foundation, 1994.

40. F. Batmanghelidj, M.D., *Your Body's Many Cries for Water;,* Global Health Solutions, Inc., 1992; also see F. Batmanghelidj, M.D., *How to Deal With Back Pain & Rheumatoid Joint Pain ,* Ibid, 1991; F. Batmanghelidj, M.D., *Prevent Arthritis and Cure Back Pain,* The Arthritis Fund/The Rheumatoid Disease Foundation, 1994.

41. F. Batmanghelidj, M.D., "Pain: A Need for Paradigm Change;" *Anticancer Research,* Vol. 7, No. 5B, PP. 971-990, Sept.-Oct. 1987.

42. Martha Christy, *Your Own Perfect Medicine,* Future Med, Inc., Scottsdale, Az 85267, 1994; also see Martha Christy, "Incredible Natural Cure That's Never Out of Reach," *Health Freedom News,* The National Health Federation, Vol. 14, No. 5, September 1995.

43. William Kaufman, Ph.D., M.D., "Niacinamide: A Most Neglected Vitamin," *Journal of the Int. Academy of Preventive Medicine,* Vol. III, No. 1, 1983; also printed in *J. Amer. Geratr. Soc.,* 3:929, 1955.

44. Carlton Fredericks, Ph.D., *Arthritis: Don't Learn to Live With It,* Grosset & Dunlap, New York, 1981.

45. Anthony di Fabio, *Flouridation: Governmentally Approved Poison,* Supplement to the Art of Getting Well, The Arthritis Fund/The Rheumatoid Disease Foundation, 1994.

46. John Marion Ellis, M.D., *Free of Pain,* National Headquarters, Natural Food Associates, 1988.

47. Michael T. Murray, N.D., *Arthritis,* Prima Publishing, 1994.

48. Personal experience of authors.

49. Reproduced by permission of Luke Bucci, Ph.D., and publishers of *Chiropractic Products* where the complete text was published in August 1988, p. 61-63.

50. Linus Pauling, Ph.D., *How To Live Longer and Feel Better*, Avon Books, 1986.

51. *Osteoarthritis Treatment News*, American College of Rheumatology.

52. Thomas J.A. Lehman, M.D., "Arthritis in Childhood and Adolescence," from Med Help International.

53. Carl Reich, M.D., *The Allergic And Auto-Immune Diseases*, also *Case History -- Osteo*, unpublished, ; used permission of author.

54. Carl Reich, M. D., Stephan Cooter, Ph.D., *Calcium and Vitamin D Deficiency: The Clinical Work and Theory of Carl J. Reich, M.D.*, Supplement to the Art of Getting Well, The Arthritis Fund/The Rheumatoid Disease Foundation, 1995; Robert Barefoot and Carl J. Reich, *The Calcium Factor,* Bokar Consultants, 1992.

55. Personal correspondence with Carl Reich, M.D, and from a large number of unpublished papers received.

56. *The New York Times*, 1995; from America Online: Ofanim, 10/6/95.

57. McDonagh, E.W., D.O., "Fractured Hips and Broken Lives," *Clinic*, n.d., n.p.

58. Jean Barilla, M.S., The Antioxidants, Keats Publishing, Inc., 1995.

59. Personal interview with Thomas Gervais.

60. Sherry A. Rogers, M.D., "One of the Best-Kept Secrets in Medicine: Osteoarthritis is Reparable," *Let's Live*, October 1995, p. 96.

61. Robert C. Atkins, M.D., *Dr. Atkins Health Revolution: How Complementary Medicine Can Extend Your Life*, Houghton Mifflin Company, Boston, MA 1988.

62. Robert M. Giller, M.D., Kathy Matthews, *Natural Prescriptions*, Carol Southern Books, 1994.

63. Barbara Sage, Acupuncture.Com; E-mail: AcuCom@aol.com.

64. "Shark Cartilage May Ease Arthritis Pain," *Women's Health Letter*.

65. Personal letter from Richard A. Kunin, M.D.

66. Personal letter from Edward Rybak received October 20, 1995.

67. Alan R. Gaby, M.D., "Orthotics for Osteoarthritis," *Townsend Letter for Doctors*, August/September 1995.

68. Pfeiffer, Naomi, "Acupuncture Relieves Knee Arthritis," *Medical Tribune*, September 10, 1992:8.

69. Dr. Tsu-Tsair Chi, N.M.D., Ph.D., *Mineral Infrared Therapy*, Chi's Enterprise, Inc., 1993.

70. Julian Whitaker, M.D., *Dr. Whitaker's Guide to Natural Healing*, Primar Publishing,1995.

71. Debbie Carson, "Kombucha Tea," *Trans*, Summer 1995, p. 14; Can be contacted at (615) 889-4701.

72. Dr. Andrew Lockie, *The Family Guide to Homeopathy*, Fireside, 1989.

73. Personal communication with Rex E. Newham, D.O., N.D., Ph.D. November 6, 1995.

74. Alan R. Gaby, M.D., "Commentary," *Nutrition & Healing*, c/o Publishers Mgt. Corp., September 1994.

75. Ricki Lewis, Ph.D., "Arthritis: Modern Treatments for That Old Pain in the Joints," *Consumer* 06/01/1991.

76. K.M. Lucero, "The Electro-Acuscope/Myopulse System: Impedance-Monitoring Microamperage Electrotherapy for Tissue Repair," *Rehab Management: The Journal of Therapy and Rehabilitation*, Volume 4, Number 3, April/May 1991.

77. D. Keith McElroy, M.D., received information through personal correspondence.

78. Alan R. Gaby, M.D., "Nutrient of the Month: The Story of Vitamin B³," *Nutrition & Healing*, Volume 2, Issue 11, c/o Publishers Mgt. Corp., November 1995.

79. Jwing-Ming Yang, *Arthritis -- The Chinese Way of Healing and Prevention*, YMAA Publication Center, Yang's Martial Arts Association (YMAA),1991.

80. Personal interview with Lori Humboldt, November 26, 1995.

81. "Back Pain, Chronic," *Alternative Medicine Digest*, Issue 8, Future Medicine

Publishing, Inc. 1995.

82. Personal interview with Jack M. Blount, M.D.

83. Personal interview with Mark Davidson, D.O., N.D.

84. Steven Foster, Herbal Remedies: Feverfew: When the Head Hurts, Alternative & Complementary Therapies, Sept/Oct 1995, p. 335.

85. Sherry A. Rogers, M.D., "Is It Chronic Low Back Pain or Environmental Illness? *Journal of Applied Nutrition*, International Academy of Nutrition and Preventive Medicine, Volume 46, Number 4, 1994.

86. Sherry Rogers, M.D., *Wellness Against All Odds*, Prestige Publishing, 1994.

87. Lita Lee, Ph.D., "Estrogen, Progesterone, and Female Problems," paper furnished by Lita Lee, Ph.D.

88. Henry Kriegel, "Memorandum," November 7, 1995, Kreigel & Associates.

89. "Boswella," paper provided by Craig T. Kisciras, Rx Vitamins™; *The Lawrence Review of Natural Products*, The Library Bastyr University, Februry 1993.

90. Agatha Thrash, M.D., Calvin Thrash, M.D., *Home Remedies*, Thrash Publications.

91. Dava Sobel, Arthur C. Klein, "Bee Venom," *Arthritis: What Works*, St. Martin's Press, 175 Fifth Avenue, New York, NY 10010, 1989; Also see *Alternative Medicine Digest*, Future Medicine Publishing, Inc.

92. Personal communication with Louis J. Marx, M.D.

92. Case history provided by Stephen Center, M.D.

93. Ben Charles Harris, *Eat the Weeds*, Keats Publishing, Inc., 1969.

94. Correspondence from Harold Babcock.

95. Jeanne F. Brooks, "Aspirin, Acetaminophen, Ibuprofen and Naproxen Cause Kidney Failure," *Health Consciousness*, Vol. 16, No. 1, January/February 1996, p. 54; from *San Diego Union -- Tribune*, November 4, 1995.

96. "Arthritis," *Alternative Medicine Digest*, Issue 10, Future Medicine Publishing, Inc. January 1996.

97. Personal correspondence with Harold R. Babcock.

98. Personal interview with Dr. Catherine Russell.

99. Information and studies provided by Lance Griffin, DNA Pacifica, 730 Summersong Lane, Encinitas, CA 92024. Studies were conducted at several different sites following a model prepared by the San Diego Clinic.

100. Karel Pavelka, M.D., Ph.D., "Osteoarthritis and Glycosaminoglycan Polysulfuric Acid," *The Experts Speak*, I.T. Services, Health Associates Medical Group, Sacramento, California.

101. Margaret A. Flynn, Ph.D., R.D., "Osteoarthritis, Folate and Vitamin B12, *The Experts Speak*, I.T. Services, Health Associates Medical Group, 1996, p. 163.

102. Sherry A. Rogers, M.D., "One of the Best Kept Secrets in medicine: Osteoarthritis is Reparable," *Townsend Letter for Doctors & Patients*, April 1996, p. 108.

103. "Topical Use of Nettle Leaves for Osteoarthritis," C.F. Randall, *British Journal of General Practitioners*, Nov:533-34, 1994.

104. Jonathan V. Wright, M.D., Alan Gaby, M.D., *Nutrition & Healing*, c/o Publishers Management Corporation, Issues 1994-1996.

105. The Academy of Traditional Chinese Medicine, *An Outline of Chinese Acupuncture*, Forcign Languages Press, Peking, 1975.

106. Jacques Staehle, "Chinese Esthetic," Acupuncture Point Chart by Jacques Staehle, CD & P Health Products, P.O. Box 53, Nutley, NJ 07110, 1981.

107. 540. "Wax on Your Fruits & Vegetables," Citzien Petition, 34 Nathan Lord Rd., Amyherst, NH 03031.

108. Jule Klotter, "Toxins in Pesticides," *Townsend Letters for Doctors*, May 1993, p. 518.

109. Zane R. Gard, M.D., Emma J. Brown, B.S.N., Ph.N. "Literature Review &

Comparison studies of the Sauna and Illness -- Part II," *The Townsend Letter for Doctors*, July 1992.

110. Alan R. Gaby, M.D., Jonathan V. Wright, M.D., *Nutrition & Healing*, September 1995.

111. Lita Lee, Ph.D., "Hypothyroidism, A Modern Epidemic," reprint from *Earthletter*, Spring 1994, 2852 Willamette St., #397, Eugene, Oregon.

104. Simon Mills, M.S., Steven J. Finando, Ph.D., *Alternatives in Healing*, New American Library, New York, 1989, p. 156.

105. George E. Meinig, D.D.S., "What Reviewers and Patients Are Saying: Root Canal Cover-up Exposed! Many Illnesses Result," Bion Publishing.

106. George E. Meinig, D.D.S., *Root Canal Cover-up*, Bion Publishing, 1994.

107. Hal A. Huggins, D.D.S., M.S., *It's All In Your Head*, Avery Press, 1990.

108. Personal letter from Richard A. Kunin, M.D.

109. John R. Lee, M.D., "Does Fluoridation Work?" *Health Freedom News*, 212 W. Foothill Blvd., Monrovia, CA 91016, June 1994, p. 13.

110. Gerard P. Judd, Ph.D., "Evidence Against Fluoride Continues to Mount," *Health Freedom News*, 212 W. Foothill Blvd., Monrovia, CA 91016, November/ December 1994, p. 29.

111. Cornelius Steelink, "Tooth Decay & Fluoride," *Townsend Letter for Doctors*, 911 Tyler St., Port Townsend, WA 98368-6541, October 1994, p. 1128.

112. Personal communication from Louis J. Marx, M.D.

113. E. Denis Wilson, M.D., *Wilson's Syndrome*, 2nd Edition, Cornerstone Publishing Co., 1993.

114. Lita Lee, Ph.D., "The 24-Hour Urinalysis According to Loomis," reprinted from *Earthletter*, Vol. 2, Summer 1994.

115. David W. Schnare, Max Ben and Megan G. Shields, "Body Burden Reductions of PCBs, PBBs and Chlorinated Pesticides in Human Subjects," *Ambio*, Vol. 13, No. 5-6, 984, p. 378. Also see Shields, Megan, M.D., "Hubbard Method of Detoxification Requires Niacin for Increased Effectiveness," *Townsend Letter for Doctors*, July 1989; Tretjak, Ziga, Shields, Megan, Beckman, Shelley L., "PCB Reduction and Clinical Improvement by Detoxification: An Unexploited Approach," *Human and Experimental Toxicology*, 1990; Norman Zucker, M.D., "Hubbard's Purification Rundown: A Workable Detox Program," *Townsend Letter for Doctors*, January 1990; "Human Detoxification -- New Hope for Firefighters," *California Firefighter*, Federated Fire Fighters of California, No. 4, 1984; Foundation for Advancements in Science and Education, Park Mile Plaza, 4801 Wilshire Blvd., Los Angeles, CA 90010; Zane R. Gard, M.D., Erma J. Brown, B.S.N., P.H.N., Giovanna DeSanti-Medina, "Bio-Toxic Reduction Program Participants (Condensed) Case Histories," *Townsend Letter for Doctors*, June 1987.

116. Agatha Thrash, M.D., Calvin Thrash, M.D., *Home Remedies*, Thrash Publications, 1981.

117. Bernard Jensen, D.C., Ph.D., *Tissue Cleansing Through Bowel Management*, Bernard Jensen, D.C., Ph.D., 1981.

118. Roger Jahnke, O.M.D., books, *Qigong: Awakening and Mastering the Medicine Within, The Self Applied Health Enhancement Methods*; *The Most Profound Medicine*; tape, *Deeper Relaxation for Self Healing*, Health Action Publishing.

119. L. Ron Hubbard, Dianetics: *The Modern Science of Mental Health, Science of Survival; Research and Discovery Series*, and other books and publications, Bridge Publications.

120. . L. Ron Hubbard, *The Volunteer Minister's Handbook*, Op.Cit., Bridge Publications, 1959-1984. Hubbard has also described antithesis characteristics, the social personality, which are not listed here. Inquire at the nearest Church of Scientology for full text.

121. Wallace Sampson, "Alternative Reading," *Science News*, March 4, 1995.

180 ANTHONY DI FABIO, M.A. & GUS J. PROSCH, JR., M.D

122. Assessing the Efficacy and Safety of Medical Technology," *U.S. Office of Technology Assessment*, U.S. Government Printing Office, 1978.

123. Joseph D. Campbell, Ph.D., "Safety: Supplements vs. Drugs," "A Question of Health," *Townsend Letter for Doctors*, December 1993; from *Nevada Sentinal*.

124. James P. Carter, M.D., Dr. PH, *Racketering in Medicine: The Suppression of Alternatives*, Hampton Roads Publishing Company, Inc., 1993.

125. *SW News*, Church of Scientology, Religious Technology Center (L.Ron Hubbard quotation taken from LRH ED 348 INT, issued on LRH's Birthday, 1983), Issue 46.

126. Julian Whitaker, "The American Dietetic Association Must Be Stopped in its Tracks," Phillips Publishing, Inc., January 1995 Supplement.

127. Richard G. Foulkes, B.A., M.D., "The `Cost' of Fluoridation," *Townsend Letter for Doctors*, 1993, p. 1068.

128. Kirkpatrick W. Dilling, "FDA -- Friend or Foe?" *Townsend Letter for Doctors*, June 1993.

129. "'Put the Head in the Bed and Keep it There'," *Business Week*, October 18, 1993.

130. John Finegan, "Case Study: How the FDA Blocks Products With Possibilities," *Health Freedom News*, March 1994.

131. Anastasia Toufexis, "Dr. Jacobs' Alternative Mission," *Time*, March 1, 1993.

132. "Coenzyme Q10 Seized in Texas," *Townsend Letter for Doctors*, Dec.,1992; Catherine J. Frompovich, Ph.D., "CoQ-10 on FDA's Hit List," July 1991.

133. Damon Runyon-Walter Winchell Cancer Research Fund (DRWWCRF), *Annual report*, 1990 (New York: DRWWCRF, 1990).

134. Tori Hudson, "Tamoxifen: Adjunct Treatment? Preventive Medicine? Substitution of One Disease for Another? *Townsend Letter for Doctors*, May 1993.

135. James T. Bennett, Thomas J. DiLorenzo, *Unhealthy Charities*, BasicBooks, Quoting AHA, *Annual Report*, 1991, pp. 2,13 and Engelking, "American Cancer Society Patient Service Programs."

136. "Dr. Linus Pauling: One of the Greatest Scientists of Our Time," *Prescription for Health*, Vol. 5, No. 1, January 1993.

137. Saul Green, Ph.D., "The JAMA Critique of the Gerson Program & The Reply JAMA Refused to Publish," *Townsend Letter for Doctors*, April 1944.

138. L. Ron Hubbard, *Dianetics and Scientology Technical Dictionary*, Op.Cit., Bridge Publications, 1975; **Overt Act, 1.** an **overt act** is not just injuring someone or something; an **overt act** is an **act** of omission or commission which does the least good for the least number of dynamics* or the most harm to the greatest number of dynamics (HCO PL 1 Nov 70 III) **2.** an intentionally committed harmful **act** committed in an effort to resolve problem. (SH Spec 44, 6410C27) **3.** that thing which you do which you aren't willing to have happen to you (1SH ACC 10, 6009C14). (See *Dianetics and Scientology Technical Dictionary*, footnote 13 above.)

* (**Dynamics** are defined by Hubbard as the urges, drives, or impulses to life, those activities that motivate us along the desire for survival through our self, children/ sex, our group, mankind, animal life, physical universe, spiritual world, and a Supreme Being. See *Dianetics and Scientology Technical Dictionary,* above.); **Overt-Motivator Sequence, 1.** if a fellow does an **overt**, he will then believe he's got to have a **motivator**. (AHMC 2, 6012C31) 2. the **sequence** wherein someone who has committed an **overt** has to claim the existence of **motivators**. The **motivators** are then likely to be used to justify committing further **overt** acts. (*PXL* Gloss). (See *Dianetics and Scientology Technical Dictionary* above.)

139. Joel D. Wallach, D.V.M., N.D. transcript of taped presentation.

140. H. Vasken Aposhian, "DMSA and DMPS -- Water Soluble Antidotes for Heavy Metal Poisning," *Ann. Rev. Pharmacol. Toxicol*, 1983, 23:193-215.

141. Joel D. Wallach, D.V.M., N.D., *Rares Earths: Forbidden Cures*, Double

Happiness Publishing Co., Bonita, CA 91908.

142. C. Norman Shealy, M.D., Ph.D., *Miracles Do Happen: A Physician's Experience with Alternative Medicine*, Element Books, Inc.

143. V. Rejholec, "Long-Term Studies of Antiosteoarthritic Drugs: An Assessment," *Seminars in Arthritis and Rheumatism*, Vol. 17, No. 2, Suppl. 1 (November), 1987, pp. 35-53.

144. Personal interview with Professor Werner Schiedl.

145. Michael T. Murray, N.D., "Glucosamine Sulfate vs. Other Forms of Glucosamine," *Health Counselor*, Vol. 8, No. 3, p. 57.

146. *Arthritis & Rheumatism*, 1996; 39:648-656.

147. *Chemical Marketing Reporter*, January 2, 1989.

148. Bruno Chikly, M.D., *Lymph Drainage Therapy*, The Arthritis Society of America, 5106 Old Harding Road, Franklin, TN 37064.

149. "The Color of Stress," *Discover*, May 1997, P. 16.

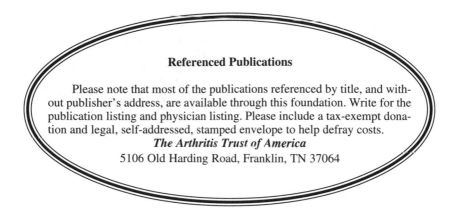

Referenced Publications

Please note that most of the publications referenced by title, and without publisher's address, are available through this foundation. Write for the publication listing and physician listing. Please include a tax-exempt donation and legal, self-addressed, stamped envelope to help defray costs.
The Arthritis Trust of America
5106 Old Harding Road, Franklin, TN 37064

Chapter II
Rheumatoid Arthritis
The Case of Jack M. Blount, M.D. and the Two Authors
Another "Incurable" Disease

"I don't really know when it started," Jack M. Blount, M.D. of Philadelphia, Mississippi, said. "but I was a young medical student when I was first told that I had rheumatoid arthritis."[7]

As with so many who've been afflicted with this painful, disfiguring problem, Dr. Jack M. Blount's story is an emotionally gripping account of a man who has been to the very depths of hell and has come back to tell us how he escaped it's fires. Keep in mind that he is cured of the ravages of rheumatoid arthritis, that he has sucessfully treated better than 17,000 patients, and that, until he retired, he freely gave of his knowledge.

Dr. Blount was reduced to total invalidism and took to alcohol, morphine-containing drugs, barbiturates and was a terminal case. He had to give up his medical practice in March 1974 having taken steroids such as cortisone for more than twenty years.

In his youth, Dr. Blount was active physically, although his arthritic symptoms began as a systemic (throughout the body) illness in his teens with muscle pain, pain in the foot, pain in the back, between ribs pain, inflammation of eye (iridocyclitis), and skin lesions, (psoriasis). Eventually he got pains in the joints, generalized arthritis with fluids into joints, compression of nerve in the wrist (carpal tunnel syndrome), inflammation of the colon, (ulcerative colitis), death of a femoral head for which a steel and plastic joint was inserted, and numerous other problems.

"I cured myself and more than 17,000 others of an incurable illness -- rheumatoid arthritis -- which is a disease of the entire body, not of just the joints although most of the pain and destruction seems to be in and around the joints. I was hopelessly ill."

In the Spring of 1974 Dr. Blount developed complete destruction (aseptic necrosis) of his right hip socket and femoral head. He had to quit his private medical practice and take to bed. The only thing that would help to walk was a hip replacement with a steel and plastic joint (prosthesis)."

"Despair set in, I could only lie in bed and stare at the ceiling. The cure of my illness was hopeless. No one knew the cause. No one knew anything useful to do for it."

While lying in bed Dr. Blount's arthritis became complicated by colitis (inflammation of the colon) with diarrhea of sometimes up to twenty times a day, kidney stones, alcohol, and drugs. He was in and out of hospitals repeatedly. He thought he'd surely die. Friends kept sending word that they were praying for him, and he often thought of committing suicide. The pain and agony was unbearable.

One morning, after he had accumulated about forty sleeping pills, he swallowed them all. Four have been known to kill. " I didn't want to kill myself, but I couldn't endure such perpetual agony. After some hours my wife found me unconscious and on finding the empty bottle, she knew what I had done. I awoke very groggy and tied to a hospital bed."

Having given up his medical practice, now an alcoholic and on powerful drugs, Dr. Blount, an otherwise spiritual person, continued to hope for a miracle, which at last came.

He discovered the work of Professor Roger Wyburn-Mason, M.D., Ph.D., an English nerve specialist, who'd written an interesting book titled *The Causation of Rheumatoid Disease and Many Human Cancers.* Apparently Professor Roger Wyburn-Mason was curing folks of rheumatoid arthritis.

Dr. Blount found a way to obtain a chemical compound related to the one used by Dr. Roger Wyburn-Mason in treating arthritics, and Dr. Blount's miracle, at last, occurred -- he was free of rheumatoid arthritis, although the permanent damage done to tissues, cartilage, sinew, and bones still remained, just as the ending of a war leaves behind scattered debris, everywhere wasted.

"I decided to find out if some of my former rheumatoid arthritis patients were brave enough to try the same treatment. I telephoned them and invited several of them to my home, one at a time. To each I explained the treatment. Every single one was eager to try it. Nothing else had ever helped. Why not? During the Summer of 1977 about thirty of them were treated and most of them had the same good experience that I had."

Dr. Blount, reinvigorated, reopened his medical clinic. Swiftly by word of mouth, thousands from throughout the United States visited him seeking the same treatment and wellness from rheumatoid arthritis and related diseases, including the authors.

Dr. Blount writes, "I pray that the entire world will soon know and people everywhere can receive the same relief that I have. What a joy I know now! I thank God!

"Galloping" arthritis means that rheumatoid arthritis and its symptoms are progressing very rapidly. Although both of us greatly benefitted from a new treatment for rheumatoid arthritis developed by English physician Roger Wyburn-Mason, M.D., Ph.D., one in particular, Anthony di Fabio, suffered from what his family doctor described as "galloping" rheumatoid arthritis.[7]

It began at age 53. The first pangs of rheumatoid arthritis were passed off as simply unimportant, transitory pains in toes, fingers, and groin of unknown origin. Later visits to medical specialists suggested that persistent shoulder pains were from "degenerative arthritis." This diagnosis of osteoarthritis was confirmed by medical doctors at the

Veteran's Administration Hospital.

During the following year fatigue sapped strength making for hopeless despair. Excessive work and responsibility, increasing pain, apathy, and the knowledge that there would be no relief -- no cure -- from this new burden conspired to precipitate divorce.

Which was it? Rheumatoid arthritis? Osteoarthritis? Or both?

There's little question that various physical exercises kept the joints fluid, although painfully so at times, but the greatest puzzle was that within two years of the   initial   diagnosis of "degenerative" arthritis, the small finger on the right hand began to turn sidewise, and a typical rheumatoid arthritic hard nodule had begun to form there. It was only later that we learned from Professor Roger Wyburn-Mason, M.D., Ph.D., an English nerve disease specialist who developed the first consistently successful treatment for rheumatoid arthritis, that all forms of arthritis should be rested, as joint activity increases inflammation and pain and prevents healing.

Pains continued to increase at various joints, and finally, about three years into the disease, the hands began to flush red and hot and to swell, especially on arising early mornings. A great number of like symptoms in other joints lasted throughout the day.

Now the little finger on the left hand began to twist, and all the joints at the hands began to almost glow a fire-red. Under such swelling and pain, have you tried to open ordinary bottles: catchup, pickle jars, soft drinks?   Lifting pots and pans becomes an exceedingly painful chore. Changing a tire without help is excruciatingly difficult. Everything becomes a carefully choreographed ritual to avoid incurring more pain.

A pall of hopelessness extended from this sufferer to family and friends, and   finally even to   passing   acquaintances who could instinctively sense the unhappiness carried about by this rapidly aging man.

How could one make fast friends when daily the body changes, and daily one becames weaker and much more ineffective? How could long-range committments be kept, or strong personal relationships be acknowledged? How fair is it to impose such burdens -- future helplessness and twisted grotesqueness -- on those you love ? As must be true with thousands of other arthritics in similar circumstances, the thought is there -- that death is preferred over the condition of   helpless crippling endured in persistent pain.

A kind of miracle occurred, just when it was most needed. We both discovered Jack M. Blount, M.D., a physician in Philadelphia, Mississippi who had also been a victim of rheumatoid arthritis, but was not only cured, but was curing thousands of people with a new treatment. One of us (Gus J. Prosch, Jr., M.D.) was cured of a long-standing back pain as well as a swollen knee. The other of us (Anthony di Fabio) was cured within weeks:

• After two weeks the puffiness and redness of fingers disappeared for the first time in a half year.

• After four weeks the pain, depression and fatigue ended.

• After seven weeks the redness of finger joints nearly disappeared; his attitude toward life and people changed remarkably, and again life was worth the effort, and so were people and personal relations. Daily he could turn more bottle tops, and lift heavier loads, and wrestle playfully with another without screaming bloody murder! Best of all, extreme apathy was gone, as was middle-of-day fatigue!

During the next two years the importance of stress reduction, proper nutrition, observing food allergies, chelation therapy, and sustaining a yeast-free body were learned and utilized; and these were but a beginning -- and still disease free nineteen years later, at age 72!

In advising other physicians, one of us (Gus J. Prosch, Jr., M.D.) Birmingham, Alabama, pleads: "If you're sincere and truly desire to relieve the agony and suffering of your arthritic patients, I beg of you to give our recommended treatments a trial on several of your rheumatoid arthritis and osteoarthritis patients. I promise that you will receive superior results in relieving your patient's pain, suffering, and disability more than anything you've ever used before."

You'll be treating the cause of the rheumatoid disease and not simply the symptoms.

You can now offer these severely neglected patients far more than the simple 'hope' of finding relief which conventional methods of treatment cannot even offer. You'll be offering them total relief which will literally change the entire lives of these patients and their families.

"You'll never find the satisfaction and pleasure of helping your fellowman any more than by using these techniques to treat your arthritic sufferers. You'll totally and thoroughly understand what I mean when certain patients come to you in a wheelchair and after receiving your treatment and injections by our recommended techniques, they refuse to use the wheelchair to leave your office, but walk out instead!"

Contrary to mythology stemming from traditional practicing rheumatologists, there are very good treatments that will bring about remission or actual cure of rheumatoid arthritis.

What Joy! What contentment! What satisfaction!

Good luck and God be with you!"[181]

What is Rheumatoid Arthritis?

The symptoms of rheumatoid arthritis are: destruction and deformity of joints; lethargy and depression; may affect every body tissue; presenting symptoms with differing names; increasing number of painful joints; joint tenderness with limitation of movement; increasing number of painful joints; swollen and heated joints; and symmetric joint deformities

Not knowing the cause or causes, traditional medicine considers rheumatoid arthritis as a chronic inflammatory disease that affects symmetrically placed joints, and usually also affects other organs and systems. There is a recognition that rheumatoid arthritis can be a disease of the whole body, that is, act systemically.

Rheumatoid arthritis can simmer for years, with marginal symptoms, and then flare up suddenly, creating serious problems, flaring down just as abruptly. More often than not, it continues unabated, destroying joints and other organs, leaving the victim crippled and depressed.

Distribution of Rheumatoid Arthritis

Arthritis and related "auto-immune" or collagen tissue diseases are among the most prevalent chronic conditions in the United States, affecting perhaps 40 million people in 1995 with a projected 60 million to be affected by 2020.[250] According to the *Textbook of Internal Medicine*,[1] every population on earth has citizens who suffer from rheumatoid arthritis. In the United States, it has been estimated that there are about 6-6.5 million. About 1% to 2% of all populations are affected, with women 2 to 3 times more frequently than men.

Yakima Indians and urban South African blacks have unexplained higher incidence of the disease.

Onset may be at any age, but normally occurs between ages of 35 and 45, peak age of onset being between 25 and 55 years.

Embryos and newly born children may show signs of rheumatoid arthritis, called "Still's disease." Older children, with the same disease, also can have rheumatoid arthritis, called, "juvenile arthritis."

Clinical Symptoms

First signs of rheumatoid arthritis are usually joint stiffness -- particularly fingers -- on arising in the morning. This early sign may also occur with other diseases, such as osteoarthritis.

Although other diseases may develop first, such as a compression of nerves in the wrist producing numbness, tingling or pain, called "carpal tunnel syndrome," or "polymyalgia rheumatica," a generalized inflammation of the large arteries characterized by aching and stiffness, most will develop sweating at night, generalized and transient muscle pains, undue fatigue, lethargy, and episodes of pain and stiffness in the shoulders, knuckles, wrists or other joints.

Often the onset will follow after severe trauma, such as emotional problems, surgery or pregnancy.

Over time, an increasing number of joints will become painful, and there may be weight loss and loss of appetite.

There will be joint tenderness, often heated, swollen and quite painful.

Eventually, left untreated, joints become disfigured and, in many cases, crippling may be permanent, or require prosthesis, that is, joint replacement.

Associated Conditions

Rheumatoid arthritis has been associated with about 80 differently named diseases. There are two kinds of classifications among these 80 diseases: (1) auto-immune diseases, and (2) collagen tissue diseases.

According to English Professor Roger Wyburn-Mason, M.D., Ph.D.,[8] nerve specialist and author of *The Causation of Rheumatoid Disease and Many Human Cancers* (precis available through this foundation) and other books, all of the auto-immune diseases and the collagen tissue diseases grade into one another in a continuous spectrum, with one person having more of one uniquely named condition than another. "Rheumatoid arthritis," Professor Wyburn-Mason has said, "is just one among the 80 that are all related to each other depending upon the organ or system affected." Professor Wyburn-Mason named these 80 diseases "rheumatoid disease."

Rheumatoid arthritis -- as one of the 80 rheumatoid diseases -- is traditionally viewed by both victim and their doctor as a "joint" disease. Although much pain, swelling and destruction appears in the joint, that is only the visible portion of the disease, as the disease is actually manifesting itself throughout the whole body. It is both an auto-immune disease and a collagen tissue disease acting upon all systems of the body.[8]

****

Tissues Affected by Rheumatoid Disease

Arteries: Periarteritis

Bone: Paget's disease, cysts, myelomas

Brain and Cord: Tremors, seizures

Bronchi: Bronchitis, intrinsic asthma

Cardiac: Dysrhythmias, myocardial disease, pericardial disease

Cecum: Appendicitis, mesenteric adenitis

Colon: Ulcerative colitis

Endocrine: Thyroid, parathyorid, thymus, pituitary, adrenal, gonads

Esophagus and Stomach: Atropic mucosa (pernicious anemia), webs

Eyes: Iridocyclitis, expohthalmias

Fascial Planes: Bursitis

Female Genitals: Ovarian cycsts, fibroids, salpingitis-sterility, tubal pregnancies

Functional Central Nervous System: Neuroses, psychoses, senility

Hemopoetic: Systemic lupus erythematosus, polycythemia, purpura

Joints: Arthritis
Kidneys: Pyelonephritis, calculi
Liver: Hepatitis, cholangitis, gallbladder disease
Lower Small Gut: Regional enteritis, Crohn's disease
Lungs: Alveolitis
Lymphatics: Lymphomas, splenomegaly
Meninges: Headache, meningomas
Muscles: Myositis
Nerves*: Trigeminal neuralgia*, mutliple sclerosis*
Nose and Throat: Rhinitis, eustachian salpingitis, enlarged tonsils & adenoids,
etc.
Ovum: Fetal deformities, abortions
Pancreas: Pancreatitis, maturity diabetes, noninsulin dependent diabetes
Salivary & Tear Glands: SICCA syndrome, Sjogrens syndrome
Skin: Psoriasis, alopecia, erythemas, urticaria
Spine: Degenerated discs, low back syndrome
Tendons: Tendonitis, ganglion
Upper Gut: Coealic disease

---

* Professor Roger Wyburn-Mason, M.D., Ph.D. cautioned against using the specific anti-microorganism drugs for nerve diseases that are recommended for the other above conditions, as the presence of toxins in a sensitive subject as evidenced by tissue antigens can cause violent exaggeration of symptoms due to action of the drugs against the organisms.
※※

Genetic Marker

According to the *Textbook on Internal Medicine*,[1] the following genetic factors or relationships are associated with the possibility of having rheumatoid arthritis: (1) There is a slight increase in rheumatoid arthritis among those of first-degree relatives, where one has developed it; (2) Thirty percent of one of the identical twins will develop the disease if the other twin develops it, as opposed to 5% in nonidentical twins; (3) In Asian, Indian, Swiss and Ashkenazi Jews, the disease is associated with a noticeable percentage of those who carry certain genes, called genetic markers; (4) In those who have rheumatoid arthritis, there are five identifiable subtype genes (genetic markers) -- as measured by mixed white blood cell culture -- that seem to be related to inheritance of genes which are adversely affected by an infectious agent; (5) In a rather imprecise test called "Rheumatoid Factor," or "RF test" somewhere between 50-95% of those who have rheumatoid arthritis have specific measurable proteins, called "immunoglobulins," in their blood that act as protective antibodies to foreign invaders. There is a noticeable association of a particular gene with a positive measure of this Rheumatoid Factor (RF). (Rheumatoid Factor is misnamed, as many other disease conditions will also show a positive reading, when measured.)

Diagnosis
There are seven criteria used to identify rheumatoid arthritis, according to the American Rheumatism Association[1], as follows:

1. On arising in the morning, there is stiffness in and around the joints lasting at least an hour before best improvement. This is the customary "first sign" of rheumatoid arthritis, but it can also apply to many other conditions. Later, the following remaining factors also apply:

2. At least three joints have simultaneous soft tissue swelling or fluid, rather than only bony overgrowth. Fourteen areas affected may be the right or left finger joints closest to the nails (distal interphalangeal), the second joints from the end of the fingers (proximal interphalangeal) (also affected by osteoarthritis), and the knuckles (metacarpophalangeal joints), wrist, elbow, knee, ankle and, from the toe nails, the second toe (metatarsophalangeal) joints. (See Figure 1: "Names of Joints of Right Hand," Chapter I, Osteoarthritis.)

3. At least one joint is swollen.

4. There is simultaneous involvement of joints on opposite sides of the body, although not necessarily matching joints.

5. There are observable subcutaneous nodules over bony prominences or other related joint regions.

6. Positive Rheumatoid Factor (RF) -- a non-specific immunoglobulin laboratory test -- as measured from the patient's blood. Many other diseases also have a strong "Rheumatoid Factor" without also involving rheumatoid arthritis, or related rheumatoid diseases, and so this sign must be evaluated only in association with many other factors.

7. X-ray (radiographic) changes that show erosions or bony decalcification, excluding osteoarthritis.

When rheumatoid arthritis begins after age 60, it is twice as likely to come on suddenly, and most often will resemble a generalized inflammation of the large arteries, especially of the temple and back of the head. This condition, called "polymyalgia rheumatica," often resembles an influenza-like attack, with low-grade fever, malaise, loss of appetite and weight loss. There will be aching and stiffness involving mainly the trunk and muscle groups nearest the center of the body.

Usually headaches are severe, with throbbing pain in the temple with redness, swelling, tenderness and nodulation -- little knots -- of the temporal artery, whose pulsations may be strong, weak or even absent.

Older rheumatoid arthritics who display symptoms of polymyalgia rheumatica may also suffer from inflammation of the shoulder and hip membranes (synovitis), but may have an absence of the Rheumatoid Factor, subcutaneous nodules, and elevated Red Blood Cell Sedimentation Rate (ESR), a test which evaluates the extent of tissue response to inflammation and other factors.

In older people, joint stiffness of a severe and crippling nature with severe pain is the normal set of symptoms.

What Causes Rheumatoid Arthritis?

The Immunological Response

There are many factors that cause rheumatoid arthritis which will be discussed briefly in this chapter.

Whatever the cause for rheumatoid arthritis, something triggers an immune response to the synovial membrane, the lubricating fluid of the joints, resulting in antibody production against it. Antibodies play a key role in immunity. These large protein molecules (antibodies), formed by blood and lymph cells in response to foreign protein invaders (antigens), bind to the foreign invaders (antigens) and enhance the foreign body's removal from our bodies. The antibodies do their job by combining with antigens, forming immune complexes, called "immunocomplexes."

The immune complexes, in turn, bind complement, a natural component of our blood that assists in killing bacteria.

The immune complex-complement unit is then destroyed by roaming cells called phagocytes that search out these immune complex-complement particles.

Several cell-toxic chemicals are produced during this entire process which causes significant joint and other tissue damage. Often referred to as "free-radicals," these biochemicals are lysosomal enzymes (enzymes that dissolve), superoxide radicals (chemicals with active oxygen), lymphokines (secretions from activated T cells), and activated complement enzymes -- all of which can damage cells and tissues by means of destruction of the molecular integrity of the chemicals that make up the cells.

Multiple Causation

Rather than one source-cause, we find that inflammatory and destructive sequences found in rheumatoid arthritis is a manifestation of a diseased condition of the body from multiple sources, among which are (1) an inadequate or weakened immunological system; (2) a developed internal allergic response to unknown allergens; (3) candidiasis, effects of a yeast/fungus and other organisms-of-opportunity, (4) external allergies such as pollens, chemical sensitivities, and food allergies;[15,16] (5) lack of appropriate nutrition, including vitamins, minerals, and essential fatty acids; (6) hormonal imbalances and metabolic problems; (7) stress; (8) trauma and infections from sports injuries and surgery; (9) exposure to infectious organisms; (10) pollution, metal toxicities, intake of harmful chemicals, etc.; (11) other unknown factors.[5]

English Professor Roger Wyburn-Mason, M.D., Ph.D.,[4,5,7] pioneer in rheumatology, cancer and the nervous system, taught that until the discovery of the syphilis spirochete, *Treponema pallidum*, this

dreaded disease, syphilis, would have been classified by medicine as
an ideal example of a defective immunological system — just as
many rheumatologists now view rheumatoid disease.

Had the syphilis spirochete not been discovered, billions of ineffective dollars would have been spent searching for a way to "modulate,"
that is, "change," the immunological system, just as is being done today
for rheumatoid arthritis.

Medical researcher Thomas McPherson Brown, M.D. -- also a
pioneer in the treatment of rheumatoid diseases -- based on experiences
similar to those of Roger Wyburn-Mason, M.D., Ph.D., wrote that, with
the exception of osteoarthritis, "all the many and varied types of this
affliction [arthritis] have an inflammatory component, they all show
connective-tissue damage, and they all are under the aegis of a process
which resembles the autoimmune reaction."

In a real autoimmune reaction the body destroys its own cells. The
primary target of attack in rheumatoid arthritis is not ones' own cells.
What is called the autoimmune reaction in all these forms of arthritis is
actually the body's natural defense against an infection in the connective
tissues. The body attacks disease agents that cling to the cells or are
embedded within them. The infectious agent and the body's reaction
cause the inflammation, pain, and eventual disfigurement of rheumatoid arthritis. When the body makes that response, it also attacks the cell
to which the disease agent is connected. But if the agent is taken away,
the body immediately stops the attack.

According to Dr. Brown, "This process differs from true autoimmu-
nity in that one important aspect. It can be stopped, and true autoimmu-
nity cannot."[109]

Prior to the discovery of the tubercle bacillus, *Mycobacterium
tuberculosis*, there were perhaps 100 different names (and therefore
presumed to be 100 different diseases) for external symptoms
observed by physicians.

After the discovery of the syphilis spirochete and the tubercle
bacillus — single source-causations — syphillis was no longer viewed
as a defect of the immunological system, but rather an infectious
disease; and those one hundred tuberculosis names collapsed into one
name: tuberculosis of the spine, of the lung, of the skin, of the bone, and
so on.[4,5,7]

Historically, rheumatoid disease seems to represent characteristics of both syphilis and tuberculosis in that:

• like syphilis, nearly all pharmaceutical research is aimed at
proving that the individual's immunological system is defective and
therefore needs changed (modulated) by some drug that damages the
immunological system even further;

• like tuberculosis, there have been created many different names
-- eighty -- on the viewing of differing reumatoid disease symptoms, but

in fact all of the different names belong to the same disease process --
rheumatoid disease.

Seldom are the eighty or so named rheumatoid diseases found pure
and isolated, but rather there will be components of many distinctly
classified diseases found in the same patient, indicating an underlying
commonality, now newly named under the cluster heading of "rheumatoid disease."[8] All eighty rheumatoid diseases have a commonality in
that they are all collagen tissue diseases or appear to be "auto-immune"
diseases which are pervasive, affecting every portion of the anatomy
as described in a long listing of diseases described by Professor Roger
Wyburn-Mason, M.D., Ph.D. in the preceeding pages. (See, "What is
Rheumatoid Arthritis?")

Theories as to Causation of Rheumatoid Arthritis and
Related Rheumatoid Diseases

During the inflammatory process which we call rheumatoid arthritis, there is formed lysosomal enzymes (enzymes that dissolve), superoxide radicals (chemicals with active oxygen), lymphokines (secretions from activated T cells), and activated complement enzymes, often
referred to under the general heading of "free-radical pathology."
Rheumatoid arthritis results from the damage done to our tissues by
"free radical pathology."

Elmer M. Cranton, M.D. and James P. Frackleton, M.D.[171] have
outlined how reactive chemicals inside the human body bring about
diseased conditions and premature aging. These chemicals usually are
atoms or molecules that have the power to attach to or displace other
normal atoms or molecules in our tissues, thus bringing about improper
or inappropriate functioning of an organ or tissue. A simple example is
the aging of rubber which, after time, or through exposure to various
chemicals or by means of the disassociating effects of ultraviolet light,
will crack and no longer stretch as it once did. In an analogous manner,
our body cells, tissues, organs and systems may not respond for repair
and other normal functions as before, because of the effects of free
radical pathology.

Corazon Ilarina, M.D.[14], of the Bio Medical Health Center, in Reno,
Nevada, basis her medical practice on the idea that toxins are "trapped"
in collagen (connective) tissue, and that these toxins may be from virus,
bacteria, fungi, chemicals, foods and drugs. Helping the body to clean
out these toxins produces wellness.

Other physicians, of course, have other approachs, such as rebalancing an unbalanced hormonal system. [195,196]

There is truth in all of the above theories, as well as substance in
the practices derived from the theories, and, insofar as they lead to
wellness, none of them can be faulted.

Two Accepted Theories of Causation

Medical textbooks provide two theories that stand out from all others:

(1) Something has gone wrong with our immunological system, and the cells designed to protect us are attacking good tissues.

(2) We were born with, or develop a tissue sensitivity to toxins, or proteins of foreigns invaders, microorganisms such as bacteria, protozoa, yeast/fungi, mycoplasmas (bacteria without cell walls), and viral. This tissue sensitivity can also extend to external sources, such as foods, airborne chemicals, and pollens. When antigens from foreign invaders attach themselves to our synovial (and other) tissues, our immunological system sends in fighters to destroy them, and inadvertantly also destroys our good tissues.

Although both theories are acceptable to the established medical profession,[1] only the first receives the majority of funding from pharmaceutical companies who have an interest in convincing us that their patented, "immuno-modulating" or anti-inflammatory drugs are better than someone elses. "Immuno-modulating" is a general term referring to attempts to somehow change our defensive system in some unknown biochemical manner.

Considering the billions of research dollars already expended in defense of the "something's-wrong-with-your-immunological-system" theory -- its abysmal lack of success in bringing about cures -- and the striking successes in pursuing the second theory, one can only wonder at the motivation of those who administer research funds.

How the Body Defends Itself

Writing in *Scientific American*, Sir Gustav J.V. Nossal, M.D., Ph.D.,[212] Director of Walter and Eliza Hall Institute of Medical Research and Professor of Medical Biology at the University of Melbourne, Australia, explains that each of us are protected by a wide diversity of cells and molecules that form an army of agents whose ultimate target is against substances called "antigens." These are usually foreign molecules from a micro-organism, or other foreign substances.

Special cells in our bodies called "macrophages" roam about searching for these antigens, ingesting them, and fragmenting them into "antigenic peptides," compounds formed by the union of two or more amino acids which are building blocks for protein.

Pieces of these newly formed peptides are joined to another kind of molecule -- "major histocompatibiility complex" (MHC) -- and are then displayed on the surface of our cells.

Other white blood cells, "T lymphocytes," have receptor molecules that enable each of them to recognize a different peptide-MHC combination.

When T cells recognize a match, they become activated, they divide, and they secret a substance called "lymphokines," chemical signals that mobilize other components of the immune system.

One set of cells that responds to this new signal is the B lymphocytes, which also have on their surface receptor molecules of a single form and shape, a single specificity.

Unlike the receptors of T cells, these B cells can recognize parts of antigens that are free in solution without the major histocompatibiility complex (MHC) molecule attached.

When activated, the B cells begin dividing to increase their numbers and differentiate into "plasma cells" that can secrete "antibody" proteins, which are a soluble form of receptors.

These antibodies bind to antigens that they encounter, and neutralize them -- or precipitate their destruction by means of "complement enzymes," or by scavenging cells.

Some T and B cells have a memory that persists while they circulate in our blood stream, and this is a kind of watchguard in the event the same kind of antigens appear in the future.

Immunization therapy is based on the principle that repeated encounters with the same antigens will prepare us to have quick response and protection against the same foreign invader.

Unfortunately for arthritics, complement enzymes and scavenging cells can also create the damage which we call arthritis. Reasons for doing so are many, but not at all complex to understand and to handle.

The Causations of Rheumatoid Disease

According to the *Textbook of Internal Medicine*[1], the exact cause or causes of rheumatoid arthritis are unknown, but the "possibility" is ventured that multiple agents may initiate rheumatoid arthritis. "Rheumatoid arthritis," they write," is a chronic inflammatory disease of . . . joints that is frequently accompanied by an involvement of other organ systems."

Professor Roger Wyburn-Mason, M.D., Ph.D.,[8,9] has shown in *The Causation of Rheumatoid Disease and Many Human Cancers*, that virtually every organ in the body is involved with the afflictions that accompany rheumatoid arthritis. His nomenclature is most appropriate so we will often refer to "rheumatoid disease," rather than simply to the more limited term "rheumatoid arthritis," the latter referring only to joint dysfunction that may accompany the rheumatoid disease condition.

The proper question, therefore, is "What causes rheumatoid disease?"

The following list is not intended to be all-inclusive, but rather to name those factors that have been found to be important in treating rheumatoid diseases. Also, these factors do not necessarily operate independently, but rather interact in a multitude of different paths. According to Michael T. Murray, N.D.,[211] leading researcher and author in the field of natural medicine, and co-author of *A Textbook of Natural Medicine*, and other books, "Microbial factors, ... , definitely contributes to the disease process of rheumatoid arthritis, but at this time it appears highly unlikely that there is a single causative microbe in rheumatoid arthritis. . . . ." While there are a large variety of bacteria in the bowels composing as much as 60% of the feces, the magnitude of the task set for our immunological system is suggested by the fact that the numbers of *Escherichia coli* bacteria alone surpass the numbers of all humans that have ever lived.[248]

Physicians who have been consistently successful in helping their patients to become well from so-called "incurable" rheumatoid arthritis have paid serious attention to the factor of infection, and to other factors as well, depending on the special requirements of each patient.

Suspected Causes of Rheumatoid Arthritis, and Related Rheumatoid Diseases or Factors that Help to Precipitate the Disease

Type	Source
Dietary Deficiencies	Enzyme deficiencies, insufficient food, unbalanced diet, avoiding good fats and eating wrong fats, vitamin and mineral deficiencies, etc.
Allergies and Chemical Sensitivities	Environmental chemicals: perfume, hair insect sprays disinfectants, et. al. Pollens and plants: eggplant, pepper, potatoes, tobacco, tomatoes, et. al. Chocolate, coffee, milk, soybeans, sugar corn, wheat, et. al.
Genetic Predisposition	Inherit genes similar to those of foreign microorganisms, contribute to enzyme deficiencies, et. al.
Microorganisms	
Amoeba	*Entamoeba histolytica; Limax amoeba*
Bacteria	*Bacillus aerogenes; Borrelia burgdorferi; Brucellae; Campylobacter jejuni; Chylamydiae; Clostridia difficle; Clostridia perfringens* corynebacteria; diptheria bacilli (*Clostridia perfringens*); enterococci; *Escherichia coli; Eysipelothrix rhusiopathiae Gonococci; Haemophilus influenzae; Klebsiella pneumoniae* Meingococci, mycoplasma (pleuro-pneumonia-like); *Mycobacterium tuberculosis; Mycoplasmas pulmonis, Mycoplasmas hyorhinis; Mycoplasmas gallisepticum); Proteus vulgaris; Pseudo monas aeruginosa; Salmonellae; Shigellae; Streptococcus (fecalis, hemolyticus I, infrequens, ignavius, mitis, moniliformis, pyrogenes, non-hemolyticus I, non-hemolyticus II, salivarius; sub-acidus)*[221], *Treponema pallidum; Trepenema pertenue; Yersinia enterocoliticia; Yersinia pseudotuberculsis*
Pleomorphic	Organisms that survive despite stripping off of their cell-walls; and, organisms that can revert to more primitive forms, passing through various structural stages -- protozoal, bacterial, mycoplasmic, yeast/ fungal, even viruses so small that they cannot be filtered out of a solution. These organisms, under a

	suitable environment, can also restructure themselves into any of their prior forms.
Portions or fragments of microorganisms	All of those listed
Rickettsial	An organism occuping a niche between viral and bacterial; require cells for growth; can be filtered; transmitted by lice, fleas, ticks, mites, et. al.
Virus	Epstein-Barr; German measles; hepatitis; influenza; mumps; parovirus rubella, Fifth disease (children's rashes); varicella
Yeast/Fungi	*Candida albicans,* others
Hormonal imbalances and metabolic problems	From dietary deficiencies (prolonged fasting), genetics, stress, use of prescription drugs such as cortisone
Pollution, Metal Toxicities	Automobile exhaust, fluoride, teeth fillings water and air impurities, herbicides and pesticides, et. al.
Sports Injuries and Surgical Operations	Weaken/unbalance immunological system; interfere with meridian flow lines; place exceptional stress on joint members open door for invading microorganisms
Stress	Weaken/unbalance immunological system; unbalance hormonal system; upset appetite, thus nutritional factors
Weakened Immunological System	Sports injuries, surgical operations, stress illness nutritional deficiencies, et. al.

Summary of the Above factors

One, some, or all of the following factors cause rheumatoid disease, operating separately, or in cooperation with other factors.

1. Genetic predisposition.
2. Stress.
3. Dietary deficiencies.
4. Sports injuries and medical operations.
5. Infectious organisms.
6. Allergies and chemical sensitivities.
7. Pollution, metal toxicities, intake of harmful chemicals, etc.
8. Hormonal imbalances and metabolic problems.
9. Weakened immunological system.

1. Genetic Predisposition

Although all of the specific mechanisms are not yet known, it's generally accepted that genetic factors influence susceptibility to rheumatoid arthritis. Embryos have been born with the disease, and small babies can suffer from the disease, called "Still's disease." Children who've been raised under identical circumstances will differ as to which one is subjected to arthritis and which one is not. One identical twin will have a greater probability of acquiring the disease if the other identical twin has acquired it. In certain of the rheumatoid diseases such as ankylosing spondilitis, it is known that the arthritic's gene arrangement bears similarity to gene arrangement of a commonly infecting organism, *Klebsiella pneumoniae.* Certain races and also certain families have a propensity for the disease.

However, if you've once been well, and now are not, it's unlikely that your genes are forcing you to be sick, but more probably you've acquired the disease through associated living conditions of nutritional deficiencies, stress, and the influence of all or many of the above named factors. According to Joel Wallach, D.V.M., N.D., "There are literally dozens of human 'genetic' diseases that can be prevented and in the early stages reversed or 'cured' with minerals."[249]

That one is genetically predisposed, does not necessarily mean that you will suffer health consequences if all other factors are properly controlled. Most of the important factors are within your control. For example: schizophrenia is a group of mental disorders involving disturbances in thinking, mood, and behavior associated with an altered concept of reality. Although schizophrenia and rheumatoid arthritis are usually mutually exclusive; that is, one does not normally find both conditions in the same person, both of these illnesses can occur in the same family.[256]

Researchers have found that the two diseases result from blockage of an enzyme, preventing conversion of the amino acid tryptophane from converting to niacin (B_3). Depending upon where in the bio-chemical conversion chain this blockage occurs, a person may develop either schizophrenia or rheumatoid arthritis, but not both.

As will be described in the section on *Allergies, Biodetoxification, and Chemical Sensitivities*, a proper food elimination diet can solve both problems.

<h2 style="text-align:center">2. Stress</h2>

No subject is more important to wellness than stress management. It's also the subject that physicians tend to ignore, and patients to avoid.

Generally, physicians are not taught the skills of teaching stress management in medical school, most of them being heavily oriented toward drug treatments. Even those who later specialize in mental, emotional and psychic disciplines are not provided with techniques that work effectively, and so, having at best a failed technology, psychiatrists resort to the use of damaging, mood-altering drugs. In like manner, rheumatologists, having at best a failed technology, resort to damaging drugs that also create further stress.

The best that continual reliance upon drugs can do for a distraught mental/emotional state is to temporarily occlude its painful effects, and delay the individual's need to confront "real-world" stimuli. A continuous drugging of sensitive mental/emotional problems continually delays solutions to problems. Meanwhile, the physical aspect of the problem -- which is the opposite side of the mental/emotional state -- continues seeking resolution, that is, restoration of the normal state. Failing this, a "disease" process is established.

In like manner, a continued reliance upon traditional, damaging "immunomodulating" and anti-inflammatory drugs hide rheumatoid arthritis symptoms while the disease rages onward unsensed -- until it becomes too late and permanent damage is evident. (See "Stress," Chapter I, Osteoarthritis.)

3. Dietary Deficiencies

Dietary deficiencies which will later be covered in more detail may be categorized as follows: Eating foods,

(a) that lack appropriate vitamins, enzymes, essential fatty acids and minerals of sufficient quantity and quality that are necessary for the specific individual at a particular time in their life.

(b) that are the wrong foods, and which produce, or generate, an acidic systemic condition, rather than an alkaline condition.

(c) that are non-foods (packaged, processed, frozen, canned, et. al.), as opposed to eating genuine food direct from the garden.

(d) to which an individual has developed an allergy, or developed an allergic response to its components.

(e) to which an individual has developed a chemical sensitivity, or has been genetically endowed with such a response

(f) that support organisms of opportunity, such as *Candida albicans*.

There are and have been many diets to ease the pain and swelling of arthritis, among which has been the Dong diet, based on an age-old Chinese diet of fish, vegetables, rice and small amounts of chicken; the Norman F. Childers, Ph.D. 'no-nightshades' diet, which excludes all members of the nightshade family such as tomatoes, peppers, and tomatoes; low-fat, mainly vegetarian diet; the macrobiotic diet; Pritikin and McDougall diets, and many more.

Many physicians have developed or recommend dietary regimens based on the clinically demonstrated fact that if allergy inducing foods are eliminated, and if the individual has the proper kind of nutritional support, the body will recover and health will ensue. Usually it is through complete, close cooperation with physicians who've made a special effort to learn fundamental nutritional biochemistry beyond their medical school training, that patients obtain fast benefits.

Unfortunately, commonly used medical books, such as *The Merck Manual*,[2] baldly state that diet does not seem to be a factor in producing rheumatoid arthritis.

Physicians who have success in curing rheumatoid diseases know that these books are in error. Dietary factors are very important in producing rheumatoid arthritis, and also dietary factors are very important in achieving wellness from rheumatoid arthritis.

4. Surgery and Sports Injuries

While there has been seldom, if ever, a direct link noted between injuries suffered from surgical procedures or sports accidents and a condition of rheumatoid disease, there have been numerous anectdotal reports linking the two. Usually the arthritic victim reports that "Right after having my operation, I came down with rheumatoid arthritis;" or, "Just after my skiing accident, I began having trouble in my knee, and then it spread, and I was told I had rheumatoid arthritis."

Clearly operations or sports accidents can stretch or tear at tendons and ligaments, and these can result in osteoarthritis that can be healed by the body with the aid of a treatment known as Reconstructive Therapy.[40] (See Chapter I, Osteoarthritis, "Structure.") However, what has been frequently reported is not the relatively simple stretching or tearing of ligments or tendons, but rather the precipitation of active systemic rheumatoid disease.

There are two likely explanations   for this phenomenon, not necessarily mutually exclusive:

(a) The stress created by the accident or operation sufficiently weakened or unbalanced the immunological system to hasten the rheumatoid disease systemic process; and,

(b) The accident or operation permitted the entry, or activation (growth and spread), of microrganisms to which an individual has developed (or been genetically endowed with) a susceptibility to its toxins or protein products, resulting in the manifestations of systemic rheumatoid disease. Changing the bio-chemical balances of the body via stress, antibiotics, and surgery also permit organisms to change forms, known as "pleomorphism." Organisms-of-opportunity prolifer- ate. Some of these various forms are associated with rheumatoid diseases.

5. Infectious Organisms

Describing the search for causative organisms in the condition of rheumatoid arthritis, the erudite publication, *Textbook of Internal Medicine*, states, "Despite intensive search for an initiating microbial agent(s), none has yet been convincingly identified."[1]

Whether or not a microbial source(s) has been found as the causative agent(s) for rheumatoid arthritis depends chiefly on how the disease symptoms are defined. A physician must be sufficiently astute to be able to distinguish symptoms that are "similar to," or "the same as" other symptoms, yet stemming from differing causative stimuli, includ- ing various microorganisms. In addition to food allergies, symptoms of or symptoms similar to rheumatoid arthritis can be created by each of the following organisms:

(a) Yeast: *Candida albicans.*

(b) Bacterial: *Borrelia burgdorferi, Brucella, Gonoccous, Meingococcus, Mycobacterium tuberculosis, Pneumococcus, Propi- onibacterium acnes, Streptococcus, Staphyloccus, Salmonella, Strep- tobacillus moniliformis, Treponema pallidum, Treponema pertenue*, and others.

(c) Rickettsial, an organism that fills the niche between virus and bacteria.

(d) Viral: Mumps, Rubella, Viral hepatitis, and others.

(e) Mycoplasmas, bacteria without cell walls.

A further complication in identifying microbial sources of "arthritic" symptoms is the almost total avoidance by the practicing medical profession of the fact that microorganisms can change size, shape and function depending upon the nature of their surrounding environment; that is, some microorganisms are "pleomorphic."

Microorganisms can also survive antibiotics by stripping off their cell walls, and thereafter pass throughout our bodies as unrecognized interlopers, as it is the cell wall that communicates to our defenses that an invader is present. The facts of pleomorphism and cell-wall deficient organisms are accepted as standard scientific fare by microbiologists and protozoologists, but hardly known to traditional medical practitioners who administer ineffective "modern" medical treatments.[23]

Historically, the gigantic pharmaceutical industry -- and thus the modern medical profession -- is built upon a flawed assumption, which is that for each disease there is one organism which, while living out its own unique life cycle, nonetheless sustains its shape and form, and thus function. A one-to-one correspondence is presumed to be established between components of the life-cycle of this single organism and its influence on our bodies. By ascribing wholly to this sometimes true assumption, billions of dollars are expended by the pharmaceutical industry, and thus medical profession, in attempting to determine a single organism for each named disease.[42,43] Also, although all organisms do not have such complex life cycles, no one knows how many different organisms can create the same set of symptoms in the human body. There may very well be a many-organism to one-set-of-disease symptoms; or, equally, one organism to many different disease symptoms, as, for example, the nearly ubiquitous mycoplasmas, the smallest and simplest self-replicating bacteria also without a cell membrane to separate its inner workings (cytoplasms) from its environment. Mycoplasmas cause arthritis in at least six mammalian avian species: cattle, goats and sheep, pigs, rats, chickens and turkeys.[252] There are reports of similar isolations from humans. But, are these causative? The only cause? Or, one of many causes?

The success of antibiotics over some microorganisms, stemming from the initial use of sulfa drugs during world war II, has further inadvertently reinforced the false assumption that for every disease there is a unique causative organism. But even this success has its dark side. Gerald J. Domengue, Professor, Department of Surgery, Section of Urology and Department of Microbiology and Immunology, Tulane University, School of Medicine, New Orleans, Louisiana,. presented in 1975 to the 75th Annual Meeting of American Society for Microbiology, Enterobacteriaceae Roundtable, New York, New York, in 1975, definitive proof that antibiotics such as penicillin, erythromycin, and other antibiotics destroy the walls of bacteria without killing bacteria, thus making the bacteria invisible to the human defense system. Then later the bacteria restructure themselves, making themselves visible to the human defense system -- and also restoring the body's symptomatic response to the disease. "You've gotten reinfected," the unknowing doctor tells the patient.

Treatment of mycoplasmas with tetracycline and erythromycin appear to reduce disease symptoms, but this is usually not accompanied by eradication of the organisms from the infected host while also building up resistant mycoplasmic strains, according to Shmuel Razin, Department of Membrane and Ultrastructure Research, Hebrew University-Hadassah Medical School, Jerusalem, Israel.[251] Those who have come to rely on long-term usage of tetracycline for and its derivatives (minocycline) should take care.

Although some knowledge of pleomorphism and cell wall deficient microorganisms began with Professor Antoine Bechamp, contemporary of Louis Pasteur, a scientific report published in *Microbia* in 1976 by Gerald J. Domengue et. al.,[43] among many other earlier scientific reports, should have set the stage for revision in thinking as it applied to medical research and the relationship of microorganisms to their surrounding environment, but did not do so. Lida Mattman, Ph.D.,[23] Professor Emeritus, Department of Biology, Wayne State University, Detroit, Michigan, author of *Cell Wall Deficient Forms: Stealth Pathogens*, writes that "Cell Wall Deficient organisms [and pleomorphism] play an important role in many aspects of rheumatology. Wall-deficient gonococci, Mycobacteria, Clostridia, Salmonella, and Corynebacteria have been found in acute arthritis."

Arthritis by Organisms-of-Opportunity

Some microorganisms are well-known, and emminently dangerous to us. A systemic yeast/fungus infection, such as *Candida albicans* and related organisms, often harms us for years, unrecognized as other than localized infection by traditional medicine, such as the many women who are treated for a vaginal yeast infection without understanding or being told that this is a visible symptom of an overall systemic problem, that the whole body needs treated, not simply the vagina.

Candida albicans is found everywhere. It invades various parts of bodily tissues resulting in localized infections. Common sites of infection arc the mouth in infant thrush, gastrointestinal tract, vagina, urinary tract, prostate gland, skin, fingernails and toenails.

Under normal conditions our bodies are able to resist this invasion, as it does other germs. However, whenever various substances weaken the immunological system especially by knocking out our intestinal micro-flora -- as happens with the use of antibiotics -- the yeast/fungus organism begins to spread, and in the spreading creates virtual havoc throughout the body parts and systems.

A chief problem with infestation by candida is that its effects are systemic, and within that systemic invasion symptoms presented can mimic many other diseases, including that of rheumatoid arthritis.

A second primary problem is that candida sufferers will unknowingly become sensitive to an increasing number of foods, presenting with more and more food allergies, and also will become increasingly sensitive to environmental chemicals.

Candida albicans is known to have   six   survival switching mechanisms, that is, different forms and functions, as well as a cell-wall deficient form. Each of these forms, and the seventh cell-wall deficient form, are it's survival response to a changed environment. Like invasive bacteria that have been stripped of their cell walls via routine use of antibiotics, later to reconstruct themself whole, the seventh cell-wall deficient form   passes totally unrecognized by our immunological system, thus forming a reservoir for persistent reinfection.[36]

Once a good population of *Candida albicans,* or similar organisms, have taken root in the human body, especially in the fungal form, it or its toxins can and do invade every tissue, and the results are that it can mimic every form of disease, including various rheumatoid diseases which includes rheumatoid arthritis.

Over time, and in its fungal state, intestinal fungal infections also produce an ever-increasing number of food allergies, the results of which can and do also mimic many different diseases such as rheumatoid diseases which also includes rheumatoid arthritis.

Candida specialist Marjorie Crandall, Ph.D., says, "The existence of the yeast syndrome should have been predicted *a priori* by the medical profession based on well-known microbiological and immunological reactions to yeasts. To deny the existence of chronic candidiasis is to deny . . . patients effective medical care and self-help counseling, and condemn them to needless suffering and disability."[156] (See*Conquering Yeast Infections*, S. Colet Lahoz, R.N., M.S., L.Ac.; *Dr. Crook Discusses Yeasts and How They Can Make You Sick*, William G. Crook, M.D.; *The Yeast Syndrome*, John Parks Trowbridge, M.D., Morton Walker, D.P.M.; *Allergies and Biodetoxification*, Anthony di Fabio; *Candidiasis: Scourge of Arthritics*, Anthony di Fabio; *The Yeast Connection Cookbook*, William G. Crook, M.D.)

Relationship Between Candidiasis and Rheumatoid Disease

Rheumatoid   disease   spreads   with   a   weakening   of   the immunological system. *Candida albicans* spreads with a weakening of the immunological system.

Rheumatoid   disease   as well as candidiasis seems to   lead   to increasing food allergies and chemical sensitivities over time.

Both   diseases   produce, or can produce,   similar   symptoms   in many   bodily tissues.

Both diseases are systemic in nature.

A candidiasis victim does not necessarily have rheumatoid disease, but a rheumatoid disease victim almost certainly suffers from some degree of candidiasis.

Candidiasis spreads with the use of almost any kind of surgery where an antibiotic was used, or if given antibiotics for any purpose one will probably suffer from some degree of candidiasis. Why? Because the antibiotics kill off the "good-guys" bacteria required in your intestinal tract for good nutrition and protection against microbial organisms, whence yeast/fungus spreads taking the "good-guys'" place and sending rootlets into your intestinal mucosa -- the fungal stage -- helping to age your total system. When this happens serious treatment against candidiasis should begin and the "good guys," *Lactobacillus acidophilus*, need be replaced.[53]

More often than not, all rheumatoid disease sufferers, including rheumatoid arthritis victims, unknowingly suffer from an invasion from organisms-of-opportunity, among which, and often most referenced, is the yeast/fungus organism named *Candida albicans*.[36,55,56,57,58,59,60,61,62]

According to Richard A. Kunin, M.D., San Francisco, California, "Intestinal flora are an important factor in arthritic disorders, particularly in cases of chronic inflammation and mucosal barrier damage. The leaky bowel permits antigen to penetrate into the blood stream, where it can excite a condition of immune activation, thus relapsing arthritic joints. In addition, certain organisms, such as Kelbsiella (*Klebsiella pneumoniae*) species, are known to induce joint inflammation. It is a good idea to perform a comprehensive bowel flora study as well as laboratory testing of bowel competency."[129]

Testing for Candidiasis

The normal clinical assessment for candidiasis is a questionaire filled in by the patient, and given to the doctor for review. If a score of a pre-determined value is achieved, it's assumed that the patient is at high risk with candidiasis.[36]

Some physicians have begun to use sophisticated laboratory analysis called "Enzyme-linked Immunosorbant Assay," or "ELISA," coupled with another test called "Candida Immunodiffusion."

Foreign substances derived from yeast/fungus, bacteria, their toxins, or foreign blood cells, when introduced into the human body, are called "antigens." These antigens cause our bodies to produce protein defenses, called "antibodies," or "immunoglobulins."

In the ELISA test, dilutions of a patient's blood are incubated and when certain *Candidia albicans* particles bind to certain protein antibodies, [immunoglobulins (IgG)], the test indicates the presence of candida.

In the Immunodiffusion test, antibodies are detected for specific antigens.

Test reports are provided in a computerized personalized printout for each patient. ELISA tests are reported as an antibody standard of strength per volume tested (titer), while the Immunodiffusion results are reported as either positive or negative. One laboratory capable of performing delicate tests for Candidiasis and Food Allergies is Immuno Laboratories, Inc., 1620 W. Oakland Park Blvd., of Fort Lauderdale, FL, 800-231-9197.[79]

6. Allergies and Chemical Sensitivities

How Allergies Create Inflammatory Arthritis

According to Paul Reilly, N.D.[74] of Tacoma, WA,

• Diet affects bowel flora and gastro-intestinal tract permeability; that is, leakage.

• The nature of bowel flora and gastro-intestinal permeability determine the amount of bacterial toxins released from dying bacteria (endotoxins).

• When these toxins (endotoxins) are absorbed, they become potent activators of biochemical pathways that promote inflammatory processes, including antigen/antibody combinations called immune complexes.

• The liver is the chief organ for eliminating immune complexes, including those from the gut. When the liver has been overloaded, is functioning weakly, or has been damaged, these undegraded antigens are released into the blood system where they lodge in various tissues creating further inflammation.

• Inflammation caused by allergic reactions also contribute to free-radical pathology (an excess of chemicals with power to combine with and disrupt otherwise stable tissue), and that extra burden on the body can contribute to arthritic symptoms as well. After all, free-radical damage is the end product of what arthritis is all about. Cleaning up or preventing the development of extra free-radicals, even temporarily, should give some relief to the arthritic.[75]

Food allergies and tissue sensitivities to environmental chemicals can produce symptoms so similar to rheumatoid arthritis that the normal practicing rheumatologist cannot distinguish between them. Indeed, there may be no difference!

Lendon H. Smith, M.D.[208] of Portland, Oregon, who has written a Foreward to *Dr. Braly's Food Allergy & Nutrition Revolution*, highlights three principles: (1) allergic reactions to foods can be responsible for bedwetting, stomach aches, headaches, colic, arthritis, muscle aches, and, in short, just about any symptom the body is capable of producing -- even obesity; (2) "Food sensitivities can't do everything, but they can do anything;" (3) "Eighty percent of those people with food sensitivities have hypoglycemia." (See James Braly, M.D., *Dr. Braly's Food Allergy & Nutrition Revolution*.)

There are two kinds of allergies: extrinsic (exogenous) and intrinsic (endogenous). Extrinsic allergies are caused by substances external to the human body, such as pollens, house dust, cat fur, and so on. Intrinsic allergies are those caused by substances internal to the human body, such as toxins from microorganisms or the protein products from microorganisms.

There are also two kinds of chemical sensitivities, those which are extrinsic, such as gas fumes, herbicides, pesticides and so on, and those which are intrinsic, minute   substances -- metabolites -- stored in the fatty (lipids) parts of the cells, and also the toxins and protein products of dead microorganisms that have taken up residence in the body.

Sometimes there is a blurred line between allergies and chemical sensitivities, as the body will often respond with one as though the other were present. In either case, with either type of substance, internal or external, allergy inducing or tissue sensitivity to chemicals and toxins, various forms of diseases can be mimicked, including various forms of rheumatoid diseases, including rheumatoid arthritis.

Allergies and chemical sensitivities can also be strongly related to the presence of organisms-of-opportunity, such as the yeast/fungus, *Candida albicans*, and related organisms.

While chemical sensitivities may be distinguishable in most cases to an "allergic" response, food allergies are hardly bio-chemically distinguishable from drug addiction. Warren Levin, M.D. of New York City, New York, calls this a "new concept to the medical profession, but one of great importance to the healing arts, . . . You will notice that I do not speak of allergy or addiction nor of allergy and addiction, but rather of a single entity -- allergy/addiction."[37]

7. Pollution, Metal Toxicities, Intake of Harmful Chemicals, etc.

Tens of Thousands of Pollutants in Air and Water

Gregory S. Ellis, Ph.D., C.N.S. and Allen M. Kratz, PharmD,[254] writing in *Alternative Health Practitioner*, explain that, "Based on our 17 years of experience, we have found that chemicals and metals are the two most pervasive and deepest toxicities. Currently there are 70,000 chemicals in commercial use; 25% are known hazards. Recent reports from the Environmental Protection Agency demonstrated that 100% of the samples of human body fat contained toxic doses of chemicals . . . ," styrene from styrofoam, 1,4-dichlorobenzene from mothballs and house deodorizers, xylene from paints and gasoline, DDT although banned in 1972, cadmium, mercury, lead, beryllium, and antimony, these five metals [are] involved in "at least 50% of the deaths in the United States, and much of the disabling diseases."

It should be clear from the following recital that pollutants, metal toxicities and the intake of other harmful chemicals are pervasive throughout our modern world. Although thousands of studies have shown how the overburdening of our various physiological systems produce or contribute to every form of disease -- including rheumatoid arthritis -- due to external pollutants, there is relatively little control over them.

These pollutants and toxins clog up the lymph system faster than we can drain the debris, and they also create damage to arteries, causing the arteries to narrow, and to distribute ever-lessening nutrients to tissues.

The body must work harder than ever before in man's history to repair damage from unnatural sources. Enzyme systems -- which Professor Hector del Rio Solorzano, M.D., Ph.D., D.Sc., Coordinator of the Program for Studies of Alternative Medicine, University of Guadalajara, Guadaljara, Mexico, describes as the fundamental keystone to life itself -- are constantly immobilized by pollutants.[154] Without properly functioning enzymes systems many disease states are brought into being, including rheumatoid arthritis. (See *Systemic Enzyme Therapy*, Hector E. Solorzano del Rio, M.D., Ph.D., D.Sc.; *Who is Looking After Our Kids*, Harold E. Buttram, M.D., Richard Piccola, M.H.A.)

The Case of Irene Thompson

Dr. John Mansfield,[122] author and allergy specialist in Connecticut, described Irene Thompson from Switzerland, who suffered from many different joint pains and swelling so severe she'd been on cortisone treatment.

When Dr. Mansfield put her on a low-allergy food elimination diet of five foods, she had great improvement in a week, but even so, she still had only 70% improvement of her joint pain and swelling.

Later, when visiting her mother in Zurich, she learned that her joint pains had disappeared 100 percent, but when she returned home her pain and swelling returned.

Dr. Mansfield deduced that it was her gas cooker and gas-fired central heater that created her problem; i.e., chemical sensitivity to the gas and its products.

When Irene turned off her gas line at the main street connection, her joint pain disappeared completely again, thus verifying Dr. Mansfield's deduction.

Irene moved her gas heater to an outhouse. Irene's joints have been as operational and pain-free for five years as they had been while visiting with her mother in Zurich, where her mother had an all-electric flat.

Dr. Mansfield was able to help another women, by discovering that she'd become sensitive to the chlorine in her tap water, and could tolerate the water when it was boiled, and the same occurred with Tony, a farmer, who had become sensitized to chlorine because of his years of use on the farm when sterilizing his dairy equipment.

Dental Poisoning and Root Canal Infections

As has already been discussed in Chapter I, Osteoarthritis, mercury and fluoride contribute greatly to weakening of the immunological system, and to destroying essential enzymes necessary for proper utilization of food. Weakening of the immunological system promises entry for destructive pathogens that may lead to rheumatoid arthritis, and other diseases. Destruction of enzymes means mal-functioning biochemical systems that may lead to rheumatoid arthritis and other diseases.

Sam Ziff and Michael F. Ziff, D.D.S. report that "Within the industrialized world, mercury holds the unique distinction of being the only poison routinely implanted in over 65% of the population. In the United States, this represents approximately 144,000,000 people who are subjected to the chronic inhalation of mercury vapor and the swallowing of corroded particulate 24 hours a day, 365 days a year, as long as the mercury remains implanted in their teeth."[143]

Removing mercury fillings is a growing movement. Keith W. Sehnert, M.D., Gary Jacobson, D.D.S., and Kip Sullivan, J.D.[126] -- based on completed studies and clinical practices -- believe that we often overlook the single most important source of auto-immune disorders -- the toxic mercury fillings in our teeth. They say, "The use of mercury amalgams has been banned and are on a scheduled phaseout in Germany, Austria, Denmark and Sweden." Mercury toxicity, they feel, leads to generalized morning stiffness, skin rashes, dry eyes and mouth, joint pain, immune dysfunction, lymph node swelling (axillary), skin bumps (subcutaneous nodules), ringing in the ears, burning and numbness sensations, chronic fatigue, depression and/or environmental sensitivities. Of great pertinence, these are the same symptoms one finds with those suffering from one or more of the eighty auto-immune/collagen tissue diseases, including rheumatoid arthritis.

It would be well to find a dentist sympathetic to the problem of mercury toxicity, and have yourself tested to determine if mercury leakage has reached a level of possible damage, in which case, replacement of the fillings by a more neutral substance might very well result in complete remission of whatever the disease appears to be. A word of caution: unless the dentist is especially trained, as would be a "biological dentist," the willy-nilly removal of mercury amalgams may very well cause the inhalation and absorption of more organic mercury then before. Some who have endured amalgam removal by an untrained dentist developed other diseases related to mercury, such as chronic fatigue syndrome. Although biological dentists are not located near you, it is worth the travel and additional expense to have the work performed properly.

The Case of Connie Anderson

Connie Anderson suffered miserably from muscle and joint aches, headaches, and overall, extreme lethargy, with repeated infections from yeast, colds and flu. After more than a year of ineffective antibiotics prescribed by various physicians, Connie read a book by Hal Huggins, D.D.S., *It's All in Your Head*.[191] She traveled 250 miles to consult with biological dentist Stephan Cobble, D.D.S., who, after testing, began Connie on a planned program of mercury fillings replacement.

Almost immediately Connie's immunological system recovered. During the past five years Connie has not had her otherwise persistent muscle and joint aches, headaches or lethargy. She's seldom been sick since that moment forward.

In another teeth-related poison, the effects of municipal fluoridation of water systems are, by themselves, long-ranging, enigmatic and monstrous, covering the range of diseases which include osteoporosis, fluorosis, broken bones, weakened immunological system, and more.[153] (See *Fluoridation: Governmentally Approved Poison*, Anthony di Fabio.)

Volatile Organic Compounds (VOCs)

Tissue sensitivity that produces arthritis symptoms derives from chemical and metal pollutants. According to Harold E. Buttram, M.D. and Richard Piccola, M.H.A., authors of *Our Toxic World: Who's is Looking After the Children*,[263] Quakertown, Pennsylvania, "Volatile Organic Compounds (VOCs) consist of a very large class of commercial chemicals which tend to evaporate into and contaminate indoor air of buildings. They enter the human system not only by inhalation but also through skin absorption. . . . 70,000 chemicals are used in commerce, of which several hundred are known to be toxic . . . less than 10% have had any testing for neurotoxicity, and only a handful of these have been evaluated thoroughly."

In one study conducted on 400 residents of New Jersey, North Carolina, and North Dakota,   10 volatile chemicals were commonly found in indoor air, drinking water, and exhaled breaths.

Since a vast majority of the pollutants are fat soluble, and the brain consists mainly of fat, the pollutants or their metabolites get stored in brain tissue as well as other fatty cells. Acute symptoms include dizziness, forgetfulness, headaches, mental fogginess, difficulty concentrating, and poor coordination. In a University of Pittsburgh study findings included social alienation, poor concentration, anxiety, and impairments in learning and memory as compared with those not exposed. Children may be up to 10 times more vulnerable to chemical toxins than adults.

William Crook, M.D., Jackson, Tennessee, author of *The Yeast Connection* and *Solving the Puzzle of Your Hard to Raise Child*, commented that when he first went into practice in Tennessee in the 1950's, he could not recall that he ever observed a hyperactive child during those years. Now they are found in every classroom, as any teacher will attest. It is more than coincidental that the present epidemic of hyperactivity and behavioral problems among school children has coincided with steadily increasing levels of Volatile Organic Compounds (VOCs) found in modern buildings. Just as coal miners once carried canaries into their mines to provide an early warning of poisonous gases, we have sent in our children. Standard texts in neurotoxicology point out that behavioral problems may be the earliest sign of chemical toxins.[130]

The Drugging of America

The American drug/medical treatment business is nearly a trillion-a-year industry.[246] "Internationally, the illegal narcotics industry has estimated annual revenues of between $500 billion and $1 trillion."[246] The order of magnitude of drug usage (legal and illegal) -- and drug dependence -- and unnatural adversely affecting biochemicals produced by commercial interests and unwittingly experienced or consumed by humans in America ranks with at least our war military budget totals, if not the national debt![246]

Socially Accepted Drugs

According to Robe B. Carson's[246] report on the *Proceedings from the Sixth International Conference on Drug Policy Reform* of the Drug Policy Foundation, "America's biggest drug problem is not street drugs but legal medical drugging which attacks symptoms while ignoring the cause of disease, which is never caused by a lack of a synthetic pharmaceutical. Also ignored is the fact that the symptom (e.g fever) is often the body's wise, proven way of dealing with a problem (e.g., proliferating germs). Thus the symptom-chasing drug subverts the body's own curative efforts, the only ones that work safely. With its cause left unaddressed, disease persists and becomes deeply entrenched generating repetitive demands for symptom-oriented drugs."

Socially Unaccepted Drugs

The economic facts of just one illegal narcotic, cocaine, is staggering:[246]

An estimated 30 to 60 tons of cocaine worth $55 billion is imported into the United States yearly; 3,000 try it for the first time each day; 600,000 young people ages 12-17 have used cocaine wthin the past year; 20 to 40 million Americans have tried cocaine within the past year; over 1.1 million young people have tried cocaine;

Cocaine, in all of its commonly used forms including 'crack', has been associated with sudden heart attacks in people under the age of 30, some of whom had used the drug for the first time; babies exposed to cocaine in the womb often don't cuddle or nurse well and may be generally irritable and unresponsive, making them hard to care for, with additional serious problems for their future and also society's.[246]

Pesticides and Herbicides

The proof that pesticides and herbicides can produce arthritis and related symptoms lies with the successful use of detoxification programs. Repeated testing of lipid-stored (fat-stored) toxins show a decrease in levels as arthritic symptoms decrease.

In addition to prescription and street drugs, the human being is burdened with increasing intolerable commercial chemicals.[246]

Found in retail store waxed produce are fungicides benomyl, benzflor, botran, carbendazim, diphenyl, imazilil, orthophenylamine, orthophenylphenate, orthophenylphenol, sodium orthophenylphenate, and thiabendazole.

The FDA has tested less than 2/10ths of 1% of domestic food production. It does not regularly test for a number of pesticides, so don't count on all food stuffs being safe.[246]

According to James P. Carter, M.D., Dr. PH, Tulane University, Louisiana, "There is almost no toxicity data for 80% of the 49,000 commercially-used chemicals; data is inadequate or non-existent for 64% of 3,400 pesticides and inert ingredients; they are also inadequate or non-existent for 74% of 3,400 cosmetic ingredients, for 61% of 1,800 drugs, and for 80% of 8,600 food additives. In the work-force, 20%-35% of workers are affected by chemicals in building materials, chemicals which cause illness, absenteesim, and low productivity."[246]

Even the inert ingredients in pesticides are not inert. According to Jule Klotter in "Toxins in Pesticides," *Townsend Letter for Doctors*, "Forty of the ingredients that fall under the 'inert' category are considered toxic by the Environmental Protection Agency (EPA) and probably cause cancer, brain/nervous system poisoning, and reproductive effects. Another 60 are 'potentially toxic' because of their similarity to known harmful compounds. Inert ingredients make up 85% of most pesticide formulas. Why the EPA has not required inert ingredients to be listed is a puzzle, especially when it leads to the following bizarre situation: one of the inert ingredients of the lawn herbicide Roundup® is polyoxiethleneaminc (POEA), which is more toxic than glyphosate, the listed active ingredient."[246]

Impure Drinking Water

As rheumatoid disease, including rheumatoid arthritis, is linked to various microorganisms, as well as to environmental toxins, source of entry into the human body is also from drinking water. Americans are ingesting such noxious pollutants as bacteria, viruses, lead, gasoline, radioactive gases and carcinogenic industrial compounds.[246]

Pathogens that may bring about arthritic symptoms include bacteria, mycoplasma, viruses and protozoa. Clear evidence of public exposure from our drinking waters is seen with the cryptosporidium outbreak that struck Milwaukee, Wisconsin.

Nationwide various microorganisms sicken 900,000 people a year, . . . usually those with weak immune systems, such as arthritics, the very young and very old, AIDS sufferers and organ-transplant patients.[139,140]

Milk and Meat Poisoning

Danila Oder writes that Bovine Growth Hormone (BGH) may be perfectly safe for the cow while biochemically forcing the cow to provide more milk (on an already milk-gutted market) but the health problems associated with its use have been wholly overlooked by the FDA. These include increased udder infections by the cow, and therefore increased usage of antibiotics. The antibiotics are sure to enter into the milk supply, thus adding tremendously to an already overburdened immunological system.[144] Increased use of antibiotics in our food supply also means the creation of more cell wall deficient or pleomorphic organisms accompanying our nourishment, which can lead to rheumatoid arthritis and other diseases. Cell-wall deficient infections, of course, cannot be recognized by healthy or weakened immune systems, and later when the cell-wall deficient bacteria reconstruct themselves, there is no clue to the relationship between the initial infective source and the presently identified disease.

However, without any consideration for either the weakened immune system, or the creation and passing along of more pleomorphic organisms, according to Carl L. Tellen, "Studies by the Centers for Disease Control (CDC) determined food borne illnesses from meat and poultry cost Americans 4-8 billion dollars annually."[145]

Iron Overload

Iron supplementation, or any product containing iron supplements such as fortified breakfast cereals, is not recommended for the arthritic without complete testing by a knowledgable physician for the following reasons, as reported by Adeena Robinson[264] in *Iron -- A Double Edged Sword*:

An excess of iron can enhance or even create symptoms of arthritis; it causes damage to joints and exacerbates the inflammatory process. Usually -- but not always -- those with rheumatoid arthritis who also have a negative (Rheumatoid Factor) RF factor suffer from an excess of iron. Given either orally or by injection, inflammation can worsen within 24-48 hours; conversely -- assuming iron overload -- inducing a mild deficiency in iron through phlebotomy (blood-letting or donation of blood) or intravenous chelation by deferoxamine can reduce or eliminate inflammation. In one study, six of nine patients reported complete remission of symptoms while the remaining three reported at least 50% improvement. (See Chapter I, Osteoarthritis, "Chelation Therapy.")

Other diseases, such as heart, diabetes, of the pancreas and endocrine system, sexual dysfunction, multiple sclerosis, cystic fibrosis, and neurological disorders can also be intensified or traced to iron overload.

One mechanism by which iron overload progresses various diseases, such as rheumatoid arthritis and cancer, is that the component related to invasive microorganisms is intensified. Many microorganisms thrive on excess iron. When our body produces a fever, it is simultaneously moving iron into safe storage where microorganisms have less opportunity to obtain it.

Signs and Symptoms of Iron Overload

• Chronic fatigue usually present; abdominal pain often severe and of undetermined origin; gastrointestinal disorders, peptic ulcer, gastritis, bouts of diarrhoea and/or nausea and vomiting, not due to any known cause; hair loss; skin color changes common: gray-white or slate gray color; headaches including migraines; progressive hearing loss; memory loss and confusion; dizziness, loss of balance and coordination; weakness, shortness of breath on exertion; abnormal fluid retention; bone and joint pain; lethargy, weakness, and malaise; and visual disturbances: blurred or failing vision, difficulty focusing, and eye pain.

8. Hormonal Imbalances and Metabolic Problems

Pollutants, faulty nutrition, microbes, pharmaceutical drugs, genetics -- to name a few factors -- can all affect hormones, their utilization, and our health. Denis E. Wilson, M.D., Orlando, Florida, in *Wlson's Syndrome*, has shown that insufficiency of sleep, sustained stress, use of drugs such as cortisone, and many other factors can create a condition whereby our thyroid system is stuck in an emergency state leading to thyroid mis-utilization, or hypothyroidism. Hypothyroidism, in turn, decreases proper utilization of enzymes, which, in their turn, create many defective biochemical pathways that lead to 60 different disease states, including various forms of arthritis.

Thyroid is the master regulator of other hormones, and will frequently determine the rate at which we heal or don't heal. Writing about iodine which is used by the thyroid, Richard A. Kunin, M.D. says, "This remarkable mineral is not only anti-inflammatory, it also can inactivate immune complexes, thus reducing auto-immune activity." Immune complexes are formed when antigens are combined with our protective antibodies for the purpose of inactivating microorganism invaders. Iodine "is a broad-spectrum antibiotic, particularly against fungi and yeast organisms, most viruses and almost all bacteria. A few days on potassium iodide can turn off an acute attack of arthritis, especially if there is an antigen or an organism involved."[129]

Pituitary determines how fast we grow, and also relates to healing factors.

Parathyroid determines how well we utilize calcium and where we place it in our bodies.

Dehydroepiandrosterone (DHEA) is a precursor to many other hormones, and is often necessary in conjunction with sex hormones, testosterone, progesterone and estrogen.

While the subject of hormonal replacement therapy is quite complex, and should not be attempted without adequate medical help, it is a growing practice that promises, along with other therapies, to bring us great benefits.

Summary

We haven't covered all factors that cause or contribute to rheumatoid arthritis and related diseases -- no book this size could do so; and further, no one doctor or writer could have the complete range of knowledge necessary to do so. But, we believe that we've covered the major share of causative and contributing factors. Our proof is simple: when treatments based on these factors are placed into practice with the help of cooperating patients, arthritics get well.

Traditional Treatments

Traditional treatments are predicated upon an assumption which has never been demonstrated, and may be false. There is the belief that those suffering from rheumatoid arthritis have primarily a defective immune system.

Because the immunological system is defective -- it is assumed -- the treatments prescribed have become more and more damaging, the use of cytotoxic drugs (methotrexate) being the latest in a long line of non-rational forms of treatment.

While it is true that there are genetic markers in specific forms of rheumatoid disease (ankylosing spondilitis, rheumatoid arthritis), there has been little scientific proof that the sole causation of rheumatoid arthritis is the result of an inherent genetic defect affecting the immunological system that needs to be "modulated," changed, or damaged further.

The idea of single causation in the form of a "defective immunological system," or that the immunological system attacks itself, is not scientifically established, and is probably nonsense, especially in view of the fact -- as all practicing rheumatologists know -- that none of the traditional treatments based on this assumption have ever been shown to effect a cure.

The greatest indictment against present practices for rheumatoid arthritis, simply stated, is that traditional practices make no attempt to cure the disease.

As is also true in the treatment of cancer, a professional, opaque sack, has been placed over the eyes of those practicing rheumatology that prevents them from looking elsewhere to assist their patients. There seems to be a professional lethargy against reviewing and trying treatment regimens that fall outside of the scope of traditional practices, even though these practices have long failed.

The late orthopedic Surgeon, Robert Bingham, M.D. , Desert Hot Springs, California, wrote, "Of course you realize that the specialty of rheumatology is narrowest of all medical fields, the fewest disease, the fewest treatments and the fewest facts on which to make clinical and therapeutic decisions. In spite of its certification as a specialty, any physician with an interest, whether it be a general practitioner, internist, orthopedic surgeon, or physiatrist (certification specialty in physical and occupational therapy), could master the field as well as any Board Certified specialist in a year's study. That is why the majority of cases of arthritis are not, and never will be, treated by rheumatologists."[17]

Whether administered by a rheumatologist or general practitioner, traditional treatments for rheumatoid arthritis address themselves to easing pain and lengthening the time of patient mobility. Normally, traditional treatments include rest, use of analgesics and non-steroidal anti-inflammatory drugs, cortisone, gold compounds, D-penicillamine, and cytotoxic drugs. According to some statistics, on the conservative treatment to be described, 75% "improve" (not become cured), during the first year of the disease, while 10% are eventually disabled, despite full treatments.[2]

Overall, traditional treatment does not bring about more cures than the placebo effect, which are improvements that would be expected by chance alone. About 30% of rheumatoid arthritis patients -- at least for the time being -- will "improve," regardless of what, within reason, has been done to them. Patient follow-up over a longer time span usually indicates that most of these relapse. Just as occurs in the treatment of cancer where damaging surgery, radiation and chemotherapy are used, despite extremely aggressive traditional treatment against rheumatoid arthritis, the long-term course of rheumatoid arthritis appears to be unaffected.[8,9,29]

What's wrong with traditional treatments for rheumatoid arthritis is very easy to describe, and quite shocking to those afflicted. Except for the advice to rest -- which is usually good advice for all diseases -- the body needs to recuperate its ability to repair and to heal -- all the remaining treatments address themselves to symptomatic relief while the disease rages onward, destroying tendons, ligaments, joint capsules, other bodily tissues, and an otherwise beautiful life.

"English rheumatologists tracked 112 rheumatoid arthritis patients receiving [traditional] 'aggressive' drug treatment over 22 years. . . . More than half either died or became severely disabled. The authors concluded that it was fallacious to believe that [traditional] arthritic drugs of any sort cause a remission in patients." They said that with current treatment "the prognosis of rheumatoid arthritis is not good."[125,170]

In another study conducted by Vanderbilt University, Nashville, Tennessee, 75 patients undergoing traditional rheumatology treatments were tracked over nine years. Twenty had died and ninety-three percent of the remaining survivors had lost "significant functional capacity," that is, the ability to grip well and move about -- although when they had enrolled in the program at the beginning they had been reasonably ambulatory, with 85% still at work.[125,170]

Retail sales of traditional arthritic drugs is estimated to cost the American arthritic about $3 billion per year.[170] Standard medical treatment is estimated to be a $10-billion-a-year business.[170]

Several years ago these traditional treatments were conservatively oriented by starting the patient with the least harmful of all possible drugs, primarily to alleviate pain. That has changed in recent years, with many rheumatologists beginning their patients with the most damaging, most toxic treatments, as will also be explained.

The "conservative" treatment program is (or was) as follows:

Rest and Nutrition

During the acute flare-ups or active stages of the disease, rheumatologists may advise bed rest and the consuming of "ordinary" nutritious foods. Many times the patient is wrongfully told to ignore other food and diet programs recommended for rheumatoid arthritics because "Food and diet quackery is common and should be ignored."[2]

When doctors advise their patients to ignore other food and beneficial diet programs, but rather to eat "ordinary" nutritious foods, they often fail to define, or to define correctly, what is "ordinary" and what is "nutritious." Considering the billions of bucks dedicated to brainwashing the buying public (including naive doctors) into believing that a particular packaged food is nutritious or healthful, and convincing us that everyone is using a particular brand therefore we should use it too, "ordinary" huckstered pre-packaged, pre-prepared, in-any-way-processed foods are both non-nutritious and non-healthful.

Nutritional advice normally given to rheumatoid arthritis patients, if any, is tragic and exceedingly damaging. The very best of medical books will wrongly advise physicians that nutrition is not a factor in rheumatoid disease. This advice has never been subjected to the test of scientific scrutiny, and is as wrong as general blood-letting was wrong during earlier centuries in efforts to "strengthen" a patient, or rid him/her of disease.

Medical students have exceedingly tiny amounts of training in medical school regarding nutrition, vitamin and mineral supplementation, and the use of herbals. Their academic courses are so loaded, and their time so taken with "important" courses, that, unless the physician is self-trained after graduating, their minds are left vacuous regarding nutrition. Such an untrained physician then tends to accept authoritarian dogma, actually religious-like beliefs. Gaduating physicians read such statements as "Food and diet quackery is common and should be ignored," in prestigious, authoritative publications, and then detrimentally pass this anti-pearl of anti-wisdom on to their patients.[2]

Nutrition, of course, is the most complicated set of bio-chemical activities taking place in the human body, and ought to consume the major portion of the medical student's hours.

The advice, that nutrition is unrelated to the progress of rheumatoid arthritis, is simply criminal advice, leaving millions in crippled, painful agony.

Julian Whitaker, M.D. has said it best: "The known outcomes of conventional treatment are the best argument for employing the natural approach. What I recommend may not be as 'easy' as taking aspirin or popping pills. A serious, habit-changing intervention for individuals with rheumatoid arthritis is the best course, starting today."[159] Julian Whitaker, M.D., *Dr. Whitaker's Guide to Natural Healing*, Prima Publishing, PO Box 1260BK, Rocklin, CA 95677, 1995.

Any successful farmer can report on the beneficial effects of proper nourishment and vitamins and minerals on their hogs, milk cows and chickens. Unless they pay attention to these important requirements, the meat is less, milk of poor quality, and eggs of decreased quantity and quality. Their animals may also suffer from other debilitating diseases, altogether resulting in serious economic losses.

Although most agree that the human being is both spirit and animal of origin, with a body that cannot function with less vitamin and mineral supplementation and proper dietary factors than do other animals' bodies, we've somehow lost our perspective.

There are physicians -- such as Warren Levin, M.D. of New York City, New York, Jonathan Wright, M.D., of Kent, Washington, Rex Newham, N.D., D.O., Ph.D. of Cracoe, England, Hector E. Solorzano del Rio, M.D., Ph.D., D.Sc., of Guadalajara, Mexico and hundreds of other holistic minded physicians -- who have dedicated their lives to studying the relationship of nutrition to good health, including that of rheumatoid arthritis. There is no question in their minds, and in the body's of their patients, that well-defined, appropriate diets, with proper vitamin and mineral supplementations, will often turn around a diseased condition, including that of rheumatoid arthritis.

How do they know?

They've seen it happen time after time!

Aspirin: Cornerstone of Drug Therapy for Arthritics

Salicylates, or acetylsalicylic acid -- aspirin -- was the drug of first choice, and the afflicted was told to take a certain number of aspirin each day. Aspirin was described as the "cornerstone" of drug therapy for rheumatoid arthritis.

Aspirin was prescribed, <u>in writing</u>, in doses sufficient to produce mild symptoms of intoxication, that is, ringing in the ears (tinnitus), and diminished hearing.

Four small "balanced" meals per day were also recommended, the last a bedtime snack, was also prescribed <u>in writing</u>. Gastric buffering action of the various foods was explained, as well as the use of antacids between meals to counteract the gastrointestinal effects of the aspirin.

Patients who awoke at night with severe pain were prescribed choline salicylate, which produced less harmful gastrointestinal effects than did aspirin, but also did not have quite the same amount of anti-inflammatory effects.

Non-Steroidal Anti-inflammatory Drugs (NSAIDS)

When the pain, swelling and heated joints reached the point where aspirin was no longer effective, stronger non-steroidal anti-inflammatory drugs were prescribed. Among these were indomethacin, ibuprofen, phenylbutazone, naproxen and others. Often the above compounds are found under many different brand names, some in strengths over-the-counter, and others in heavier dosages under physician prescriptions.

Indomethacin, for example, has some analgesic, anti-inflammatory and anti-heat (antipyretic) activity. Small amounts were given with or after meals usually three to four times per day, and then the daily dosage increased at daily and weekly intervals depending upon severity of the disease.

After it was perceived that the acute phase of the disease was under control, the dosage was leveled off to about 3 or 4 times starting dosage.

Later, dosage was reduced until the patient was weaned away from the drug entirely.

All of the non-steroidal anti-inflammatories were considered to be substitutes for aspirin, the drug of first choice.

What's Wrong With Aspirin and Non-Steroidal Anti-Inflammatory Drugs (NSAIDS)?

Aspirin and non-steroidal anti-inflammatory drugs are temporarily useful for alleviating symptoms while addressing the systemic causation of rheumatoid arthritis. Their extended usage, however, can result in several serious problems. The death rate for those using NSAIDS, compared to those who do not, is seven times greater, accounting conservatively -- according to some investigators -- for at least 2,600 deaths each year, and 20,000 hospitalizations each year.[125]

The United States Food and Drug Administration estimates about 200,000 cases of gastric bleeding occur each year from the use of aspirin and non-steroidal anti-inflammatory (NSAID) drugs, with their estimates of deaths being between 10,000 and 20,000 per year.[125]

Non-steroidal anti-inflammatory drugs (NSAIDS) have been reported in the *British Journal of Rheumatology* as a possible cause of infertility -- "induced lutenized unruptured follicle syndrome," a phenomena long observed in medical practices, but never before ascribed to arthritis treatment.[255]

Salicylates (aspirin), for example, can erode the lining of the stomach, leading to bleeding ulcers and other gastrointestinal problems. Enteric coated and buffered aspirin is of little use except for those who have peptic ulcers or hiatus hernia.

The FDA now requires a warning with each non-steroidal anti-inflammatory (NSAID) prescription, saying, "Serious gastrointestinal toxicity such as bleeding, ulceration and perforation can occur at any time, with or without warning symptoms, in patients treated chronically with NSAID therapy."[125]

In a study reported in *Clinical and Experimental Rheumatology* by

Dr. R. Myllykangas-Lugosujarvi,[414] Rheumatism Foundation Hospital, Finland, "Complicated diverticular disease (inflammation in the intestinal tract), probably related to antirheumatic medication, is a more important cause of death in patients with rheumatoid arthritis than is generally recognized."

Sustained-release tablets might provide longer relief for some patients, and may help an individual through pains that awaken them at night.

Aspirin is usually discontinued when indomethacin or ibuprofen is used.

Non-steroidal anti-inflammatory drugs such as ibuprofen (sold over the counter) can be given for those who do not tolerate aspirin. Although less of a gastrointestinal irritant than asprin, it can produce gastric symptoms and gastrointestinal bleeding. Although this drug has a supposed "safety" record, it can cause inflammation of the colon (colitis).[125]

With hydrooxychloroquine usage, repeated eye tests are required by an opthalmologist before and every 2 to 3 months during treatment. Hydrooxychloroquine should be taken under close medical supervision as it may create irreversible retinal degeneration.[21]

Indomethacin has both analgesic and anti-inflammatory properties, and, unlike corticosteroids, has no effect on pituitary or adrenal glands.

Adverse effects of the usage of indomethacin are headache, dizziness, lightheadedness and gastrointestinal disturbances such as nausea, loss of appetite, vomiting, epigastric distress, abdominal pain and diarrhea.[21]

Indomethacin, naproxen and a sustained release preparation of ketoprofen may cause perforations of the colon, because, by decreasing the mucosal prostaglandins -- very active biological substances -- they compromise the intestinal integrity, according to Dr. J. Hollingworth of Selly Oak Hospital in Birmingham, England.[125]

Joel Wallach, D.V.M., N.D. reports that indomethacin can cause confusion and headaches in older patients, and that rather than take this drug, the patient should take calcium, magnesium, boron, copper, selenium, lithium and chondroitin sulfate (Knox® gelatin).[249]

Gastrointestinal bleeding may also result from use of indomethacin.

Indomethacin should not be given to a patient with active peptic ulcer, gastritic, or ulcerative colitis, conditions which can easily accompany rheumatoid arthritis.

Occasionally fluid retention is a problem.

Central Nervous System effects may be transient and disappear altogether on continued usage with dose reduction, but occasionally the effects are of such severe nature that therapy must be discontinued altogether. Patients who show signs of Central Nervous System symptoms should not operate automobiles or other hazardous equipment.

Non-steroidal anti-inflammatory drugs may also cause blurred or diminished vision, Parkinson's disease, hair and fingernail loss, and also damage the liver and kidneys, to name just a few more human insults.[125]

Phenylbutazone has an anti-inflammatory effect but rarely helps rheumatoid arthritis. Phenylbutazone cannot be considered a simple analgesic, but should be used under careful medical supervision. It's usage can result in serious side affects of anemia and loss of certain leukocytes (agranulocytosis). Through it's use, there is an incidence of 2.2 deaths per 100,000 exposures from the above named conditions. The risk increases with age and long-term usage, especially women, to 6.5 deaths per 100,000.[21]

Other side effects of phenylbutazone include gastrointestinal, skin, heart, kidney and other serious effects.

As the major share of pharmaceutical drug research is aimed at relieving symptoms for arthritics -- not cures -- there are always new analgesic, non-steroidal anti-inflammatory drugs being huxtered as "break-throughs." None of these help our bodies to heal.

Cortisone -- Corticosteroids

The most dramatic, short-lived relief of symptoms comes from corticosteroids (cortisone or steroids)   a variety of related drugs that quickly relieve pain, swelling, and heated joints for a short period. When first discovered, it was hailed as the panacea for the arthritic, and then it's many damaging effects became known.

Steroids, or their analogs (triamcinolone hexacetonide; prednisolone tertiary-butylacetate) were, and are, given orally as prednisone, into the joints themselves (intra-articular), or at specific sites, especially near connections of tendons, ligments, and other locations near joints.

Although corticosteroids temporarily dampen down the clinical symptoms and permit freedom of movement without pain, it's usage is, or should be, greatly restricted because of many damaging side effects.

What's Wrong With the Use of Cortisone?

Although pain relief is nearly instant, on use of cortisone, prednisone and dexamethasone, and their chemical variants, none of them will halt the progression of joint destruction. Cortisone merely suppresses the symptoms or "clinical manifestations," of arthritis, acting at the cellular microscopic level.

Corticosteroids inhibit the early phenomena of the inflammatory process which includes swelling, blood clotting, capillary expansion, capillary and fibroblast proliferation, deposition of collagen tissue and later scar tissue formation, migration of white blood cells into the inflamed area, and phagocytic activity. All of the described inhibited functions are required by the human body for protection, growth and repair of tissue.

Cortisone impairs wound healing and provides the grounds (predisposition) for infection. It has major effects on the monocyte/macroph-age systems, preventing the release of a substance that aids in fighting infection (interleukin I).

Large doses of corticosteroids results in a deficiency of lympho-cytes in the blood, leading to deficiency of lymph cells (lymphopenia). Large blood cells (leucocytes), called "monocytes," show an impaired ability to kill invading microorganisms.

Corticosteroids interfere with a variety of functions, not mentioned here, and the result of all of the adverse phenomena is an increased incidence of infection usually controlled by cellular immunity, which means an increase in infections: mycoplasmal, yeast/fungal, bacterial, protozoal, and so on. These are many of the same organisms associated with, or suspected as causative agents, in various forms of rheumatoid disease.

The list of invading or growing microorganisms resulting from the use of corticosteroids resembles the agents to which patients with Hodgkin's disease, a condition of enlargement of lymph tissue, spleen and liver, and other tissues, or the agents to which acquired immune deficiency syndrome (AIDS) are vulnerable.

Steroids are also widely used in organ transplants involving kidney, heart, liver and bone marrow. In part, subsequent deaths that are news-media-wise blamed on infections after transplantations are a direct result of use of the corticosteroids as well as other immunosuppressive drugs.

When cortisone is administered in the joint for the purpose of relieving pain, not only does the joint continue eroding (often faster), but the cortisone is placed at the wrong site of pain causation, a fact which nerve specialist Professor Roger Wyburn-Mason, M.D., Ph.D. and surgeon Dr. Paul Pybus were able to demonstrate more than thirty years ago. An effective treatment based on the knowledge, called "Intra-neural Injections," was further developed by Dr. Pybus and one of us (Gus J. Prosch, Jr., M.D.). The sources are lesions in nerve cells in nerve ganglia that lie along uninsulated (unmyelinated) "C" nerve fibers that lead to the joint. A small amount of a type of non-damaging, non-systemic cortisone deposited, called "depot," at that remote location will halt the swelling, pain and heat at the joint immediately, lasting for up to three weeks, with no adverse erosive effects to the joint or other bodily systems. During the interim, actual causes of arthritis can be properly tackled without undue pain.[22] (See *Intraneural Injections for Rheumatoid Arthritis and Osteoarthritis and The Control of Pain in Arthritis of the Knee*, Dr.Paul K. Pybus.)

When the body receives hormones from external sources it lowers its own production. Some arthritics reach the point of reliance on external cortisone to such an extent that their body refuses to produce any, and the patient is now totally dependent upon periodic shots for life itself. While this is an ideal drug-dependency state for improving the profit status of those who produce cortisone (having a human hooked on a drug for which life itself is dependent), it is a life of misery for the patient -- knowing that the disease rages onward and that symptom relief comcs only from a drug company who demands dollars for symptom-free -- but not disease free -- life to continue.

Other problems result from the extended use of cortisone, but the foregoing should explain some of the major dangers.

It is no wonder that some arthritics take to drink or other harder drugs!

Gold Compounds

Often, in addition to salicylates and after aspirin and non-steroidal anti-inflammatory drugs begin to fail in easing symptoms, gold compounds were considered the drug of next choice.

While gold compounds are not effective against joint inflammation, they are thought to be helpful in those with advanced joint destruction having minimal inflammation, and may decrease the formation of new bony erosions.

There is evidence that, even when gold compounds appear to produce remissions, symptomatic relief lasts for no more than thirty months, and then usually fails.[18]

Water-soluble gold compounds (sodium thiomalate or thiosulfate) are often given intramuscularly at weekly intervals, up to a specific limit, or until significant "improvement" is apparent. The gold shots are then tapered down to a minimum level, but if no further gold shots are given, relapse usually occurs.

When toxic symptoms are observed in the patient resulting from the toxicity of gold, the drug is discontinued, but now often the patient has rheumatoid arthritis symptoms coupled with gold toxicity symptoms, and often the two conditions are not distinguished for the patient by the physician. "My arthritis is getting worse," the patient will say, and the traditional rheumatologist will reach for a new drug.

What's Wrong With Gold Compounds?

Toxic reactions to gold lie in the patient's sensitivity to the compound, its vehicle of delivery, or to heavy metal toxicity (poisoning). The adverse effects include severe itching, dermatitis, gastrointestinal problems, renal impairment (proteinuria), blood in the urine, loss of white blood cells (agranulocytosis), blood leakage into the skin, mucous membranes, internal organs and other tissues (thrombocytopenic purpura), and destruction of blood-producing cells in the bone (aplastic anemia).

There may also be other signs of toxic manifestations.

While there may appear to be improvement through the use of gold, the improvement is almost always temporary at best, the maximum length of time that symptoms are suppressed being about 30 months (on average), after which the disease symptoms begin anew, but this time with the added burden of gold toxicity disease, added symptoms that are wrongly confused by the patient and some few doctors as being manifestations of additional rheumatoid arthritis symptoms.[18]

D-Penicillamine

It is believed, but never has been demonstrated, that D-penicillamine, called "penicillamine," has beneficial effects similar to gold, and that this substance should be used after gold fails.

Penicillamine is first given orally in a smaller dosage, and then the dose doubled, which is taken for 30 days. If no improvement occurs, the dose is then tripled from starting dosage for 60 days.

When the patient appears to respond, there's no further increase in dosage.

Cordell Logan, M.D., North Carolina, felt that the patient's apparent good response, if any, to penicillamine, after the usage of gold, was in penicillamine's ability to chelate out, that is, remove, some of the gold, and the gold's terrible toxicity, not in reducing the course of rheumatoid arthritis or its symptoms.[19]

What's Wrong With D-Penicillamine?

In that the use of D-penicillamine has never demonstrated the ability to heal, the best that can be said about it's use is that it might -- as Cordell Logan, M.D. has said -- "Take out (chelate out) some of the gold from the body," thereby decreasing the effects of the toxicity of gold. As symptoms of rheumatoid disease and gold toxicity are confused in both the patient's and the physician's mind, relieving some of the gold toxicity burdens then appears to "improve," the patient's arthritis.

D-Penicillamine can cause bone marrow suppression, possible renal impairment, (proteinuria), inflammation and degeneration of kidneys (nephrosis), rashes, a foul taste, and other serious toxic effects.

Fatalities from the use of this drug have been reported, and its usage must be very carefully monitored.

Immunosuppressive Drugs

After the failure of salicylates, non-steroidal anti-inflammatory drugs, gold and penicillamine, the next attempt to change the course of an immune system presumed to have gone awry, was the usage of cytotoxic drugs. These are drugs that are routinely used in the treatment of cancer, usually also vainly so, and also for the suppression of the immune system during and following transplanted organs.

At one time cyclophosphamide and azathioprine, and other cytotoxic drugs, were used experimentally in rheumatoid arthritis as a last treatment attempt, irrationally so because of their exceedingly damaging effects, especially in their proven ability to produce malignant cancers.

In recent years, rheumatologists have reversed the normal

process. Instead of advising a moderate treatment of aspirin, then non-steroidal anti-inflammatories, corticosteroids, gold, penicillamine, and finally cytotoxic drugs, many modern day rheumatologists now begin with the exceedingly dangerous and damaging cytotoxic drugs, even when the patient has but early signs of rheumatoid arthritis. This new trend has as much scientific validity as does the use of electro-therapy in psychiatry, or beating up an automobile engine with a sledge-hammer to "fix" it.

What's Wrong With Immunosuppressive Drugs?

Unsuccessfully and widely used for the treatment of cancer, cytotoxic drugs are now being used by rheumatologists as treatment of first choice for those afflicted with rheumatoid arthritis.

"Despite over twenty years of research, with billions of dollars spent each year, the conventional medical establishment's 'war on cancer' has been a dismal failure."[24] Why an unsuccessful drug, such as methotrexate, should be extended to another disease where success is no better has not been adequately explained and appears to be part of the insanity that accompanies a profession that refuses to look outside of its own recommendations even when failing it's self-appointed mission.

Methotrexate is an example of cytotoxic drugs now used for arthritics whose adverse effects are legion.

According to the *Physicians Desk Reference*,[21] the most frequently reported adverse reactions with the use of methotrexate include: ulcerative inflammation of the mouth (stomatitis), decrease in certain blood cells (leukopenia), nausea, abdominal distress, malaise, undue fatigue, chills and fever, dizziness and decreased resistance to infection.

The skin may be affected by skin rashes, itching, pale wheals (urticaria), sensitivity to light, pigment changes, loss of hair, large blotches starting as blue-black but changing to greenish brown or yellow (ecchymosis), dilation of capillaries and sometimes arteries (telangiectasia), acne, and boils (furuncolosis).

Affects on the alimentary system may be inflammation of the gums (gingivitis), inflammation of the pharynx and mouth (stomatitis), loss of appetite, nausea, vomiting, diarrhea, vomiting of blood, stools that look like tar due to action of intestinal juices on blood (melena), gastrointestinal ulceration and bleeding, and inflammation of the intestines.

In the urogenital system there may be severe kidney disease (nephropathy) and renal failure, presence of increased nitrogenous bodies in the urea (azotemia), inflammation of the bladder (cystitis), blood in the urine (hematuria), defective egg or sperm (oogenesis or spermatogenesis), temporary deficiency of sperm (oligospermia), menstrual dysfunction and vaginal discharge, infertility, abortion, and fetal defects.

In the pulmonary system, there can be chronic pneumonia and

deaths due to pneumonia (interstitial pneumonia).

In the central nervous system there can be headaches, drowsiness, blurred vision, loss of memory, one-half of body paralyzed, full body paralyzation, and/or convulsions.

Other rarer reactions are joint/muscle aches (arthralgias/myalgias), metabolic changes, precipitating diabetes, osteoporosis, shock or collapse and even sudden death.

Methotrexate is used in dosages of 1/100 the amount employed in the "treatment" of cancer. It appears to provide a miracle within the first month or two of use for many people. Some of these continue to improve steadily as treatment progresses over several months, and may even stay the apparent course of the disease for a fraction, for years. However, the moment dependency on the drug stops, the likelihood of quintupled morning stiffness and other arthritic problems return.[205]

Cyclosporin, an immunosuppressant developed to halt the body's natural rejection of foreign tissue during transplants, acts by lowering the immune system T-cells, and should be used only under dire emergencies.

Other immunosuppressents include azathioprine and cyclophosphamide. Each have very high risks, indeed.

Clearly cytotoxic drugs are not recommended!

Conclusion

We believe that it is absolute mal-practice to continue with traditional treatments, after what we've seen work on arthritics. Traditional practices do not get better results than a placebo effect. If you give 100 patients traditional treatments, and 100 patients get a sugar pill, the number of patients who will improve will be the same in both groups. Mind you, we say "improve," not "well."

Traditional medical practices knock the immune system out. Our recommended, non-traditional practices build the immune system up.

It would be criminal to go back treating patients by traditional means taught in medical school! How can any honest man practice medicine knowing that his results are going to be the same as a sugar pill?

Unfortunately, damage that has already been done to arthritic joints may be irreversable. In the section to follow, we'll provide details of a successful treatment protocol which, from the 1970s, has routinely cured 75-80% of those rheumatoid disease victims who have not already been mis-treated by traditional means. If they have been so mistreated, the success rate reduces to about 50%, and the balance can also be cured, but with considerably more effort and attention to details. The relatively small percentage who do not immediately get well, would do so, we believe, if he or she will explore all alternatives, and will stay with a knowledgeable alternative medicine physician.

The treatments to be described consist of these steps: (1) A regimen of specifically prescribed broad-spectrum anti-microorganism drugs; (2) probable treatment for candidiasis, a yeast/fungus infection; (3) treatment for food allergies; (4) corrective diet; (5) and other selected treatments as required for each individual, such as Intraneural Injections, chelation therapy, and so on. Additional penetration into causes involves willingness to get rid of mercury, herbicides, pesticides, and to complete proper colon detoxification, This treatment program is known as The Roger Wyburn-Mason and Jack M. Blount treatment protocol, or, The Arthritis Trust of AmericaThe Rheumatoid Disease Foundation treatment program.

The Professor Roger Wyburn-Mason, M.D., Ph.D. Treatment for Rheumatoid Arthritis

First Consistently Successful Treatment for Rheumatoid Disease

During the seventies English Professor Roger Wyburn-Mason, M.D., Ph.D.[7,8] became the first physician to develop a demonstrated cure for most of the eighty or so rheumatoid diseases, whether they are classified as "auto-immune" or "collagen tissue" disease. Physicians who have followed his methods have had a consistent success rate in curing their patients of rheumatoid arthritis varying from 70 to 80 per cent unless the patient has been treated by traditional methods, in which event success of this treatment drops to about 50%. Fifty percent is not good, but is still considerably higher than the 30% placebo-effect rate of "improvement" obtained through traditional rheumatology practices. "Placebo-effect" percentage is the number who will respond to pretended treatment containing no active substance.

It is believed that nearly 100% of all patients will achieve wellness, regardless, if they will stay with an alternative medical professional until all personally relevent avenues -- too numerous in the aggregate to mention herein -- have been explored.

With the assistance of world-renown protozoologist, Vice-Admiral Stamm, Professor Wyburn-Mason concluded that common protozoal organisms were the basis to rheumatoid arthritis. No one since has been able to isolate these organisms, but Wyburn-Mason's theory led him to try anti-amoebics -- bile salts or copper sulfate -- which effectively cured rheumatoid arthritis, but which were too toxic for other than experimental use.

As will be described, Professor Roger Wyburn-Mason, M.D., Ph.D., and other physicians later discovered new uses for non-patented prescription drugs which safely cured rheumatoid arthritis.

Dr. Wyburn-Mason's research and analysis of many cases led him to conclusions that began -- at last -- to make sense of so-called "auto-immune" or "collagen tissue" diseases:

• Diseases such as rheumatoid arthritis are systemic in nature. Although the pain and deformation appears in the joint, rheumatoid arthritis is principally a condition of the whole body, not just in the joint.

• Since the disease is systemic -- throughout the body -- every tissue in the body can be affected, thus manifesting different disease symptoms from a single source-cause. This explains the overlap of many disease symptoms classified as "auto-immune" or "collagen tissue" conditions.

• Although the 80 or so diseases -- systemic lupus erythematosus, psoriasis, rheumatoid arthritis, etc. -- are given different names, based on differing symptoms, they can all be manifestations from the same causation. Differing causes may affect tissues in the same way, thus producing the appearance of the same disease. However, causations of rheumatoid disease, including rheumatoid arthritis, can also affect all tissues, as shown in the following table:

Tissues Affected According to
Professor Roger Wyburn-Mason, M.D., Ph.D.

Arteries: Periarteritis
Bone: Paget's Disease, cysts, myelomas
Brain and Cord: Tremors, seizures
Bronchi: Bronchitis, intrinsic asthma
Cardiac: Dysrhythmias, myocardial disease, pericardial disease
Cecum: Appendicitis, mesenteric adenitis
Colon: Ulcerative colitis
Endocrine: Thyroid, parathyroid, thymus, pituitary, adrenal, gonads
Esophagus and Stomach: Atropic mucosa (pernicious anemia), webs
Eyes: Iridocyclitis, exophthalmias
Fascial Planes: Bursitis
Female Genitals: Ovarian cysts, fibroids, salpingitis-sterility, tubal pregnancies
Functional CNS: Neuroses, psychoses senility
Hemopoetic: Systemic lupus erythematosus, polycythemia, purpura
Joints: Arthritis
Kidneys: Pyelonephritis, calculi
Liver: Hepatitis, cholangitis, gallbladder disease
Lower Small Gut: Regional enteritis, Crohn's disease
Lungs: Alveolitis
Lymphatics: Lymphomas, splenomegaly
Meninges: Headache, meningomas
Muscles: Myositis
Nerves: Trigeminal neuralgia, multiple sclerosis
Nose and Throat: Rhinitis, eustachian salpingitis, enlarged tonsils, & adenoids,etc.
Ovum: Fetal deformities, abortions
Pancreas: Pancreatitis, maturity diabetes, noninsulin dependent diabetes
Salivary & Tear Glands: SICCA syndrome, Sjogrens syndrome
Skin: Psoriasis, alopecia, erythemas, urticaria
Tendons: Tendonitis, ganglion
Upper Gut: Celiac disease

• Since every tissue can be affected, the disease conditions such as rheumatoid arthritis seldom appear in "pure" form. If the astute physician will look carefully, he'll find that each condition can grade gradually into another, or several, of the eighty or so "auto-immune" or "collagen tissue" diseases. Professor Roger Wyburn-Mason concluded the following as published in 1978 in his *The Causation of Rheumatoid Disease and Many Human Cancers.*[8,9] (See *The Causation of Rheumatoid Disease and Many Human Cancers a Precis.*)

• The principal causation of the eighty or so rheumatoid diseases is a tissue sensitivity -- often a genetic susceptibility -- to the toxins or proteins derived from microorganisms internal to but foreign to the body.

• Kill the invading organisms -- which results in a massive concentration of toxins or dead protein products -- and the result is a "Herxheimer effect," a temporary intensification of the disease symptoms.

• When the body clears out the toxins or dead protein products, the Herxheimer effect and the rheumatoid arthritis and related diseases, disappear.

He taught, ". . . from the above considerations it is apparent that the various 'collagen' and 'auto-immune' diseases, including rheumatoid arthritis, show every combination and gradation from one to the other. It seems that the various manifestations are those of one disease. Every tissue of the body may be affected or the brunt of the disease is born by only one or two organs. Joint disease is but one manifestation of the spectrum and may be absent."[8]

The Herxheimer Reaction

To fully understand, and to follow-through with adequate compliance of Roger Wyburn-Mason's successful treatment protocol, it's essential that both the treating physician and the patient fully understand a phenomena related to achieving wellness called "The Herxheimer Effect."

Your physician will recommend certain prescription drugs be given in a quantity according to body weight, and then he and you will observe to determine if you have a temporary intensification of your disease symptoms. If so, then the treatment will most likely be successful. If not, and if the disease does not remit, another prescription drug or a combination of them should be tried.

Of course, all this time treatment (1) with proper nutrition and supplements, (2) against candidiasis, (3) for food allergies, and (4) with other important processes will be started and on-going. The object is to halt the disease process as swiftly as possible, after which good nutritional practices, and other requisite treatments employed rebuild the immune system, and strengthen tissues, organs, and systems.

Understanding the Herxheimer effect[4,5,7,8,9.48.49] is a key to understanding The Arthritis Trust of America's treatment based on the discoveries of Professor Roger Wyburn-Mason, Dr. Paul K. Pybus, and one of us (Gus J. Prosch, Jr., M.D.).

The important Herxheimer effect applies as well to many treatment and healing processes that are not necessarily related to rheumatoid arthritis. In 1902 Doctors Adolph Jarisch Herxheimer and Karl Herxheimer, studied the treatment of syphilis using various kinds of relatively dangerous medicines such as mercury. They learned, and concluded, that whenever an organism more complex than a simple bacterium was killed inside the human body, one had "flu-like" symptoms. This phenomena was later named the Jarisch-Herxheimer effect, or simply "The Herxheimer." It's called "The Herxheimer Effect" when treating tuberculosis, rheumatoid diseases, including rheumatoid arthritis, the "Desert Storm Disease," leishmaniasis, and some other tropical diseases. When treating leprosy it's called "Lucio's Phenomenon." When treating candidiasis, it's called "The Die-Off Effect." Some call it "The Healing Crisis."

During treatment for rheumatoid arthritis one kills invading organisms which produces a Herxheimer effect. The Herxheimer is a phenomena that results from either the dead protein products of dying microorganisms, or their toxins. If an individual infested with these organisms has a susceptibility to the proteins or toxins -- which is likely for the arthritic -- their sensitive internal tissues will react with a temporary intensification of disease symptoms.

Once the germs are dead, and the patient's body has detoxified -- or cleaned out the damaging proteins and toxins -- the patient is improved or well, excepting damage that is irreversable.

Often while enduring through the Herxheimer during treatment, it appears to many as if they have the flu, and so is described as "the patient having flu-like symptoms." "Flu-like symptoms" is an over-simplification of what happens with different patients, as, in the case of rheumatoid arthritis, there is often a large "flare-up" of the disease symptoms during the Herxheimer.

In all cases of the Herxheimer, there is the appearance of a war or tussle going on inside the body akin to the antigen/antibody warfare experienced from various kinds of allergies, where the body produces fever, sweat, aching and swollen joints, diarrhea, nausea, and so on, in varying proportions with varying degrees depending upon state of metabolism, genetics, source of disturbance and so on.

When using the prescription medicines to be described, it's necessary that a physician guide the patient, and that the physician fully comprehend the distinctions between specific drug toxicities, the Herxheimer effect, and also understands possible allergic responses. These distinctions probably can come only through experiences obtained during applied clinical practices.

Those physicians who fully understand the distinction between the Herxheimer effect, drug toxicities, and allergies find themselves with a guiding clinical tool that permits physicians early in the treatment regimen to determine the probability of success for a given patient, as, through the work of Dr. Paul Pybus, Chief Medical Advisor Emeritus for The Arthritis Trust of America (formerly The Rheumatoid Disease Foundation), it was learned that, generally, the more severe the induced Herxheimer, the more probability of wellness — which is not to say that one who has a very light Herxheimer may not also get well.

Case Histories[4,5,7,8,9,173]

Successful treatment -- cure -- of rheumatoid arthritis for Jack M. Blount, M.D. and the two authors has already been described, using metrondizole. The following case histories by Professor Roger Wyburn-Mason, M.D., Ph.D, Research Fellow at Royal College of Surgeons of England, and other physicians, are among thousands of cases where patients have been successfully cured of this terrible, crippling disease.

Following these case histories are summaries of clinical studies performed by several physicians, showing their patients' rates of cures.

Successive Cases Treated With Furazolidone and Metronidazole

Furazolidone is an antibacterial and antiprotozoan drug effective against a wide range of common intestinal "parasite" infections, both bacterial and protozoan, such as *Giardia lamblia* and *Entameoba histolytica.*

Allopurinol has been reported as being an effective treatment of the protozoan diseases Leishmaniasis ("Desert Storm" disease) and Trypanosomiasis and it shows promising results in the treatment of *Trypanosoma cruzi* infections and diseases due to other blood infections (haemoflagellates).

Metronidazole is anti-yeast, antibacterial, and antiprotozoan most often used for treating vaginal trichomonas, and also as an intravenous infusion in hospitals for bacterial infections. Intravenous infusions are not useful for treating rheumatoid disease, as the metabolite of metronidazole is the active substance, which must be metabolized by our natural intestinal flora.

The following are the details of successive cases of active rheumatoid disease treated by Professor Roger Wyburn-Mason, M.D., Ph.D. with furazolidone in doses of 100 mg four times a day for 7 days. (One of us, Gus J. Prosch, Jr., M.D. treats using furazolidone for 3-4 months.)

The Case of Alice Blackthorne

Sixty two year-old Alice Blackthorne's, mother, one brother and two sisters all suffered from rheumatoid arthritis while one brother and one sister were free of the disease. A nephew and one sister suffered from diabetes. Alice's menstrual periods ceased at the age of 40 years.

Ten years previously Alice noticed painless thickening and stiffness of all joints of the fingers and thumbs gradually increasing in degree. Her knees were also affected and her symptoms became so severe that she was unable to use her hands.

Four months later the right knee and both elbows became painful and swollen, movements were restricted, and she developed bursitis of both elbows followed by pain and restricted movements of the right shoulder. She was treated with numerous anti-inflammatory drugs, including steroid (cortisone) injections into the shoulder joints and elbow (olecranon bursae).

Five months previous to being seen by Professor Wyburn-Mason, she developed carpal tunnel syndrome, a compression of a nerve (median) for which an operation was undertaken. X-rays showed some slight loss of disc space in a fingerjoint, but otherwise the appearances were within normal limits.

In the serum blood test, the so-called, Rheumatoid Factor (RF) was strongly positive, and other blood tests were consistent with rheumatoid arthritis.

Alice was taking 3 Naprosyn® tablets a day with little relief. There was morning stiffness and stiffness after sitting. Examination showed marked rheumatoid deformity of hands and thumbs and of some of the finger joints (metacarpohalangeal). She could not make a fist. The changes of rheumatoid arthritis with heat and swelling were present in both wrists. There was restriction of the shoulders, neck and foot joints (midtarsal), and some swelling of the feet was present.

Alice was treated with furazolidone, which produced dark yellow coloration of the urine, stiffness and swelling of the affected joints on waking, but less pain in the shoulder joints.

On the fifth day, the symptoms had all increased in severity with increased swelling and pain in the knees with limitation of flexion, but no free fluid. The symptoms (Herxheimer effect) persisted for the next week when they gradually subsided, and after one month had completely disappeared. She was now able to make a fist on both sides, but there was no tenderness of any joint.

Two months after beginning treatment she had been able to give up taking Naprosyn, and all joint movements were full, free and painless. There was only minimal bony swelling in her fingers which had been present for 10 years. Blood examination was now normal.

Alice remained well for the next eight months of observation.

The Case of Carrie Stringfellow

Sixty three year-old Carrie Stringfellow's past history included hysterectomy for fibroids and ovarian cysts at age of 49 years.

Three years previously, she developed pain, heat, hotness and restricted movements of the fingers, wrists, neck, elbows, shoulders, hips, knees and ankles. There was pain under the balls of the feet on weight bearing. There were headaches and nocturnal sweating. In addition she had all the symptoms and signs of proven ulcerative colitis, a chronic inflammation of the colon. She also had considerable weight loss though her appetite was good. She had been treated elsewhere with Indocid®, Feldene®, brufen, penicillamine, myocrisin, and salazoprin for diarrhea.

Examination showed a high color in the cheeks, mildly pale muco-
sae, pain and swelling of the fingers and wrist joints with deformities
of the wrists, left elbow (olecranon) bursitis, pain, and restricted movements of the shoulders making it impossible for her to feed herself or
to raise her arms above 45° from the body. Both knees showed fatty
tumors (lipomata) below the knee cap, though the movements were
reasonable and full, but painful on the left side. There was slight pain
on extreme movements of the left ankle with foot joint (midtarsal) movements painful and restricted. She was tender on pressure under the balls
of the feet.

Carrie was treated with furazolidone as above. On the fourth day,
the Herxheimer effect occurred, the joints of the upper limbs were
stiff and painful. There was pain in the neck and head. The left hip was
painful and movement restricted. The left knee became swollen and
stiff, but not hot. These symptoms persisted for six weeks and then
suddenly disappeared and on examination six weeks later the only abnormal physical sign to be made out was some slight fluid above the
right knee (supra patellar bursa); otherwise she was without evidence
of rheumatoid disease.

Carrie went on a journey to Australia and New Zealand and back
lasting six months without any recurrence of symptoms and remains
well.

The Case of Harriet Simpson

Harriet Simpson, aged 68 years had a past history of cholecystec-
tomy -- removal of the gall bladder -- for inflammation of the gall
bladder (cholecystitis) without gall stones. She also had had a ten year
history of pains in the neck and shoulders with moderately restricted
movements of the neck and shoulder joints. The neck pain tended to be
severe on waking and occurred especially on the left side. Later it
extended down both scapulae, along the course of the suprascapular
nerves. The joints of both middle fingers became hot, swollen, painful
and the movements restricted, especially of the middle interphalangeal
joints.

Examination showed moderate restriction of all movements of the
neck with pain at extremities and tenderness on pressure over the cervical spine. There was audible noise (crepitus) on the neck movements
and tenderness on pressure over the shoulder joints with some slight
restriction and pain on movements in all directions. The interphalangeal
and metacarpal-phalangeal joints of both middle fingers were hot swollen and flexion restricted, so that the tips could not voluntarily reach
the palms which showed redness over the skin of the palm. X-rays of
the fingers and shoulder joints were normal, but those of the neck
showed mild narrowing of the disc space between C4 and C5 vertebrae.

The blood count correlated with rheumatoid arthritis.

Harriet was given furazolidone in the above dosage with no effect for 4 days when she began to develop influenza-like symptoms with general malaise and aching pains in most of her joints, increased pain in the neck and shoulders, and increased signs of inflammatory changes in her middle fingers, all of which became markedly painful. Her movements were further restricted and joints more swollen. She sweated slightly and ran a temperature of 102.2° Fahrenheit for 4 days. The urine became dark yellow in color. The exaggeration of symptoms of rheumatoid disease (Herxheimer effect) persisted for two days after cessation of treatment. The exaggeration of symptoms then rapidly died down and within a week all symptoms and signs of rheumatoid arthritis had disappeared and remained absent over the next six months of observation, at the end of which time blood signs became normal.

She now feels extremely well.

The Case of Joan Tremont

Joan Tremont, aged 43 years, had a mother who suffered from rheumatoid arthritis and diabetes.

Joan's rheumatoid disease began some 5 months before being seen with pain in the balls of the feet on weight bearing, the feet swelling and the midtarsal joints becoming painful. The toes were painful on flexion and the ankles painful on any movement. Two years previously, she had pains across the lower abdomen and lumbar spine, which have persisted. In the last three months pains and swelling had spread to the fingers, thumbs, wrists, shoulders and neck, which was stiff. She suffered from night sweats. There was marked morning stiffness. Blood samples showed the Rheumatoid Factor (RF) positive. She had been treated elsewhere with aspirin, Indocid and exercise with some relief.

Examination showed warmth, tenderness, swelling and restricted movements of the wrists, finger joints, thumb joints and both foot (midtarsal) joints with tenderness on pressure under the metatarsals. X-rays showed no bony changes.

She was treated with metronidazole 2 gm on two successive evenings which was followed by generalized joint pains after 24 hours with sweating, headache, and a temperature of 101.5° Farhenheit -- the Herxheimer effect.

Seven weeks later, there was marked improvement in Joan's symptoms, but the thumb and first finger joint on both sides remained hot and swollen and the tips could not be flexed into the palms. Otherwise there were no abnormal physical signs.

Joan's symptoms persisted over the next two months when the dose of metronidazole was repeated with a similar result.

After a further two months, her only symptoms were pains in the fingers (dorsum) and tenderness of the right joint of the sternum and clavicle (sternoclavicular joint).

Five months later she noticed some return of pains and swelling to the fingers and wrists and hotness and tenderness of the right sternoclavicular joint, and hotness and tenderness on the inner side of the left foot which could not be inverted fully without pain. The symptoms remained unchanged requiring treatment with aspirin for the next year.

Joan was treated with furazolidone. After three days, this caused aching in the fingers, elbows and shoulders and the midtarsal joints with generalized influenza-like symptoms and tenderness in most of the other joints. She sweated and her temperature rose to 100.8° Fahrenheit for 3 days -- Herxheimer effect. Her symptoms rapidly disapppeared three days after cessation of treatment when she complained of only occasional sharp pains in various joints, but there were no physical signs of rheumatoid arthritis to be made out.

Four months after being treated with furazolidone, blood signs became normal. Over the course of the next three months, she became completely symptomless and has remained so for eight months since the course of furazolidone.

The Case of Peter Dickson

Peter Dickson, age 53 years, had a grandmother and mother both suffering from rheumatoid arthritis. For 15 years, he had suffered from pain in the back of the right wrist with swelling, hotness and difficulty flexing. There was occasional similar pain in the left wrist.

Some of his blood signs indicated rheumatoid arthritis, while others did not.

X-rays of the wrists and hands showed no bony changes. He had been treated with Inodcid, 25 mg twice daily, which controlled the swelling but did not completely relieve the pain and had no affect on the restriction of wrist movement.

He had also been treated by acupuncture and some kind of electrical stimulation of the area without benefit, and with various unknown herbal remedies without effect. A notable feature was that the pain and swelling were worse in the morning after taking alcohol of any sort.

The right wrist (dorsum) and neighboring region of the hand was markedly swollen, hot and tender in one small area. No flexion of the wrist was possible and palmar flexion and lateral deviation of the wrists was somewhat limited. No rheumatoid changes were found elsewhere in the body.

Peter was treated with furazolidone and this was followed by a marked increase in the swelling in the right wrist lasting 14 days -- the Herxheimer effect. He also had slight symptoms affecting the left wrist.

Three weeks after taking the tablets, pain and swelling had ceased and the movements of the wrists had returned to normal for the first time in 15 years.

He was followed for six months without return of symptoms or signs.

The Case of John Benson

Two months before John Benson, aged 59 years, was seen he noticed an onset of marked weakness of the arms with stiffness of the wrists and fingers, which could not be extended fully, and an inability to make a fist on either side. He also had tingling in the inner side of the thumb, index and middle fingers and the outer side of the ring finger on both hands. The neck was somewhat stiff, and there was marked pain and restricted movements of both shoulders and in the elbows, especially the left, and these could not be extended fully. There was also some pain and restricted flexion of the right knee. There was marked sweating of the palms of the hands, especially on the right. All the symptoms were worse after sitting. X-rays at another hospital showed no abnormalities in the joints. The weakness of the upper limbs were so severe that he was unable to carry on his work as a pianist. Blood signs were mildly indicative of rheumatoid arthritis.

John had been treated at another hospital for four months with indomethacin, 25 mg three times daily, without benefit.

Examination showed marked weakness of all muscles of the arms and of movements of the wrists and fingers with inability to lift his arms above an angle of 75° of the body at the shoulders. He was unable to dress or undress because of this weakness. The palms were sweating profusely and on both sides there was evidence of nerve dysfunction. The finger joints and wrists were swollen, hot and markedly restricted. He was unable to flex the index and ring fingers into the palms. Both elbow joints were hot and tender and the movements restricted and there was marked tenderness and pain on attempted movement of the shoulder joints. Movements were partly restricted by severe weakness and pain. There were no abnormalities in the lower limbs. The CNS (central nervous system) was normal, but tests indicated the presence of muscular weakness (myasthenia gravis) in addition to some nerve dysfunction evidently associated with the rheumatoid condition.

He was treated with furazolidone as above. This produced a headache on the second day when all his joints became painful and there was general malaise, aching and morning stiffness. He sweated during sleep, but nine days after commencing treatment there was a rapid improvement in the joint pains and weakness of his upper limbs, though three weeks later he was still unable to close his fingers fully and full extension of the right wrist was not completely possible. There was also slight weakness of extension of the right elbow.

Two months after treatment, John still complained of stiffness on waking and after sitting, with occasional pain in the right shoulder, both elbows and the middle interphalangeal joint of the right index finger. He was not quite able to make a fist and the medial nerve disturbances were still present. The middle interphalangeal joints of both index fingers were slightly swollen and tender with restricted flexion.

The course of furazolidone was then repeated for 7 days again with mild increase in pains in the upper limb joints with hotness and swelling of the wrists and elbows and increased pain in the right shoulder joint (Herxheimer effect) lasting for 5 days, after which the muscle weakness symptoms had completely disappeared and the symptoms of nerve dysfunction were absent.

All joint pain and swelling had now ceased. He was followed for a further six months and has remained symptomless.

Successive Cases Treated With Allopurinol or Metronidazole

The following are the details of successive cases of active rheumatoid disease treated by Professor Roger Wyburn-Mason, M.D., Ph.D. .

The Case of George Stanopoulis

George Stanopoulis, age 66 years, had a fifteen year history of pain, swelling and restricted movements, particularly of knees, but also of hips, ankles, wrists and hands. He had been treated by many anti-inflammatory drugs including aspirin, Naprosyn, indomethacin, Motril®, brufen and others. None of these helped the pain and swelling of the joints.

On examination, there was heat, swelling and restricted movements, especially affecting the knees but also the ankles, feet (midtarsal) joints, elbows, wrists, both shoulder joints and the neck. The finger joints were swollen, hot and tender and he could not make a fist on either side. Blood signs correlated with rheumatoid arthritis.

George was treated with allopurinol 300 mg, three times daily for 7 days without any reaction until the 4th day when he began to get shooting pains in most of his joints. The temperature rose to 102.6-103.0° Fahrenheit for 5 days accompanied by shivering chills and on the 6th day by profuse sweating. Severe stabbing pains affected the whole lower limbs, but also in various other parts of the body. This Herxheimer effect lasted for 9 days when his temperature settled and remained normal.

Five weeks after the initial rise in temperature his symptoms and signs of disease had completely disappeared according to him "in a most extraordinary way."

He has been followed for eight months during which time he has had no return of rheumatoid symptoms. He is playing golf, tennis, squash racquets and swimming.

The Case of Larry Owens

Larry Owens, aged 22 years, had a grandfather who suffered from rheumatoid arthritis.

Three years previously Larry's right knee became painful and swollen and left knee, both ankles and left elbow followed within the next six weeks. These symptoms were relieved by non-steroidal anti-inflammatories during the next six months; but after two years, he developed pain in the lower back (lumbar region) and pain, swelling, hotness and restricted movements of the right elbow and wrist, and then other joints became affected on the left. Inflammation of the iris of the eye (iridocyclitis) appeared. This condition had varied in severity over the next year during which time the left shoulder and neck became painful with restricted movements, and then the hips and the heels and insteps were also painful.

Larry sweated excessively and the back of the neck was stiff. The London Hospital had informed him that he had ankylosing spondylitis, one of the eighty or so rheumatoid diseases.

Examination showed some slight painful restriction movements to right and left. All movements of the left shoulder were moderately restricted by pain. Extension of the right elbow was limited to 15° with pain. The right wrist was hot, swollen and all movements restricted. Other joints were not affected. There was no evidence of inflammation of the eye (iritis) at the time.

He was treated with metronidazole 2 gm on two successive evenings which resulted in influenza-like symptoms on the first two days, and on the second day exaggeration of the pain and swelling in both shoulder joints, right toes, balls of the feet and heels on weight bearing -- Herxheimer effect.

After this, the elbows were less painful and their movements less restricted. Other joints, however, were not infected. He had continued to take anti-inflammatories during this time.

One month after taking metronidazole, there was slight pain at the back of the neck on flexion, but movements were full. The shoulder joints were normal. The elbows were painless and would now straighten almost completely. The right wrist was cold and not tender and the movements were now full.

The treatment was repeated for six weeks, and six weeks later the only symptom was slight pain in the ball of the right foot when walking.

Larry remained well during the next two years without taking any anti-inflammatory drugs when he reported that for the last two weeks his left shoulder had begun to ache and both knees gave him some pain on walking. The right elbow became painful and could not be extended fully. His neck was stiff on waking. There was generalized morning stiffness.

Examination showed the right elbow could not be fully extended by 10°. Blood signs were normal.

He was treated with allopurinol 300 mg three times daily for 7 days. This produced mild influenza-like symptoms, slight pyrexia of 100.8° Fahrenheit, and some generalized joint pains especially for the right elbow and left shoulder joints and swelling of both wrists lasting for two days -- the Herxheimer effect.

Following this, the symptoms rapidly disappeared and within two weeks of beginning treatment he was completely symptom free without any physical signs of disease.

He has remained completely well over the last nine months.

The Case of Donna Summers

Donna Summers' (age 64 years from Barbados) family history included a mother who suffered from inflammation of the gall bladder (cholecystitis) and mild rheumatoid arthritis, and also a half-sister who suffered from a poisoned thryoid, and a second sister who had died of gastro-intestinal cancer.

Donna had had several attacks of bladder inflammation (cystitis), and two years later she suffered from mild pains and swelling of the finger joints, wrists and pains and restricted movements of the shoulder and ankles. She was treated with aspirin without benefit; and in the next year she began to suffer from severe weakness and arthropathy of almost all the joints, and an anemia requiring blood transfusions.

She was treated by repeated courses of gold injections until two years later when this was changed to prednisolone and indomethacin suppositories. She had a replacement of the right hip. Both knees had become severely affected with rheumatoid arthritis.

Four years later the pain and restricted movements of the neck became so severe that an x-ray was taken and showed severe involvement of the whole cervical spine with dislocation (subluxation) of C1 on C2 vertebra, for which she was treated with a collar. The movements of the shoulders became remarkably painful and restricted with nodules round the elbow. Within another two years, there was severe pain under the balls of the feet, and she developed nasal blockage at this time. There was a slight chest cough with brown sputum. There was pain in the right chest on deep breathing. She also complained of considerable generalized itching.

Examination showed nasal congestion and severe thinness. The chest exhibited noise in the right mid-zone, movements of the neck were impossible, and the elbows and wrists were severely painful with all movements restricted with nodules round the elbow. The fingers and thumbs were completely useless with frozen joints. The right hip movements were free and painless (the site of the prosthesis) and the left hip movements were markedly painful and restricted. The knees were knobbly without free fluid, but with severe noise (crepitus) and full movements accompanied by pain. The midtarsal joints were fixed. The toes were markedly involved with over-riding, a humping of the joints. She was unable to stand.

X-rays of the chest showed diffuse shadowing in the right lung and gross destruction of the knees, left hip joint, fingers, wrists and elbows and of the midtarsal joints with gross deformities of the toes. Blood work was strongly positive of rheumatoid disease. An ophthalmological opinion showed evidence of eye inflammation in the eye (scleritis and conjunctivitis).

In four days, she began to run an evening pyrexia of 102.6-103.0° Fahrenheit and complained of pain, hotness and swelling of most joints and pain in the neck. In addition, she developed rheumatoid nodules over the base of the vertebrae (sacrum) and on the back of both feet (dorsa). The increase in symptoms (Herxheimer effect) lasted for two weeks when the heat (pyrexia) settled and the rheumatoid nodules began to disappear slowly. The pain in the neck gradually lessened, and the hotness of the joints died down. By this time, the movements of the neck showed marked improvement in all directions, and those of the shoulders improved to such an extent Donna was able to do her hair and feed herself again. She was able to walk round the room, but this produced aching in the knee joints after five minutes. There was, however, no joint swelling and her temperature had fallen to normal.

Donna's improvement was maintained over the next eight months; and at the end of this time, blood tests returned to normal. Her eyes were markedly less dry as confirmed by tests and there was no evidence of active rheumatoid disease, though the previous joint damage, of course, persisted.

The Case of Eleanor Hays

Eleanor Hays, aged 63 years, had a past history of hysterectomy for fibroids and ovarian cystectomy at age 49 years. Ten years later, she fell and injured the right ankle and immediately developed pain, hotness, swelling and restricted movements of the fingers, thumbs, wrists, knees, elbows, shoulders, hips and ankles, pain and stiffness and restricted movements of the neck, and pain under the balls of the feet when weight bearing. This was accompanied by headaches, sweating and loss of weight.

In addition, she later developed symptoms of ulcerative colitis proven by sigmoidoscopy, radiological appearances and mucosal biopsy. She was treated by numerous anti-inflammatory substances, including indomethacin, Naprosyn, Feldene® by prednisolone and salazopyrin for the colitis. None of these produced appreciable improvement in her condition.

Her blood showed additional signs of rheumatoid arthritis.

Examination showed high facial color with mild mucosal pallor, mild rheumatoid deformities of wrists and fingers, left elbow pain, and restricted movements of the shoulders, elbows, wrists, and neck, marked grating sound during movements of both knee joints, and restricted flexion and the presence of free fluid. Movements were painful at the extremes. The left ankle showed pain on extension, and she was tender on pressure under the balls of the feet. Walking was painful at the knees and under the balls of the feet. She was tender over the large intestine.

She was treated with allopurinol. After 4 days this produced an increase in the symptoms of joint pain, with pain in the hips, knees, and ankles, the two latter becoming hot and swollen, and her neck also became painful on movement . Her temperature rose on the 4th day to 101.3° Fahrenheit, and there was general malaise and influenza-like symptoms. The muscles were tender to the touch, and she sweated profusely -- Herxheimer effect.

These symptoms continued until two days when the temperature suddenly fell to normal; and, within 5 days, there was a complete cessation of all joint swelling, hotness and pain and cessation of symptoms and signs of ulcerative colitis.

One month later her blood signs normalized. The temperature remained completely normal, and she has remained symptomless without taking any drugs over the last ten months and without any visual evidence of arthritis, bursitis, or deformities. There were no intestinal symptoms and barium enema examination was normal.

The Case of Emily Dickinson

Emily Dickinson, age 60, had no family history of rheumatoid disease. Eighteen months previously she began to notice pain, swelling, hotness and restricted movements of the fingers and wrists later spreading to the elbows, shoulders and neck and to the knees, ankles and midtarsal joints with pain under the balls of the feet on weight bearing.

She had been previously treated with indomethacin and aspirin without relief. On examination there was evidence of acute active inflammation in the fingers, thumbs, wrists, elbows and shoulder joints with pain, tenderness, heat and restricted movements. The neck movements were painful and restricted. She was unable to extend her elbows fully or to do up or undo her brassiere. She could not feed herself. The wrists, fingers and thumb joints were markedly swollen, hot and tender, and she was unable to make a fist on either side. The knees were hot, swollen with free fluid and restricted flexion, and this also applied to the ankles and metatarsal joints.

Blood work correlated with rheumatoid arthritis.

Emily was treated with allopurinol which produced on the third day a marked rise in temperature to 103.1° Fahrenheit, sweating and generalized pains in the muscles and joints which became swollen and hot and included the jaw joints (temporo-mandibular) -- Herxheimer effect. The symptoms were severe enough to interfere with sleep in spite of continuing with the Naprosyn as before treatment.

Ten days after beginning treatment, there was a sudden fall in temperature and evidence of active rheumatoid arthritis rapidly disappeared, so that after ten days she was completely free of pain and stiffness on waking, and one month after beginning treatment she showed no abnormal physical signs whatsoever.

After three months, repetition of blood tests showed absence of disease.

Emily was followed for a further six months without return of symptoms or recourse to pain killing drugs.

The Case of Maria Solorazano del Rio

Maria Solorazano del Rio, 54 years, Brazilian, had a mother who suffered from rheumatoid arthritis. Eight years previous to being seen, she began to complain of pain, hotness, swelling and restricted movements of the fingers, wrists, elbows and shoulders, both knees, especially the right, left ankle and midtarsal foot joints. This had been treated in Brazil by hot wax baths to the fingers and wrists, by massage, exercising of the upper limbs, hands and lower limbs, and by various anti-inflammatory drugs, including prednisolone 5 mg twice daily, none of which controlled the symptoms.

On examination, there were typical rheumatoid arthritic changes in the above mentioned joints with swelling and heat, and marked redness of the palm (palmar erythema) with restricted extension of the right knee. There was tenderness on pressure under the balls of the feet and elbow. Neck movements were restricted with tenderness on pressure over the cervical spine at the side of the neck. She was unable to raise her arms above the shoulder; walking was only possible with a stick.

X-rays showed a minimal loss of disc space between C5-6 vertebrae in the neck, but were otherwise normal. Blood showed strongly positive Rheumatoid Factor (RF).

Treatment consisted of gradually tapering off the prednisolone and substituting with Feldene, 2 tablets in the morning. This, however, did not control the symptoms. She was therefore treated with a course of allopurinol.

Within three days, she had a violent joint reaction with pain, swelling, hotness and restricted movements of all her joints, profuse sweating and considerable pain requiring morphine injections to control it. The temperature reached 104.0° Fahrenheit for several days. These symptoms were the typical Herxheimer effect.

After ten days, there was a sudden cessation of her joint symptoms, pain and sweating and a fall in her temperature.

Within a week, she was free of any joint symptoms and was able to walk normally.

She was observed for the next six months during which time the symptoms did not return, even after giving up anti-inflammatory drugs.

Thousands Have Already Been Cured

In addition to curing himself and one of us (Perry A. Chapdelaine, Sr.), Jack M. Blount, Jr., M.D., Philadelphia, MS, treated more than 17,000 rheumatoid disease patients. Roger Wyburn-Mason, M.D., Ph.D. successfully treated in a professional hospital/clinical setting more than 200 cases of rheumatoid diseases. One additional adult case and three children's cases are briefly summarized in the following.

Effects of Treatment With Clotrimazole

Case 1: He was suffering from painful and complete ankylosis (immobility) of the spine and other joints of the limbs. The disease had lasted 33 years. He could not move his neck or back at all, and the joints of his extremities were swollen, tender and painful. His spine, hips and knees were flexed and fixed so that his eyes were directed toward the floor when he was standing.

In 12 weeks on clotrimazole, 2 gm per day, he was able to move his spine almost normally and to stand erect. (These large experimental dosage is no longer recommended. See physician approved treatment protocol that follows.) The swelling in his hands and feet subsided, and he was able to walk with a normal gait. He is now decorating his house, digging the garden and driving an automobile again for the first time in 30 years. (See *Ankylosing Spondilitis*, Anthony di Fabio, Hector Solorzano del Rio, M.D., Ph.D., D.Sc.)

****

Pity the Children: We pity the children who have either Still's disease, or juvenile rheumatoid arthritis, both names for rheumatoid arthritis inflicted on a younger body.

We pity the children, because parents, who want the very best for them will almost invariably take them to the traditional rheumatologist with the greatest assumed prestige, often sparing no expense.

We pity the children, because their parents are unaware of the fact that even the most expensive, most prestigious rheumatologist can do nothing for their child -- and admittedly knows that he can do nothing -- except relieve some pain while the disease permanently destroys the child's tissues and joints.

We pity children who are caught in such a damning, hellish, demonized medical system that they cannot, and will not be well -- except through the meanderings of chance or the grace of God.

****

Case 2: A physician's 5-year-old daughter, had very acute painful and tender joints and night sweats with elevated temperatures continually up to 106° Fahrenheit. She was taking prednisone 80 mg per day. Her temperature fell to normal in 12 hours after beginning clotrimazole and remained down, enabling prednisone to be stopped without return of symptoms.

Case 3: Another child — 13 years of age — had the disease since she was 1 year old. Symptoms included a low hemoglobin. Her spleen was huge and the blood sedimentation rate elevated. Her hands, knees, ankles, and feet were swollen, and she was in constant pain. She had been taking prednisone, 5mg and Indocin, 50 mg per day, with only partial relief of pain. Within 2 days of clotrimazole treatment, her temperature dropped to normal for the first time in months. By the end of 3 weeks, the corticosteroid and pain-relieving drugs could be stopped, and she was walking comfortably. Her hemoglobin increased from 50% normal to 80% normal in just a few weeks. At the end of 12 weeks, all signs of active rheumatoid arthritis had subsided.

Case 4: A boy age 5, proved that the most dramatic results with clotrimazole occur in juvenile arthritis. He was completely handicapped by pain, swelling and joint deformities from onset of the disease. He had been taking prednisone, 30 mg per day. He was 9 inches too short and 20 pounds overweight for his age. In 3 or 4 days after the start of clotrimazole, 500 mg once a day, he had so much relief of pain and swelling that his actions were "lively and comfortable." He became almost uncontrollable. The cortisone was decreased at the rate of 5 mg each week, and he continued to improve. Clotrimazole was given at 500 mg/day for 5 weeks and then decreased to 250 mg/day for 7 more weeks. After 12 weeks, it appeared that he had made a "full recovery." After a year, he has remained well and is now of normal weight and height for his age.

Trials of Tinidazole Based on
Madden, J.E., B.M., B. Ch. [Oxford], and Mendel, D., M.D., B.S., Hounslow Health Centre, Middlesex, England

Introduction

Professor Roger Wyburn-Mason, M.D., Ph.D. first reported the effect of bile salts, copper sulfate, allopurinol, furazolidone, clotrimazole, and tinidazole drugs on cases of active rheumatoid arthritis. He found that in almost all cases, on first administration, these medicines caused an immediate transient exaggeration of the manifestations of the disease often with influenza-like symptoms and in the appearance of lesions in tissues not previously affected -- the Herxheimer effect. These symptoms gradually disappeared over the course of the next 2-3 months and in many cases all signs of disease activity were lost both clinically and in blood signs in the course of 8-12 months. The exaggeration of the symptoms of the disease could be lessened by the concomitant administration of an anti-inflammatory substance.

Doctors Madden and Mendel, Hounslow Health Centre, Middlesex, England, undertook a trial in an attempt to confirm this report, using tinidazole.

The cases of rheumatoid arthritis used in the trial were successive ones fulfilling the features of probable, definite or classical examples of rheumatoid arthritis according to the American Rheumatism Association classification system used in a general medical practice.

In most cases, those which were already taking anti-inflammatory drugs continued on this regimen, and the tinidazole was given as 2 gram doses on 2 successive days. An attempt at a double blind crossover trial with a placebo was unsuccessful, since in all cases taking tinidazole within 24 hours there occurred generalized malaise with influenza-like symptoms, profuse nocturnal sweating and a marked increase in the joint pain by the second or third day so that the trial was no longer blind to the observer; that is, the Herxheimer effect occurred. Therefore an open trial was used. Full investigations of each case were carried out immediately before and throughout the trial and continued for 12 months or more after the administration of the tinidazole. All patients were advised not to take alcohol during the next month and not to exercise the joints any more than essential and to avoid massage and heating the joints.

Ten cases were treated successively, all becoming well, and follow up two years later showed that wellness remained. In all ten cases, tinidazole induced sweating, pyrexia, and exaggeration of the symptoms of active disease both in the affected tissues and the appearance of inflammation in other joints, not previously affected -- the Herxheimer effect. These phenomena gradually settled down during the next few months; and after one year, joints in which no radiological damage was present were normal clinically.

Accompanying swelling of a gland and duct near the ear (parotid), and ulcerative colitis cleared permanently.

In joints with erosion of cartilage or bone deformities, symptoms persisted.

After a year, the blood changes returned to normal.

Trials of Metronidazole by
Archimedes A. Concon, M.D., Memphis, Tennessee
Introduction

Dr. Archimedes A. Concon had the experience of trying anti-microorganism drugs on a wide variety of ailments with many patients. The authors have chosen the following three examples, which includes the effect of metronidazole on the related rheumatoid diseases psoriasis, lupus erythematosus, and rheumatoid arthritis, all of which are interrelated and supposedly incurable by traditional medical practices

Cases Treated With Metronidazole (Narrated by Dr. Concon)

Case 1: "A 33-year-old white male patient came to see me with a history of psoriasis involving the hands and fingers of 12 years duration. The patient was put on metronidazole, 500 mg, 4 tablets (2 gm), after supper daily for 2 days, rest 5 days, and to repeat course indefinitely until well. At the end of 4 months, the skin on the hands were largely clear. Most of the fingernails were normal looking. At the end of 6 months, patient was clinically free."

(Psoriasis has been successfully cured and controlled, respectively, by use of anti-microorganism drugs, fumaric acid ester and pyrithione zinc. See *The Surprising Psoriasis Treatment*, Anthony di Fabio.)

Case 2: "A 61-year-old white female came in with complaints of rheumatoid arthritis involving the hands, left hip, and knees of 14 years duration. She was barely able to use her hands or walk at the time I saw her because of stiffness and pain of joints involved. She was put on metronidazole, 500 mg, 4 tablets (2 gm), after supper daily for 2 days, rest 5 days, and repeat course indefinitely until well. At the end of 3 months from the start of treatment, stiffness and pain in joints were hardly noticeable. At the end of 6 months from start of treatment, patient was clinically free. During course of treatment, patient complained of chronic nausea which was bearable. The chronic nausea disappeared after termination of treatment."

Case 3: "A 29-year-old white male patient came in with a history of Systemic Lupus Erythematosus, of 7 years duration with recent kidney involvement. His albuminuria (urinary protein) was 2+. Urinary output was adequate at start of treatment. Patient was put on metronidazole, 500 mg, 4 tablets (2 gm), after supper daily for 2 days, rest 5 days, repeat course indefinitely until well. After 1 month of treatment, his albuminuria was 1+. His urinary output was adequate. At the end of 5 months of treatment, his albuminuria was negative, and his urinary output was adequate. Patient could tolerate exposure to sunlight where before he could not. Patient was clinically free." (Systemic Lupus Erythematosus and Scleroderma have been cured by use of anti-microorganisms drugs followed with intravenous IVs of EDTA and DMSO, or IVs of hydrogen peroxide. See *Lupus and Scleroderma*, Anthony di Fabio.)

Cases Treated With Metronidazole by William Renforth, M.D., Connorsville, Indiana

Case 1: The patient was a 47-year-old white female with a diagnosis of rheumatoid arthritis at age 36. She had been treated by aspirin and weekly injections of cortisone, but had never been exposed to gold, penicillamine, anti-malarials, or anti-metabolites.

By third week of treatment with metronidazole she began to complain of mild aches and pains, but had a decrease in inflammatory swelling of wrists and ankles. By the fourth week she had marked reduction in swelling of wrists, fingers, ankles, and the rheumatoid nodules reduced in size. By the fifth week there was no evidence of acute, active rheumatoid arthritis, except nodules. By the sixth week, nodules were less prominent, and there was some correction in former deviation of her fingers.

By the 45th week rheumatoid nodules had disappeared leaving

only mild roughened areas in the tissue over the bony areas. She's resumed her usual physical activities and again does such tasks as needlework and setting her own hair. She now uses only an occasional aspirin dosage to relieve the discomforts attributed to the permanent damage.

Case 2: A 68-year-old white male had nodular rheumatoid arthritis for at least 10 years duration. He also had Sjogren's syndrome, a marked dryness of mucous membranes resulting from deficient secretion of glands. He had severe upper and lower extremity muscle atrophy, contractures of elbows and knees, inflammed and swollen joints, deformities of his hands and feet, and painful rheumatoid plantar nodules which required that he split his shoe uppers and wear bunion pads on the soles of his feet to relieve some of the pain of walking. There were changes in his lung, and chronic hepatitis. The patient literally could not raise his hands with sufficient strength to feed himself. His treatment consisted of aspirin and codeine for pain, and steroids from time to time.

As treatment progressed and the swelling and pain subsided, exercises were prescribed to recover muscular strength.

In the 24th week of metronidazole therapy, he now assists in his own personal care, drives his camper truck, is independently mobile, free of nodules, pads and painful feet. He stands about 3 inches taller now that he is free of contractures.

This patient and his wife were lost to follow-up as they have driven to Florida to resume his former occupation of fishing.

Conclusion

The above findings show that when the anti-microorganism substances in the proper dosages metronidazole, clotrimazole, tinidazole, furazolidone and allopurinol are administrated to patients suffering from active rheumatoid disease, within a few days there is caused an exaggeration of the disease symptoms -- Herxheimer effect -- which may be severe and accompanied by a rise in blood signs (ESR, eosinophilia), sweating, heat (pyrexia), all of which begin to die down after about ten days. This may be sudden and is followed by rapid and complete relief of disease symptoms, except destruction of joint cartilage or bone or permanent deformities. Muscle weakness (myasthenia gravis), psoriasis, lupus, ulcerative colitis, and other "auto-immune" or "collagen tissue" diseases likewise disappear.

In the next six months, all blood (serological) signs of infection disappear and the patient returns to health and normalization of the blood signs and, in the course of time, the rheumatoid factor (RF), if present, becomes negative.

It was fifteen years ago that the two tables below were constructed. Since then, 80% of the patients of at least one physician (Gus J. Prosch, Jr., M.D.) -- using the programs advocated herein -- have been cured

Comparative Results of Treatment With Other Drugs by Robert Bingham, M.D., Desert Hot Springs, California

Treatment	Patients Treated	Improved or Remissions	Percent of Change
Controls	22	7	30
Conventional Care	30	8	27
Copper Sulfate	12	8	66
Bile Salts	12	9	75
Clotrimazole	9	7	78
Diiodohydrooxyquinon	204	189	93
Chloroquine	12	6	50
Metronidazole	221	181	82*

*Recent cases have done better on increased dosages.

Comparative Results of Treatment With Other Drugs by Gus J. Prosch, Jr., M.D., Birmingham, Alabama

Effect	Metronidazole	%	Furazolidone	%	Rifampicin	%
None	7	3.5	23	39.0	16	5.0
Mild	9	4.5	7	11.9	5	16.0
Moderate	29	14.5	5	8.5	3	9.0
Good	56	28.0	14	23.7	5	16.0
Very Good	99	49.5	10	17.9	3	55.0
Total	**200**	**100.0**	**59**	**100.0**	**32**	**55.0**

of so-called "incurable" crippling Rheumatoid Diseases. There's good reason to believe that nearly 100% can halt the progress of their disease if they will faithfully follow all of the important recommended programs.

The Arthritis Trust of America/The Rheumatoid Disease Foundation Treatment Protocol: Anti-Microorganism Therapy

The Arthritis Trust of America's treatment protocol, developed by a committee of physicians and adopted by the Foundation in 1983, must be administered by a licensed physician, usually a Medical Doctor or Doctor of Osteopathy, or any physician (especially in foreign countries) who can prescribe the medicines that are to be recommended.

The physician must determine whether or not your body is capable of handling (metabolizing) the various medicines without danger, and whether or not interaction between various medicines that you may be taking will be safe.

Your physician must also make a determination that you do not suffer from neurological disease, such as multiple sclerosis (MS). If you have MS and should take some of the medicines described, the progress of your MS may advance — which is obviously not what is desired. (If you have multiple sclerosis, see *Universal Oral Vaccine*, Anthony di Fabio.)

In case that scares you, keep in mind that in the *Physician's Desk Reference*[21] (a collection of drug companies' package inserts) the use of some of our recommended medicines already carries warning against use by multiple sclerosis victims, and that all ethical physicians know or seek to know contents of the drug's characteristics before prescribing for a patient.

While the medicines to be described are toxic, they are nowhere near as toxic as those traditionally employed by rheumatologists when treating rheumatoid arthritis. They are to be used only for a brief period of time, just long enough to kill off vast quantities of microorganisms that seek to create rapid crippling and disfigurement. Meanwhile other programs, such as improved nutrition, anti-candida, detoxification, sterilization of foci of infection, identifying and handling allergies, and so on can be employed effectively, especially if the disease is now halted.

Medicines successfully used for the treatment and remission or cure of rheumatoid arthritis and related collagen diseases now called "rheumatoid diseases" are shown in the following table.

Table of Broad Spectrum Anti-Microorganism Drugs Used to Cure Rheumatoid Disease[7]

Generic Name	Chemical Compound Group	Brand Name	Source
allopurinol	pyrimidine	Zyloprim®	Burroughs-Wellcome
copper ions	0.005 mcg coated resins*		Dr. Seldon Nelson
clotrimazole*	imidazole	Mycelex®	Dome (Not Suitable)
clotrimazole*	imidazole	Lotrimin®	Delbay (Not Suitable)
diiodohydroxyquinon (Iodoquinol)	oxyquinoline	Yodoxin®	Glenwood
furazolidone	nitrofuran	Furoxone®	Roberts
metronidazole	nitroimidazole	Flagyl®	Searle
nimorazole	nitroimidazole	Emtryl®	Salsbury
nimorazole	nitroimidazole	Naxogin®	Erba
ornidazole	nitroimidazole	Tiberal®	Roche
rifampin	rifamycin B	Rifadin®	Marion Merrill Dow
rifampicin	rifamycin B	Rimactane®	CibaGeneva
tinidazole*	nitroimidazole	Fasigyn®	Pfizer
potassium para amino benzoate	vitamin B	POTABA®	Glenwood

*Available in USA through compounding pharmacists with prescription. Clotrimazole must be in a pure form. Tinidazole is available in Australia as Fasigyn® 500 and is known as Fasigyn or Tinidex® in Mexico without prescription. Copper ions available through Dr. Seldon Nelson, 4386 Meridian, Williamston, MI 48895.

See *Catalog of Recommended Substances and Sources* for compounding pharmacists.

Not all of the above medicines will work for everyone or against all possible organisms that can generate the conditions of rheumatoid diseases. In clinical practices usually one must start with a commonly accepted medicine or combination of medicines and make a trial, which will be described.

The English Professor Roger Wyburn-Mason, Ph.D., M.D., discovered use of most of the recommended medicines except metronidazole, whose use for rheumatoid arthritis was discovered by the Philadelphia, Mississippi physician, Jack M. Blount, Jr., M.D.; diiodohydroxyquinon (iodoquinol), to be used for these purposes, was discovered by Robert Bingham, M.D. of California; Seldon Nelson, D.O. of Williamston, Michigan developed the use of copper ions.

The treatment protocol, was designed by a volunteer committee of The Arthritis Trust of America (The Rheumatoid Disease Foundation) referral physicians. This committee was chaired by Robert M. Johnson, M.D. of Charleston, South Carolina. The protocol was subsequently modified through additional clinical findings.[7]

<u>You Must Get Off of Traditional Drugs.</u>

If you're being treated with gold, penicillamine or methotrexate, or other cytoxic drugs, then quit! Wait four months before taking our treatment, as your immunological system has already been so upset by these ineffective and often damaging treatments that your body probably will not respond well if at all to any of our medicines. DO NOT TAKE OUR TREATMENT AT THE SAME TIME YOU ARE TAKING GOLD, PENICILLAMINE, METHOTREXATE OR ANY OTHER CYTOTOXIC DRUGS. To do so simply lays the groundwork for maintaining the disease and related conditions at the same time you are attempting to rid yourself of the disease.

<u>Decrease and Get Rid of Cortisone!</u>

All of the forewarnings about cortisone were to say this: If you are hooked on cortisone, start decreasing dosage <u>under proper medical supervision</u>. Decreasing the dosage of cortisone can be dangerous if you have reached a stage where daily or weekly shots or oral pills have replaced your body's natural ability to produce cortisol (your body's natural cortisone). Except for those who no longer have any ability to produce cortisol for themselves, you MUST get off from any kind of cortisone, whether in the oral form of prednisone or given as injections, or purchased in Mexico under some brand name, or through a clinic, or found in herbs. Cortisone usage, while damping down symptoms, also permits arthritis and related diseases such as candidiasis to spread. Cortisone also interferes with the effectiveness of our treatment.

If pain is so very excruciating that you cannot be taken from corticosteroids, then have your physician consider learning the Gus J.

Prosch, M.D./Dr. Paul K. Pybus/Roger Wyburn-Mason, M.D., Ph.D. Intraneural Injections described in Chapter I: Osteoarthritis, "Structure," "Intraneural Injections." It is a very safe, tried and true method, and will tide you through until you no longer suffer.

Those patients who live near a physician trained in the Prosch/ Pybus/Wyburn-Mason Intraneural Injection treatment can most easily eliminate analgesics and other anti-inflammatories by repeated visits.

Analgesics and Non-Steroidal Anti-inflammatory Drugs

If you're on aspirin, or aspirin substitutes, non-steroidal anti-inflammatory drugs (NSAIDS) -- indomethacin, phenylbutazone, etc. -- then you may continue using any of these within safe limits. Their usage will not interfere with our recommended treatments and may not cause your immunological system to weaken. Consider, however, that continued use of these drugs can also damage you, as described in both preceding chapters under "Traditional Treatments."

When our treatments are completed successfully you should be pain free, or on minimum dosages of these anti-inflammatories until your body repairs itself.

The Successful Anti-Microorganism Treatment

Based on the knowledge that a variety of microorganisms can create rheumatoid arthritis in tissue-sensitive people, successful treatment relies on broad-spectrum medicines to rapidly saturate the body, kill the organisms, and then permit the body to sweep out the dead organisms and their products. When someone tells you that, say, metronidazole is an anti-bacterial agent, or that clotrimazole is mainly an "anti-fungal" agent, and that "everyone knows" that rheumatoid arthritis is not caused by bacteria, amoeba, or fungus, just nod and go on your way. Many of the medicines to be described can be shown under laboratory conditions to be combinations of anti-bacterial, anti-myctotic, anti-viral, viral-static, anti-protozoal or anti-yeast/fungus, under the correct conditions.

In the United States, the most frequently used first-trial medicine for rheumatoid disease is metronidazole. It's listed in the *Physician's Desk Reference,* a collection of drug packaging inserts, as being FDA approved for marketing and human use. It's easily available by prescription and is relatively well known. It's use has resulted in a large number of remissions/cures.

In this treatment protocol, and on first trial, you should take simultaneously metronidazole and allopurinol, the allopurinol during the first week. Allopurinol is normally used for gouty arthritis, but laboratory studies show that it has strong effects against certain kinds of invading organisms.

Based on a 200 pound weight, you should take 2 grams of metronidazole either in one dosage, or distributed throughout four equal treatments, per day. You should take this dosage for two days in a row, then skip for five days.

You should repeat this procedure in all for six weeks.

During the first week only, you should take 300 mg of allopurinol 3 times a day, for 7 days, then quit, taking only the metronidazole throughout the remaining 5 weeks.

For each 25 pounds you weigh over or under 200 pounds, you should increase or decrease, respectively, your dosage of metronidazole by 1/4 gram or 250 milligrams.

Five hundred milligram tablets are fine, but if your physician prescribes metronidazole in 250 mg pills, then you can easily adjust the amount taken by your weight. For example, if you weigh 100 pounds, you need to reduce the amount of metronidazole taken by 1 gram, or by four 250 mg tablets, because the difference between 200 pounds and 100 pounds is 100 pounds, which is four 25 pound units less than the treatment formula specifies for a 200 pound person. Similarly, therefore, if you weigh 250 pounds, you need to increase the dosage to 2-1/2 grams. A child, therefore, can be administered proper dosage simply by observing the weight and subtracting accordingly. Approximations to the closest 25 pound unit are acceptable.

This technique of dosage by weight is common in prescription applications, because the human body's capability of metabolizing — converting chemicals and food to usable substances, or detoxifying poisons — is often directly correlated to weight.

All cautions described by the package inserts for any of these recommended drugs should be carefully observed by your physician.

If you're an arthritic who also has candidiasis, then don't use the metronidazole first, because it will make the yeast infestation worse. In candidiasis patients one of us (Gus J. Prosch, M.D.) always uses clotrimazole, giving heavy doses two days out of the week, and then maybe a capsule morning and night the other five days of the week. Of course, you still have to receive *Lactobacillus acidophilus*, as well as the other appropriate treatments.

If you are one of the rare people allergic to allopurinol, your doctor may substitute furazolidone in the following dosage: 100 mg, four times a day for one to three months, but should any numbness of toes or fingers develop, the furazolidone should be discontinued.

Either allopurinol or furazolidone may also be taken alone as may metronidazole. However, if you are to benefit by our experiences, it is probably best to take the combination described as first trials, as the combinations act as broad-spectrum "anti-amoebics," or "anti-microbials."

In the place of metronidazole, one may take if available any of the other 5-nitroimidazoles, which includes tinidazole, clotrimazole, nimorazole and ornidazole. They may be taken in combination with allopurinol or furazolidone, or alone. The dosage is exactly the same as described for metronidazole, and the time period exactly the same.

To some extent clotrimazole is anti-amoebic, anti-viral, viral-static, anti-mycotic, anti-yeast/fungus, and anti-bacterial. It does not kill all germs, but for certain species, clotrimazole may be effective in specific dosages under specific conditions.

According to *in vitro* (test tube) research funded by The Arthritis Trust of America (The Rheumatoid Disease Foundation) and performed at Medical College of Virginia by Brian Susskind, Ph.D., Assistant Professor, Surgery and Microbiology and Immunology and Richard C. Franson, Ph.D., Associate Professor of Biochemistry, Clotrimazole also inhibits a substance inside the body known as phospholipase A_2 which is a precursor (forerunner) to production of prostaglandins (from the arachidonic acid cascade) that helps to create inflammatory responses that produce heat (pyrexia), swelling (edema) and pain in the arthritic. Phospholipase is an enzyme derived from a fatty acid containing phosphorus.

Clotrimazole stimulates the body's own production of cortisol. It acts as an "immuno-modulator" rebalancing some of the out-of-kilter characteristics of the immunological system.

Clotrimazole kills *Candida albicans*, the yeast-fungus organism that causes so many symptoms that appear to be rheumatoid arthritis, and which also creates other major medical problems, such as food allergies.

Clotrimazole is usually easier for the patient to tolerate than metronidazole — but patient tastes vary.

Nimorazole and ornidazole are available in some European countries, and perhaps elsewhere, but not in the United States. Tinidazole is available almost everywhere in the world. In the United States it can be obtained by prescription through compounding pharmacists,[52] and is easily available at any drugstore in Mexico without a prescription under the trade names of Fasigyn® or Tinidex®. Clotrimazole can be obtained by prescription through any of several compounding pharmacists in Canada and the United States, and is available in Europe.[52]

So, which is the "best" medicine in the whole treatment protocol so far as is known to date?

Answer: There is no "best." The medicine that gets you well is best, and that may also vary from person to person.

****

For a catalog listing of recommended sources, including compounding pharmacists, send a self-addressed, stamped, legal-size envelope and a tax-exempt donation to The Arthritis Trust of America, 5106 Old Harding Road, Franklin, Tn 37064.

****

Incidentally, the lower cost generic medicines in all of the drugs named are perfectly satisfactory.

If diiodohydroxyquinon (also known as iodoquinol) is used, it should be taken as 650 mg three times a day, for three weeks.

Potassium para amino benzoate, known as POTABA, should be taken as 2 grams, 6 times daily for two weeks.

Arthritics are often copper deficient, but copper ions also kill a number of microorganisms. "Copper ions" are small, resin granules upon which are deposited copper ions by a special process developed by Seldon Nelson, D.O.[52] Each granule contains but five one-hundredths of a gram of copper; these tiny granules are taken sub-lingually (beneath the tongue) in various ways: Usually the physician will start the patient with about 20 or 30 granules several times a day, increasing the amount by 10 or 20 per day, until a Herxheimer reaction is observed. Since large numbers of these small granules do not exceed the daily minimum requirement for copper, they do not require a prescription.

Used as a last resort, rifampin (or rimactane), a tuberculosis drug, should be taken as 600 mg daily for one month.

Caution on use of rifampin (or rimactane), as it is a medicine that must be administered under close supervision, and if complications occur, then the physician should take you off of it immediately.

If you have nausea with any of these medicines, your physician can prescribe an anti-nausea tablet.

It is best to start with metronidazole or clotrimazole, either with allopurinol, but not necessary.

It is certainly best to follow the dosages, and "wash-out" periods advised by the recommended treatment protocol. "Wash-out" means days when the drugs are not administered. The protocol was designed to be broad-spectrum, to saturate, and to permit drug detoxification before continuing saturation.

It is best to use the various medicines individually or in the combinations already described, but not necessary.

Usually most patients respond to the first medicines when used properly in the proper dosages, but there are a significant number that do not. Reasons they do not has already been described: their past and possibly present use of gold, penicillamine, methotrexate (cytotoxic drugs) or long-term cortico-steroids. No one should deny such patients trials with our treatment for those reasons, but they should be made to understand (1) that they should get off of cortisone if at all possible and safe — and absolutely to get off of gold, penicillamine and methotrexate or other cytotoxic drugs for 4-months prior to our treatment; (2) that their response to our treatment may not be as sure, spectacular or as swift as those not having been on such drugs; and (3) that they may need to use a number of other related and supporting treatments which, by the way, many others may also need in the long run, as has been and will be described.

Prior to taking metronidazole, the physician should insure that the patient is provided with a good supplement of intestinal microflora, such as *Lactibacilus acidophilus*. Yogurt may or may not do as it is a bulgaris species. There is medical objection to commercial Yogurt as found in most supermarkets in that such brands are often mixed with sugars and promote the growth of an arthritis-accompanying and damaging organism called *Candida albicans*, a yeast fungus that can create similar symptoms to arthritis, and other problems. There is also objection to the use of pasteurized products labeled as "acidophilus" this or that. If organisms are killed by pasteurization, then why advertise their presence?

When you look around for a good grade of intestinal microflora supplement use caution. While it does not require a prescription to purchase *Lactibacilus acidophilus* from a health food store, you may be getting a poorly performing species, or, as bad, an organism that has already been weakened by environmental conditions. Any time temperature exceeds about 74 degrees Fahrenheit, the organism may lose viability or die, as when it is transported, left on the floor or in the stockroom of the store temporarily, or inadvertently placed on non-refrigerated shelves.[53]

One of us (Gus J. Prosch, Jr., M.D.) has tried patients on a large number of the commercial probiotics (*Lactobacilus acidophilus*), settling on Vital Life from Klaire Laboratories, Inc. 1573 West, Seminole, San Marcos, CA 92069; (619) 744-09680.

Physicians who administer *Lactobacilus acidophilus*, a beneficial and symbiotic organism, usually order from a company that is known to culture a good, viable grade, and it is immediately refrigerated, which you should do also upon receiving it.

Take about 1/4 teaspoon five or six times daily. Over about three weeks, you should begin to build up proper intestinal microflora so that these organisms will metabolize metronidazole. Your enzyme system cannot metabolize metronidazole, which helps to explain why metronidazole does not always work with rheumatoid arthritics in the dosages required. Metronidazole, being also anti-bacterial, may knock out "good guys" microflora on the first six-week trials, in which case second-time trials may not be effective, as the "good-guys" microflora is not present in sufficient numbers to metabolize the medicine properly.

Supplementation with viable *Lactobacilus acidophilus* will help to normalize gut flora and reduce the concentration of certain bacteria (gram-negative), a major source of "endotoxins." Endotoxins are toxins usually confined inside the body of these bacteria until it dies, at which time the toxins are released. At the same time *Lactobacilus acidophilus* will inhibit overgrowth of the damaging yeast/fungus, *Candida albicans* (and other organisms-of-opportunity), which has itself been implicated in the disruption of immune functions as well as gastrointestinal inflammation. *Candida albicans* increases our absorption of existing endotoxins. These endotoxins also contribute to rheumatoid arthritis symptoms for those who are tissue-sensitive.

Unlike metronidazole, clotrimazole and tinidazole can be metabolized by both the human enzyme system and intestinal microflora, but it's still best to supplement your diet with *Lactobacilus acidophilus* because these medicines will assist, and will also kill off "good guys" microflora, and also for other reasons.

As a matter of good practice, after the initial few weeks of build-up of 5 to 6 one-quarter teaspoons per day of *Lactobacilus acidophilus*, it might be well to supplement with the same 1/4 teaspoon about three to four times a day until you are certain that you no longer need the organism or other probiotics that your physician suggests. In any case, it is well to take a dosage with every application of the recommended drugs. Your physician may have different dosages in mind, which you should follow.

<u>There is no evidence that metronidazole when used intravenously has any effect on halting rheumatoid disease</u>, but it might for a short period reduce some inflammation. Metronidazole is used intravenously frequently for bacterial infections, especially when the patient has been hospitalized. Temporarily reducing inflammation can be done easily by many other safe, natural means.

In any case, it is the metabolite (through the stomach) of metronidazole that kills the organisms that contribute to rheumatoid arthritis, and not metronidazole, itself. For that reason, IV-administered metronidazole is not recommended for treatment of rheumatoid arthritis.

Summary

We've showed you a way that most people suffering from rheumatoid arthritis, and related rheumatoid diseases, can quickly stop the disease process. There are other methods for achieving the same healthful goals and if one of these has worked for someone else, it may work for you. After all, your goal and ours is to see folks well, not to invest religious fervor in one particular method.

When using the treatment described in this chapter, keep in mind that future fitness depends upon satisfying your nutritional needs, staving off candidiasis and food allergies, detoxification processes, and perhaps numerous other requirements that fit your needs. Rheumatoid arthritis, and related diseases, are multi-factorial, meaning that many different conditions can and do create the same disease process.

In the chapters that follow we want you to learn about some of the other treatments that health professionals have developed for you. A few, such as dietary and nutritional recommendations, you ignore at a risk of bringing back your diseased condition. Others may not apply to you, but will to someone.

You'll be amazed at the number of ways to achieve wellness!

Diet and Supplements
Nutrition and Supplements

Inherited from our parents and from their parents, each of us is designed with a different biochemistry. There are, however, four general nutritional guidelines that must be considered for arthritics: (1) proper nutrition and supplement intake; (2) candidiasis diet; (3) food allergy diet; and (4) nutritional requirements unique to the individual, such as one suffering from diabetes. See Figure 10: "Dietary Source of Degenerative Disease."

Keep in mind the advice of Nicholas Gonzalez, M.D.,[220] who, during an interview with *Townsend Letter for Doctors*, said, "It is absolute insanity to suggest that the whole human species, as different as it is, could be put on one diet. The human species occupies every ecological niche from the arctic circle to equatorial rain forests and there are different foods available in these regions, and people have had to adjust. There is no way one diet is suitable for everybody."

According to Joel Wallach, D.V.M., N.D., we all have environmental, social, ethnic and religious limits to what we'll consume. We're all bogged down in such catch phrases as "wisdom of the body," "the Mediterranean diet," "the four food groups," "variety," and religious restrictions of various kinds.[249] A wonderful source for minerals and other essential substances, for example, are a variety of insects, but few in our modern world will consume insects.

As rheumatoid arthritis can generate irreversible tissue and joint damage faster than either candidiasis or food allergies, we normally recommend that the rheumatoid arthritis disease be halted first, before beginning the more stringent dietary aspects designed to reduce candidiasis and food allergies; although, it's entirely possible that the arthritic condition will not be fully healed until both candidiasis and food allergies are also considered. Frequently it's necessary to untangle all factors at the same time, not just one factor.

Excluding the very real possibility that the arthritic suffers from food allergies and candidiasis, there's only one proper food diet for the vast majority of us. That diet is one of fresh fruit and vegetables, whole grains and nuts, non-farmed cold-water fish, and, so on, as depicted in Figure 10: "Dietary Source of Degenerative Diseases." This diet is described by many health professionals in many different publications, often with some unimportant variations. It's chief characteristic is that food should be as natural as possible, as opposed to food that has been canned, frozen, packaged, or in any way treated for shelf-life stability or changed between the garden and the human mouth.

Figure 10:
Dietary Source of Degenerative Disease

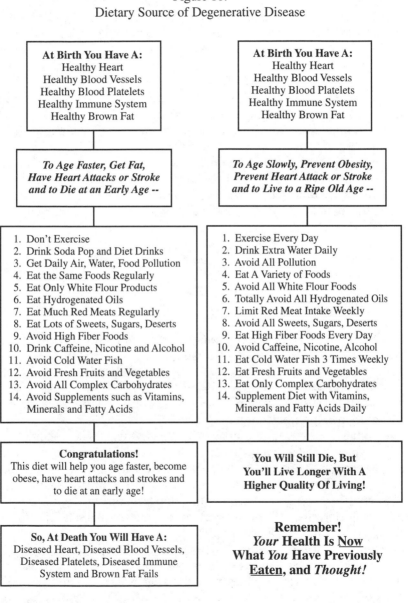

At Birth You Have A:
Healthy Heart
Healthy Blood Vessels
Healthy Blood Platelets
Healthy Immune System
Healthy Brown Fat

At Birth You Have A:
Healthy Heart
Healthy Blood Vessels
Healthy Blood Platelets
Healthy Immune System
Healthy Brown Fat

*To Age Faster, Get Fat,
Have Heart Attacks or Stroke
and to Die at an Early Age --*

*To Age Slowly, Prevent Obesity,
Prevent Heart Attack or Stroke
and to Live to a Ripe Old Age --*

1. Don't Exercise
2. Drink Soda Pop and Diet Drinks
3. Get Daily Air, Water, Food Pollution
4. Eat the Same Foods Regularly
5. Eat Only White Flour Products
6. Eat Hydrogenated Oils
7. Eat Much Red Meats Regularly
8. Eat Lots of Sweets, Sugars, Deserts
9. Avoid High Fiber Foods
10. Drink Caffeine, Nicotine and Alcohol
11. Avoid Cold Water Fish
12. Avoid Fresh Fruits and Vegetables
13. Avoid All Complex Carbohydrates
14. Avoid Supplements such as Vitamins, Minerals and Fatty Acids

1. Exercise Every Day
2. Drink Extra Water Daily
3. Avoid All Pollution
4. Eat A Variety of Foods
5. Avoid All White Flour Foods
6. Totally Avoid All Hydrogenated Oils
7. Limit Red Meat Intake Weekly
8. Avoid All Sweets, Sugars, Deserts
9. Eat High Fiber Foods Every Day
10. Avoid Caffeine, Nicotine, Alcohol
11. Eat Cold Water Fish 3 Times Weekly
12. Eat Fresh Fruits and Vegetables
13. Eat Only Complex Carbohydrates
14. Supplement Diet with Vitamins, Minerals and Fatty Acids Daily

Congratulations!
This diet will help you age faster, become obese, have heart attacks and strokes and to die at an early age!

**You Will Still Die, But
You'll Live Longer With A
Higher Quality Of Living!**

So, At Death You Will Have A:
Diseased Heart, Diseased Blood Vessels,
Diseased Platelets, Diseased Immune
System and Brown Fat Fails

Remember!
Your **Health Is Now**
What *You* **Have Previously**
Eaten, and *Thought!*

What is seldom mentioned during the advice to consume fresh fruit and vegetables is that it's next to impossible to consume a sufficient amount of any food to obtain the necessary minerals which will activate important enzymes. This factor was first reported in 1936 in a U.S. Document #264 published by the 2nd session of the 74th Congress, stating that "The alarming fact is that foods -- fruits and vegetables and grains, now being raised on millions of acres of land that no longer contains enough of certain needed minerals, are starving us -- no matter how much we eat. . . . Lacking vitamins, the [human] system can make some use of minerals, but lacking minerals, vitamins are useless."[249]

Current agriculture adds nitrogen and phosphorous to soils, producing wonderful appearing plants which appear healthy but lack over sixty essential minerals required by the tens of thousands of enzyme systems necessary for proper functioning and long, productive lives.

In a June 1992 Earth Summit Report issued in Rio, Argentina, the following depletion table was presented, according to Joel Wallach, D.V.M., N.D., author of *Rare Earths: Forbidden Cures*:[249]

Continent	% Mineral Depletion Over the Last 100 Years
Africa	74%
Asia	76%
Australia	55%
Europe	72%
North America	85%
South America	76%

According to Dr. Wallach, "Our earth is anemic! In short this means we can no longer get the 60 nutritional minerals we need from our food and if we are to sustain ourselves and our children physically and mentally we must very consciously supplement our daily intake of food with the 60 nutritional minerals just as we consciously make sure our Mercedes has the finest motor oil in it!"[249]

Collagen tissue/autoimmune disease victims, however, may require extra-special attention to certain additional nutrients, such as the proper essential fatty acids,[27] and also possible additional vitamin and mineral supplements, including the various anti-oxidants and perhaps even boron, an element once thought not to have any use by the human body but determined by the research of Rex E. Newnham, Ph.D., D.O., N.D.[28] to be vital for all arthritics.

General Dietary Recommendations for the Rheumatoid Arthritic[38]

For many years there have been numerous books written on the subject of nutrition as it relates to rheumatoid arthritis — and probably most of them are correct for some of us, with underlying common features that apply to all of us.

There are several things that stand out to be quite significant in most patients with rheumatoid diseases, which includes rheumatoid arthritis.[38]

1. The great majority of rheumatoid disease patients' body fluids are too acid in nature.

2. The great majority of these patients show signs and symptoms of a deficiency in free or ionic calcium.

3. Most rheumatoid disease patients eat margarine instead of butter and they demonstrate a lack of Vitamin A and natural D_3 plus severe deficiencies of the essential fatty acids.

In studying the nutritional status and diet of rheumatoid disease patients, one of us (Gus J. Prosch, Jr., M.D.) has made three observations that caused him to look deeper into this subject. These are that:

1. Many patients who are blood-related to arthritic patients do not develop any arthritis especially when different dietary habits were followed.

2. Often-times arthritic patients exhibited slight to significant improvement when self-administered home and folk remedies were taken, like alfalfa tablets, bone meal tablets, cod liver oil, vinegar with honey, peanut oil, . . . or cherries.

3. Some arthritic patients are more susceptible to getting reinfected after being treated with the medication that apparently eliminated the offending organisms.

Diet in rheumatoid disease does help control the severity of the symptoms. Vitamin and mineral supplementations help shorten the recovery time by strengthening the immune system. By checking the acidity of saliva and urine of arthritic patients, the great majority were considerably more acid than normal. An alkaline diet can only benefit such patients.

More often than normal, rheumatoid disease patients exhibit certain physical signs during their physical examination. Summarized, these signs follow:

1. Longitudinal ridges and increased opaqueness in fingernails.

2. Mild to moderate tenderness with strong touch (palpation) of the broad muscle of the calf or leg (soleus) or the flat, irregular, triangular muscle covering the posterior surface of the neck and shoulder (trapezius).

3. Generalized slight increase in deep tendon reflexes.

4. Generalized irritability of skeletal muscles to tapping (percussion).

5. Acid saliva of pH 4.5 to 6.5.

6. Slight to severe coating on the tongue.

Many of these signs are related to calcium metabolism in the body, and most arthritic patients wrongly drink 2% or low fat milk instead of whole milk, and eat margarine instead of butter.

• The physical signs demonstrate strong evidence of free or ionic calcium deficiency as well as a deficiency of Vitamin A and D_3 which is natural Vitamin D. Blood calcium studies are misleading as they measure the ionic calcium as well as calcium bound to proteins. Normal body fluids ideally are slightly alkaline as opposed to acid. We believe that this factor is the one primary cause of the deficiency in rheumatoid disease patients of the ionic calcium which in itself is very alkaline.(See Chapter I Osteoarthritis, "Calcium, Vitamin D_3 and Sunshine.")

• An even more important cause of this acidity is due to the diet and nutritional habits of arthritic patients. Most cellular mechanisms of the body and particularly those involving the use of ionized minerals such as the secretory glands, nerve function processes and muscle contraction, etc. proceed best in a mildly alkaline state. For this reason a diet consisting of high alkaline foods should be consumed, combined with the avoidance of acid-forming foods.

• Acid-forming foods are those which are high in one or more of three elements: phosphorus, sulfur, and chlorine; alkaline diets are those high in potassium, calcium, magnesium and sodium.

• The diet used to treat and prevent development of rheumatoid diseases should definitely avoid as much as possible the following foods: All processed and most canned foods along with caffeine, sugar in all it's forms, as well as the simple carbohydrate foods that quickly upon digestion turn into sugar, like white flour foods, crackers, many cereals, macaroni (pasta foods), white rice and corn products. Ideally nicotine and alcohol should be avoided, along with any sweets, candy, soft drinks, pastries and desserts. The "nightshade plants" (foods containing solanines) such as white potatoes, tomatoes, egg plant and garden peppers should be avoided. Tobacco is also a solanine.

Robert Bingham, M.D.,[39] who devoted his orthopaedic career to the problems of crippling, states that about 1/3 of arthritics are affected by solanines, but in a later work increased his estimate, while other physicians estimate that a higher percentage of arthritics are affected, perhaps as high as 50%.

• As a rule, most protein foods tend to be acid forming since they contain phosphorus and sulfur. Animal sources of protein — lean meat (beef, lamb, veal), poultry, fish and eggs — are definitely in this category. With the exception of shrimp, most sea food is extremely acid forming. These foods must not be avoided in the diet, however, as they provide the building blocks for all bodily functions and processes. Therefore one of these proteins should be eaten with each meal. Pork meats should be limited however. Just try not to eat an entire meal consisting of protein foods, but balance these foods with alkaline forming foods. Ideally your breakfast should always consist of some high protein foods, balanced with whole milk, fruit juices, etc. Also remember to cook protein foods at low temperatures, as enzymes and trace minerals are reduced with excessive heat and no foods should be eaten that have been deep fried.

Figure 11: Fatty Acids

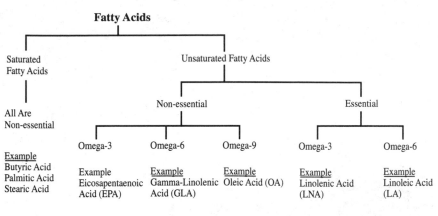

Figure 12: Unsaturated Fatty Acids

Fatty Acid	Number of Times Unsaturated	Food Sources
Omega-3		
LNA[a] (Linolenic Acid)[b]	3	Flax Seeds, Pumpkin Seeds, Walnuts, Soy Beans, Dark Green Leaves
SDA (Stearidonic Acid)	4	Seeds of certain members of the Borage family
EPA (Eicosapentaenoic Acid)	5	Cold-water Fish (Salmon, Sardine, Mackerel, Trout)
DHA (Docosahexaenoic Acid)	6	
Omega-6		
LA[a] (Linoleic Acid)	2	Safflower, Sunflower & Sesame Seeds, Wheat & Corn Germ Oils, Walnut
GLA Gamma-Linolenic Acid)	3	Evening Primrose Seed, Black Currant & Borage Oil, Mother's Milk
AA (Arachidonic Acid)	4	Liver, Brain, Meats
DPA (Docosapentaaenoic)	5	Oils of certain fish
Omega-9		
OA (Oleic Acid)	1 [c]	Olive & Almond Oil, Pecan, Cashew, Filbert, Avocado

(a) Essential Fatty Acid , (b) Sometimes called "Alpha-Linolenic Acid",   (c) 1x unsaturated = monosaturated

---

Figure 13: Fatty Acid Composition of Different Seed Oils (percent)

Name	Linolenic Acid (LNA)	Linoleic Acid (LA)	Oleic Acid (OA)	Saturated
Flax	58	14	19	9
Pumpkin	15	42	34	9
Soy Bean	9	50	26	15
Walnut	5	51	28	16
Evening Primrose		81 [a]	11	8
Safflower		75	13	12
Sunflower		65	23	12
Corn		59	24	17
Wheat Germ		54	28	18
Sesame		45	42	13
Almond		17	78	5
Olive		8	76	16

(a) Includes 9% Gamma Linolenic Acid (GLA)

Fatty Acid Tables 11, 12 and 13 used by permission of Alfred Wertheim and *Townsend Letter for Doctors*.[27]

dines, salmon, mackerel, cod halibut, herring, trout, tuna) from the Omega 3 Series. Figure 13: "Fatty Acid Composition of Different Seed Oils (Percent)", depicts the varying percentages of good fatty acids and saturated fatty acids in some common foods.[27]

• As different kinds of fats have different biological effects on the human body, both good and bad, a balance must be achieved by the arthritic in reducing various fatty acids -- arachidonic acids (AA) -- that are usually derived from red meats, dairy products and shellfish -- without also dangerously decreasing necessary protein.[27]

• See Table 12, "Essential Fatty Acids," which depicts a group of fatty acid derivatives present in many tissues, such as the prostate gland, menstrual fluid, brain, lung, kidney, thymus, seminal fluid and pancreas called the "prostaglandins." There are more than a dozen of these prostaglandins which are extremely active biological substances which affect the cardiovascular system, smooth muscle, and stimulate the uterus to contract. Those that are designated as prostaglandin II series derive from gamma linolenic acid (GLA), linoleic acid (LA), and arachidonic acid (AA), but more from arachidonic acid (AA) than from any other source. The prostaglandin II series are the chief source of inflammatory effects in arthritics.[27]

• Whereas the prostaglandin III series derived from alpha linoleic acid (ALA) and prostaglandin IV series derive from eicosapentoic acid (EPA) and docosahexanoic acid (DHA) have good biological effects, and do not support inflammation.[27]

• When the arthritic ignores good nutritional advice regarding the essential fatty acids, many different systems become weakened or defective, resulting in many different disease conditions, as depicted in Figure 15: "Do You See Yourself? Then Take Heed!!."

• Figure 14: "Essential Fatty Acids (EFA)" depicts the good and bad consequences of consuming certain common foods. Not all prostaglandins are bad or good, each having a special function in our biology. (In Table 14, read the chart from left to right to determine the effects that eating certain foods has on the physiological functions of our bodies.[27])

Additional Food Recommendations

• **Vegetables:** Most all vegetables (except corn) are highly alkaline in nature and should be emphasized in the eating program. Salad vegetables are excellent and should be eaten daily. All other vegetables are very good and when "wok" cooked or stir-fried in cold-pressed vegetable oil are even better.

• **Vegetable Juices:** Fresh vegetable juices (not canned) are nearly perfect and should be part of the diet. It's important to prepare and serve as many foods in their raw and natural state as possible.

• **Fruits and Fruit Juices:** All fruits and fruit juices (excepting cranberries, plums and prunes) are alkaline forming and are good to

266 ANTHONY DI FABIO, M.A. & GUS J. PROSCH, JR., M.D

"munch" on.

• **Milk:** Whole milk is one of the best alkaline forming foods due to its high calcium content. Raw certified whole milk is much preferable if you can find it. At least two glasses of whole milk should be taken each day, and use butter instead of margarine.

William Campbell Douglass, M.D., editor of *Second Opinion*, also emphasizes the value of raw, whole milk. According to Dr. Douglass, once milk is pasteurized it's calcium converts to a form that is not available to the human biochemistry; and, more distressing, homogenized milk can be dangerous due to release from fat globules of xanthine oxidase, which leads to increasing clogging of the arteries (atherosclerosis).[78]

One should take additional precautions to insure that the milk you purchase and consume has not been mixed with milk derived from Bovine Growth Hormone (BGH) induced sources. In addition to forcing the mammary gland into producing more milk, stimulation of increased milk-cow infections are treated with increased quantities of antibiotics which then find their way into our milk, and thence into us, with all the negative consequences described in other sections of this book.

• **Yogurt:** Plain yogurt is an excellent alkalinizing food and not only is easy to digest, but tastes great when mixed with fresh fruit such as raisins, dates, dried figs and apricots. It also makes excellent munching foods.

The recommended diet, as described above, will change one's system to be more alkaline as it should be.

Vitamin and Mineral Recommendations

• **Boron:** Rex E. Newnham, Ph.D., D.O., N.D. found that boron deficiency in soils around the globe were chief contributing factors for both ostoearthritis and rheumatoid arthritis. Through use of appropriate boron compounds he was able to achieve great improvements, remissions or cures with people in widely varying geographic locations.[28] (See Chapter I, "Boron," Osteoarthritis.)

Dr. Newnham[165] writes: "The first few cases of rheumatoid arthritis were difficult, as some patients just got better, but others seemed to get worse after 1-3 weeks. If they continued with the treatment, and took three boron tablets each day, they invariably got better."

The Case of Janet Wood

Sometimes there can be an allergic reaction to food which produces rheumatoid arthritis, as in the case of Janet Wood, aged 62, Kent, England. She was suddenly overcome with much rheumatic pain all over, shoulders, fingers, feet, knees, back.

At the Stress Centre (a clinic in England) she was found to be allergic to wheat, but it was not gluten as she could eat oats and barley without trouble. Without wheat, her pains disappeared. Every six

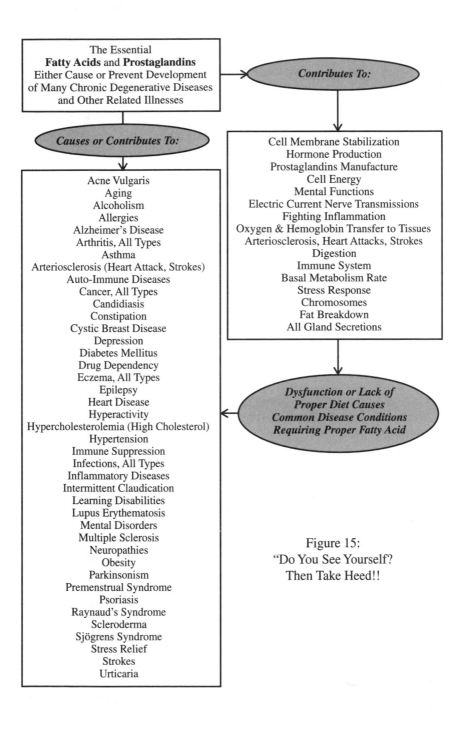

The Essential
Fatty Acids and **Prostaglandins**
Either Cause or Prevent Development
of Many Chronic Degenerative Diseases
and Other Related Illnesses

Contributes To:

Causes or Contributes To:

Acne Vulgaris
Aging
Alcoholism
Allergies
Alzheimer's Disease
Arthritis, All Types
Asthma
Arteriosclerosis (Heart Attack, Strokes)
Auto-Immune Diseases
Cancer, All Types
Candidiasis
Constipation
Cystic Breast Disease
Depression
Diabetes Mellitus
Drug Dependency
Eczema, All Types
Epilepsy
Heart Disease
Hyperactivity
Hypercholesterolemia (High Cholesterol)
Hypertension
Immune Suppression
Infections, All Types
Inflammatory Diseases
Intermittent Claudication
Learning Disabilities
Lupus Erythematosis
Mental Disorders
Multiple Sclerosis
Neuropathies
Obesity
Parkinsonism
Premenstrual Syndrome
Psoriasis
Raynaud's Syndrome
Scleroderma
Sjögrens Syndrome
Stress Relief
Strokes
Urticaria

Cell Membrane Stabilization
Hormone Production
Prostaglandins Manufacture
Cell Energy
Mental Functions
Electric Current Nerve Transmissions
Fighting Inflammation
Oxygen & Hemoglobin Transfer to Tissues
Arteriosclerosis, Heart Attacks, Strokes
Digestion
Immune System
Basal Metabolism Rate
Stress Response
Chromosomes
Fat Breakdown
All Gland Secretions

*Dysfunction or Lack of
Proper Diet Causes
Common Disease Conditions
Requiring Proper Fatty Acid*

Figure 15:
"Do You See Yourself?
Then Take Heed!!

months she was again tested and was still allergic to wheat until she started on the B-Alive® boron tablets. Then she could eat wheat bread and suffered no pains. (See Chapter I, "Boron," Osteoarthritis.)

The Case of Mary Lamb

Mary Lamb of Haxby, England, mid-seventies, had polymyalgia rheumatica, a form of rheumatoid disease that affects by inflammation the large arteries, and is often a precursor to other rheumatoid conditions, such as rheumatoid arthritis. She'd been given high doses of steroids that symptomatically relieved pain, but whenever she reduced the dosage, her pain returned. Of course, the disease progressed whether there was perceived pain or not.

When she used Dr. Newnham's recommended boron, her pain disappeared.

The Case of Mrs. E. Pedley

Mrs. E. Pedley of Coburg, England, had both rheumatoid arthritis and osteoarthritis, and for fifteen years she could hardly get about, even with supporting aids.

After using Dr. Newnham's recommended boron, she can walk freely and do her own shopping; in fact she feels younger. Her swollen joints have gone down a lot.

The Case of Crystal Malie

Crystal Malie, Honolulu, Hawaii, at 9 months of age was crying in pain and her doctor noticed that her joints were swollen. She had Still's disease. Still's disease is rheumatoid arthritis suffered by infants.

Crystal's doctor called Dr. Newnham, N.D., D.O., Ph.D. in England, who quickly sent boron tablets to Honolulu.

Crystal was given half a tablet (1-1/2 mg) 2 times daily, and in ten days she was sleeping normally, her joints were normal, and she was not in pain.

Dr. Newnham says, "This is the youngest I've ever treated. Older children get better in 2 to 3 weeks."[165]

• **Bovine Cartilage:** According to John F. Prudden, M.D., Med.Sc.D., Chairman of the Foundation for Cartilage and Immunology Research, and recipient of the Linus Pauling Award, bovine cartilage stimulates the immune system in resisting cancer and viruses but suppresses it in rheumatoid diseases. There is an abundance of evidence of the effectiveness of bovine cartilage in the treatment of arthritis. Studies have shown that bovine cartilage not only reduces inflammation, but it also provides healthy biochemical components that the body can utilize in resynthesizing cartilage. Both the oral and injectable forms of bovine trachael cartilage are effective. For bovine cartilage information write to Foundation for Cartilage and Immunology Research, 104 Post Office Road, Waccabuc, NY 10597; (914) 763-6194; Fax (914) 763-3342.

Many physicians also recommend shark cartilage, chicken cartilage.

• **Bromelin:** Reported by Dr. Christian Northrup,[166] bromelin, obtained from the skin of the pineapple plant, is a mixture of enzymes that can hasten the breaking down of proteins, called "proteolytic enzymes." Bromelin can also strengthen the connective tissue in the joints, according to Donald J. Brown, N.D.[229] It is often prescribed by holistic physicians to reduce inflammation and scarring due to joint deformity. Dr. Northrup advises taking 125 to 450 mg 3 times daily. "In addition," she writes, "try drinking raw pineapple juice."

• **Calcium, Vitamin D and Sunshine:** Emphasizing calcium, vitamin D and sunshine, Carl J. Reich, M.D., Calgary, Canada, reports that he's had many years of clinical successes treating and curing a number of diseases including rheumatoid arthritis. He's demonstrated the existence of a widespread deficiency in calcium and vitamin D_3.[83] It is most important to correct the free calcium deficiency present in most arthritics. This requires much larger amounts of vitamin A and D in their natural form than what is usually advised by the "Recommended Daily Allowances" (RDA) tables.

• Chemically manufactured, non-natural (synthetic) Vitamin A and D_2 preparations on the market simply do not work. Synthetic Vitamin D_2 does increase the calcium absorption from the small intestine but seems to be totally inadequate in regulating the use of the calcium and especially calcium excretion by the kidneys. The only preparation one of us (Gus J. Prosch, Jr., M.D.) has found to be adequate in clinical trials is the natural D_3 which is found in fish liver oils. Therefore we recommend liquid Norwegian Cod Liver Oil® by Dale Alexander as the ideal, which seems to be even better than cod liver oil capsules. It is easily taken when mixed with some orange juice and stirred rapidly. Arthritics should take one teaspoon on arising each morning and one teaspoon at bedtime. This preparation can be found in most health food stores and should be taken for at least four months, then the dosage should be cut in half.

Do not fear any Vitamin A or D toxicity with this dosage as it is less than 1/3 the toxicity level that has been reported in the medical literature. If you absolutely cannot take the liquid, you can usually find capsules at a health food store which will provide approximately 4,000 units of Vitamin D daily, but these are not nearly as effective.

Exposure to sunshine for at least 20 minutes each week will activate the Vitamin D.

• **Calcium:** Experience with many arthritic patients has taught one of us (Gus J. Prosch, Jr., M.D.) that none of the available inorganic calcium preparations are effective. Organic bone meal tablets (3-4 per day) work better than other inorganic calcium preparations but with severe reservations. The compound that works best for arthritics is calcium orotate (500 mg 4 times daily). Calcium orotate also seems to enhance the ability of the body to use and metabolize other forms of calcium ingested. It is the naturally occurring calcium in plants; but, calcium orotate has been taken off the market by the FDA. Calcium chelate or calcium aspartate can substitute as a second choice, although most any calcium is acceptable except bone meal or calcium carbonate. The above calcium preparation is also excellent for osteoporosis and it greatly strengthens the bone and cartilage structures in the body.

• **Magnesium:** We also recommend   500 mg of magnesium orotate, but this substance has also been removed from the market by the FDA, and so magnesium chelate or aspartate should be taken twice daily to balance the calcium/magnesium ratio. William Campbell Douglass, M.D.,[258] Editor-in-Chief of *Second Opinion* health newsletter, says, "We've only scratched the surface of magnesium's role in maintaining optimum health. . . . Magnesium is an essential mineral involved in more than 50 different biochemical reactions."

Other Supplements Recommended: a. Vitamin B Complex, two to three 'stress' B vitamins daily in divided doses. (These should contain 50-75 mg of each B vitamin).

b. Vitamin C, ideally 2000 mg 3 X daily (Linus Pauling, Ph.D. took 18 grams daily). William Campbell Douglass, M.D. says that "If you could take only one supplemental vitamin at all, this would be it. Vitamin C does just about everything.[258]

c. Zinc, 60 mg, once daily on an empty stomach, or again, as the orotates have been removed from the marketplace by the FDA, use zinc chelate or aspartate. (Zinc is a mild anti-inflammatory agent.)

d. Selenium, 250 micrograms daily as yeast selenium.

e. β-Carotene, 25,000 units daily.

f. Vitamin E, 400 units daily.

g. At least 6 fish oil capsules daily as MaxEPA from health food stores.

h. At least 6 Primrose Oil capsules daily. Efamol® or Natures Way® brands are recommended, as many products labled as "Primrose Oil," are actually soybean or some other form of oil. (There's no FDA control over use of the name "Primrose Oil.")

I. Rex Newnham, N.D., D.O., Ph.D., after studying the distribution of boron in soil throughout the world, and comparing it's deficiency back against forms of arthritis, concluded that these diseases all suffer from boron deficiency in addition to other nutritional deficiencies.[28] He recommends 8 to 10 mg of boron daily. (See Chapter I, Osteoarthritis, "Nutrition and Supplements.")

J. Garlic has been used for health throughout thousands of years. William Campbell Douglass, M.D.,[258] says that "there are two true wonder drugs: penicillin and garlic. Garlic will do many things penicillin can't." For the arthritic, garlic is an immune booster. But it also lowers triglycerides and cholesterol, inhibits blood platelet aggregation

-- the sticking together of blood cells that leads to clots -- increases high-density lipoprotein, which is protective against coronary heart disease, helps bronchial congestion, fever, constipation, warts, prevent cancer, cold/flu conditions, and is a great antioxidant.

Dr. Douglass says that "Any form of garlic, raw or cooked, natural or capsule, seems to be effective. I recommend eating one clove of garlic per day (or its equivalent in commercial tablets). . . more if you feel an illness coming on."

k. Enzymes are complex proteins capable of inducing chemical changes in other substances without being changed themselves during the process. There are literally hundreds of thousands of enzymes operating throughout the body. According to Hector Solorzano del Rio, M.D., Ph.D., D.Sc., surgeon, Master of Acupuncture, Professor of Pharmacology, and Coordinator of the Program for Studies of Alternative Medicines at University of Guadalajara, Guadalajara, Mexico, "When someone gets sick of any disease we can be sure that something is wrong with his/her enzymes. What we logically must do, in almost any disease, is to replace the type and quantity of required enzymes as soon as possible. Our body will automatically do the rest."

Enzyme supplementation, along with proper diet, is very important for properly digesting food, and for eliminating the inflammatory immuno-complexes (antigens/antibodies) that always accompanies rheumatoid arthritis.

Lita Lee, Ph.D., licensed nutritionist, has been able to help almost every variety of illness toward wellness by emphasizing intake of enzymes based upon a 24 hour urinalysis, a detailed questionaire, and other factors. Lita Lee, Ph.D. may be contacted at 2852 Willamette St, #397, Eugene, OR 97405; tel (541)-746-7621; fax: (541) 741-0354.

Dr. Catherine Russell and Hector Solorazano del Rio, M.D., Ph.D., D.Sc., both of Guadalajara, Mexico, use Wobenzyme™, a German proteolytic tablet, for helping to resolve immuno-complexes that contribute to rheumatoid diseases. Wobenzyme consists of pancreatin (100 mg), bromelin (45.0 mg), papain (60.0 mg), lipase (10.0 mg), amilayse (10.0 mg), trypsin (24.0 mg), quimotrypsin (1.0 mg), rutin (50.0 mg), excipiente c.b.p. (1 gragea).

They both also use the bioflavonoid Quercetin. Wobenzyme may be obtained from Hector Solorazano del Rio, M.D., Ph.D., D.Sc., Los Alpes #1022, Col. Independencia, Jal. 44340, Guadalajara, Mexico; (3) 8 23-2128; fax the same.

The above vitamin and mineral supplementations will not only help the patient's arthritis by stimulating the immune response system but will play an important role in counteracting the aging process as well as acting as a deterrent to some forms of cancer since many of these preparations act as free radical and peroxide scavengers in the body.

When the arthritic also has painful hands and feet, as in carpal

272 ANTHONY DI FABIO, M.A. & GUS J. PROSCH, JR., M.D

tunnel syndrome, an entrapment of nerves, we recommend in addition 100 mg Vitamin B$_6$.

Of the 92 natural elements, at least 79 of them are found in mammalian blood to some degree.[249] As most enzymes require trace elements for their activation as catalysts, it's clear that mineral supplements (possibly some colloidal forms as well as non-colloidial; certainly ionic forms) consisting of 60 or more elements are desirable.

Adjunctive Treatment (Supporting or Additional)

Chelation Therapy: If the patient can afford chelation therapy, we recommend a series of EDTA (Ethylene Diamine Tetracetic Acid) amino acid intravenous infusions as they will help to remove artery blockages, thus permitting the cells to be better nourished. (See Chapter I, Osteoarthritis, "Chelation Therapy.")

Candidiasis Diet

At least fifty percent of arthritis patients suffer from candidiasis, an invasion or overgrowth of yeast/fungus. Many of the symptoms attributed to rheumatoid arthritis are actually symptoms from candidiasis or food allergies.

Everyone has some degree of yeast infection, usually found in the lower bowels, vagina, and on the skin. The yeast/fungus, *Candida albicans*, among other similar organisms-of-opportunity, will spread throughout favorable body sites when the immune system has been compromised by means of stress, drugs, antibiotics, hormones such as cortisone, and for other reasons. It has seven known survival forms including one form that is -- in the blood -- cell-wall deficient, thus cannot be recognized by the immune system as a foreign invader in that form. However it's most damaging form is its fungal (mycelial) state, which occurs throughout the intestinal tract whenever our "good-guys" intestinal bacteria, *Lactobacilus acidophilus* and *Bifido bacteria,* have been killed by the use of various drugs.

As candidiasis can mimic so many other diseases due to its ability to affect so many body targets, such as organs and systems, the disease frequently goes unrecognized and untreated by traditional medical practitioners, although this factor is slowly changing.

Successful treatment of candida fungus overgrowth must follow a four-pronged attack to be effective. All four modalities of treatment must be strictly adhered to, otherwise treatment will not be effective.

We cannot emphasize this point too strongly and repeat, **that you must follow the treatment plan exactly in order to get the best results of therapy. If you want to get well, you must follow these four steps of treatment and if you neglect any one of these four important steps, your treatment will be either prolonged, or unsuccessful, when these instructions are not carried out.**

These four steps include (a) killing the fungus overgrowth with proper diet (starving out the fungus) and medication (killing the fungus), (b) nutritional supplementation and correction of vital nutrients to build up the immune system, (c) establishing a normal good bacterial flora in the intestine by supplementing *Lactobacillus acidophilus* (good intestinal germs), and, (d) avoiding stress, many forms of drugs, antibiotics, hormones, steroids and allergic foods.

There are other things a patient may do to kill candidia or to speed up the healing process such as receiving proper rest, developing an exercise routine and sometimes adding garlic, aloe vera, Pau D'Arco tea and other helpful substances, as will be descrbed.

Diet and Yeast Killing Medication

The purpose of the strict candidiasis diet is to limit the type of foods that feed the fungus.

Prescription drugs can often speed up the job of killing off unwanted yeast/fungus, but they have considerable toxicity, and can be quite expensive.

Some doctors use primarily nystatin powder, an antifungal substance, and this is thought to be an excellent medication for treating the fungus overgrowth. However, according to Virender Sodhi, M.D., N.D.,[3] Bellevue, Washington, while suppressing the fungal form, nystatin simply causes candidiasis to mutate into resistant strains while also killing off beneficial microorganisms.

Alternatively there are numerous dietary provisions along with herbs and natural medications that can be used to help eradicate the fungus. Some of these are more effective than others such as capryllic acid, tannic stearates and albuminates, fatty acids and even extracts from certain plants and vegetables, such as the herbs goldseal, Oregon grape, and barberry, as well as homeopathic remedies.

With any type of treatment of candidiasis it must be emphasized that the worst thing a patient can do is to stop the treatment before therapy is completed, no matter what medication is given. A common problem experienced many times is that patients try to 'play doctor' with their treatment and after a couple of months of therapy, they begin to feel so much better that they think they are well and stop the treatment. It's impossible to get this fungus overgrowth under control until at least four months of therapy, and when patients discontinue the treatment, the remaining fungus that have not been destroyed will simply grow back and very often will build up a resistance to the medication.

Patients who fall into this trap are always regretful so physicians should insist on emphasizing to the patient that they should never stop the treatment on their own without consultation.

Vitamin, Mineral, Fatty Acids and
Other Nutritional Supplements

In order to build up a patient's immune system, deficiencies in any vitamin, mineral or fatty acid should be corrected, because all patients who have the fungus overgrowth are suffering from some or many nutritional deficiencies.

Proper eating habits are also important to make sure that they do not develop further deficiencies of these vital elements.

One must be sure that amino acid deficiencies are corrected. This is done by supplementing with a wide variety of amino acids along with vitamin/mineral supplements, and making sure that the diet to be described is followed.

These measures are absolutely necessary to ensure that the immune system is functioning properly, and to also ensure that the patient gets well as soon as possible.

Establishing a Normal Gut Flora[19]

To build up the good germs in our gastrointestines, a special form of *Lactobacillus acidophilus* is prescribed. There are literally dozens of different types of acidophilus on the market today and the majority of them simply do not work, [insofar as potency, good quality and effectiveness], according to one of us (Gus J. Prosch, Jr., M.D.), who, after considerable search, now routinely makes available to the patient the Vital Life® brand by Klaire Laboratories, Inc., 1573 W. Seminole, San Marcos, CA 92060-2513; also Natren Inc., products are excellent, located at 3105 Willow Lane, West Lake Village, CA 91361; both are usually available at most health food stores.

It's a powdered form (absolutely essential), and contains ten billion 'good' germs per one-fourth teaspoon which equals one gram. Acidophilus in capsule form is not effective because we must build up the 'good' germs in the mouth and throat as well. Capsules simply bypass these areas. The proper manner to take the acidophilus is to take one-fourth teaspoon four times daily mixed in a small amount of water and swished a few seconds in the mouth and then swallowed. The main bottle should be refrigerated.

A good way to take the acidophilus when away from home is to get a small empty pill bottle or vial and after taking the morning dose, place one-fourth teaspoon of the powdered acidophilus in the vial. This should be carried with you, and at lunch time the powder can be dropped into a small amount of water and swished in the mouth and swallowed.

Avoidance Recommendations

According to one of us (Gus J. Prosch, M.D.) patients are advised to avoid antibiotics in any form as well as stress, some forms of drugs, hormones, steroids and foods that they are allergic to.

What To Do With Secondary Infections: When a patient gets a secondary infection from some type of germ creating, for example, a sore throat, the patient should not take an antibiotic, but instead they should go to the clinic where they can be given an intravenous infusion that will strengthen the immunological system, or kill most any germ. There are a variety of substances that will work, depending upon the physician. For example, high levels of intravenous vitamin C, or even weakened hydrochloric acid which stimulates certain components of the immune system (T cells) to fight the invader. If your physician has a large magnetic loop, lying within magnetic flux of the right polarity for about 20 minutes will eliminate the organisms by strenghtening your immune system. If your dentist prescribed antibiotics, again, these should not be taken, but rather you should visit your alternative care clinic. (Also see *Root Canal Coverup*, George Meinig, D.D.S., and *It's All In Your Head*, Hal Huggins.)

What To Do If The Patient Lives Too Far From the Clinic: Sometimes patients live a great distance from their clinic and are unable to come in for immune-strengthening injections. In such situations where they may have to take an antibiotic anyhow, they should take at least one-half teaspoon of *Lactobacillus acidophilus* every time they take an antibiotic pill, and also these patients should take at least eight thousand to ten thousand milligrams (8 to 10 grams; 1 teaspoon to a gram) of Vitamin C in divided doses each day. This will help to stimulate the immune system as well as to build up good germs that the antibiotic would be killing.

What To Do If Hormones or Steroids Must Be Taken: First advice is, don't take them. However, when unavoidable, candidiasis can be placed under control despite these hinderances, but it will take longer.

The Healing Crisis: Once therapy is initiated, the symptoms of approximately one in five patients will worsen. This is called a Herxheimer Reaction.[48] Some doctors call this a 'Die-Off Reaction' and others may even call it a 'Healing Crisis.' It occurs when a large number of candida organisms are killed off during initial stages of treatment, resulting in a sudden release of toxic substances that cause an immune response and intensified symptoms. It normally lasts no longer than a week and is frequently confused as an allergic reaction or toxicity toward the therapeutic agents. (See *The Herxheimer Effect*, this chapter.)

The use of nutritional supplements and therapeutics, as opposed to drugs, tends to lessen the intensity, duration and frequency of these symptoms. However, when symptoms are severe, treatment should be backed off to tolerable levels and built up over time. The dosage can be cut in half for a week, and then go back to original dosages.

Discontinuing Treatment: If treatment is discontinued before the patient gets the condition under control all their symptoms will usually return.

After the fungus overgrowth has subsided and the yeast are killed down to a normal level (and this takes at least three to four months) the medications and supplements are gradually decreased over a period of six to eight weeks and the patients are allowed to gradually add previously forbidden foods to their diet.

Do's and Don'ts of Candidiasis Diet
Foods You Should Avoid In Your Diet When Treating Candida

Fungus Overgrowth

General Rules: The candida fungus grows on sugar and starch and high carbohydrate foods and is fed by gluten-containing grains. Gluten grains include wheat, oats, rye and barley. The fungus also grows and is fed by other yeast molds, and yeasty foods. It is known that yeast, molds and fungi cross-react; that is, a developed sensitivity to one organism will cross over to another because of their close genetic relationship.

When taken in food or even breathed in high concentrations, they trigger symptoms and diminish the body's resistance to candida overgrowth.

Bathrooms and air vents should be kept clean and dry.

Yeast molds and fungi should be minimized in foods.

The candidiasis diet is considerably more restrictive than the recommended rheumatoid disease diet:Therefore:

1. Do not eat any sweets or desserts of any type and this includes products made with honey or molasses as well as any form of sugar or products listed on labels that end in "ose," such as fructose, glucose, maltose, lactose, etc.

2. Do not eat wheat, oats, rye, barley, or corn. Starchy foods such as rice, potatoes, buckwheat, beans and corn, should also be excluded from the diet while treatment is being undertaken. Two rice cakes each day are allowed, however. A bowl of oatmeal is allowed each day, if desired.

3. Milk (even raw) encourages candida fungus growth. Try to avoid milk, and milk products, except butter and plain unsweetened yogurt and especially avoid any yogurt that has fruit or sugar in it. Patients on this program are allowed one glass of either sweet milk or buttermilk each day.

4. Yeast is used in food preparation and flavoring in all commercial breads, rolls, coffee cakes, pastries, cakes and this, of course, includes hot dog and hamburger buns, cookies, crackers, biscuits and pastries of any kind. You must be very careful with any flour products or even meats fried in cracker crumbs as well as all cereals. All beer, wine and all alcoholic beverages contain yeast and therefore must be avoided. You should also avoid commercial soups, potato and corn chips and dry-roasted nuts. Vinegar and vinegar-containing foods such as pickled vegetables, sauerkraut, relishes, green olives and salad dressings all contain yeast and should not be used. Don't forget that soy sauce, cider and natural root beer also contain yeast. Also, all malted products contain yeast, as well as catsup, mayonnaise, pickles, condiments, and most salad dressings. The citrus fruit juices, either frozen or canned, usually contain yeast and only home-squeezed fruit juices are yeast free. All dried fruits such as prunes, raisins and dates contain yeast, as well as all antibiotics.

5. Yeast is the basis for most vitamin and mineral preparations. Nearly all vitamin and mineral preparations purchased at a drug store or from a large pharmaceutical manufacturer is loaded with yeast and should not be taken. If the patient has any doubts about other supplements it is suggested that you check with your holistic-minded health care provider before taking them. Some vitamins purchased in health food stores that claim to be yeast-free are not really yeast-free and one must be careful or they can really aggravate your fungus overgrowth.

(You may request from The Arthitis Trust of America a list or catalog of physician-approved brands and suppliers. Please send a legal-sized, stamped, self-addressed envelope along with a tax-exempt donation to help defray costs.)

6. Molds build up on foods while drying, smoking, curing and fermenting. You should therefore avoid pickled, smoked or dried meats, fish and poultry, including sausages, salami, hot dogs, pickled tongue, corn beef, pastrami, smoked sardine or other fish that have been dried or smoked. You should not eat any pork of any type as pork is usually loaded with molds and yeast. Dried fruits, such as prunes, raisins, dates, figs, citrus peels, candied cherries, currents, peaches, apples and apricots should be avoided. All cheeses (including cottage cheese), sour cream, and other milk products, such as mentioned above, should be avoided. Chocolate, honey, maple syrup and nuts accumulate mold and should be avoided.

7. Melons (especially cantelope and watermelon) and the skins of fleshy vegetables or fruits accumulate mold during growth.

8. Avoid canned or frozen citrus, grape and tomato juice. Avoid all canned or frozen foods which contain citric acid.

9. Mushrooms, truffles and many herbal products such as black tea, are loaded with yeast and should be avoided if at all possible. Don't forget that teas, including herb teas and spices, are dried foods and accumulate molds, so you should avoid these.

10. Eating fruit will boost blood sugar levels and will encourage yeast growth. But one fruit is allowed each day under this program, with the exception of melons and grapes. Bananas are probably the third highest sugar containing fruit and should be limited in amounts.

Be sure that you read through this list of forbidden foods numerous times in order to familiarize yourself with what you can and cannot have to eat. Once you're familiar with these foods, it will enable you to select acceptable foods while dining in a restaurant or while visiting friends or neighbors at meal time. You should definitely learn those foods that you must stay away from if you want to get the best results in your treatment.

It is absolutely necessary that you carefully look at all labels on the canned and packaged foods and consult the above list constantly, or you will continue to suffer needlessly the consequences of the fungus overgrowth in your body.

You can eat out in a restaurant but order very carefully. Skip the cocktails. Have virgin olive oil and lemon juice on your salads. In fact, very useful is one tablespoon of virgin olive oil each day for patients being treated for candida fungus overgrowth, because it not only has some good fatty acids in it, but the olive oil kills candida.

When dining out, order fish, chicken, turkey or lean red meats (other than pork) or other animal proteins that are prepared without sauces which might contain sugar, mushrooms or wheat as a thickener, and other harmful ingredients. Broiled or plain items are obviously the safest choice. Steamed vegetables are perfect but you must skip bread, crackers and desserts of any kind.

You must totally and absolutely avoid:

1. All sweets and desserts and sugar foods in any shape, form or fashion.

2. All breads and flour products (including whole wheat) of any kind.

3. All cheeses while on this program.

4. Any kind of alcohol beverages which are strictly forbidden since they contain sugar and yeast.

Candida Diet Allowables: What You Can Eat on This Program

Vegetables

Artichokes	Asparagus	Bamboo Shoots
Beet Greens	Broccoli	Brussel Sprouts
Cabbage	Caraway	Carrots
Catnip	Cauliflower	Chickory
Collards	Dandelion	Dulse
Egg Plant	Endive	Fennel
Green Beans (Fresh)	Green Peas (Fresh)	Kelp
Mustard Greens	Okra	Peppers
Rhubarb	Squash	String Beans
Swiss Chard	Turnip Greens	Water Cress

To wash vegetables, use one tablespoon of bleach or clorox in one gallon of cool water.

Salad Vegetables

Alfalfa Sprouts	Bamboo Shoots	Broccoli
Cabbage	Caraway	Catnip
Cauliflower	Celery	Chard
Chives	Cress	Dandelion
Dulse	Endive	Fennel
Kale	Kelp	Leeks
Lettuce	Mong Bean Sprouts	Parsley
Peppers	Rhubarb	Spinach
Squash	Swiss Chard	Water Cress

Fresh tomatoes and onions are also allowed, along with summer squash and zucchini -- all types of squash.

Meats and Proteins (All Lean Cuts)

Beef	Chicken	Clams
Crab	Eggs	Ham
Lobster	Salmon	Shrimp
Tuna	Turkey	Veal

Also all game birds and animals such as squirrel, rabbit, quail, duck goose and venison are allowed.

Nuts and Seeds

In limited amounts (one ounce) -- walnuts, sunflower seeds and pumpkin seeds.

Oils

Use only cold pressed or expeller pressed or non-hydrogenated oils. Also, you should take one tablespoon of virgin olive oil each day on your salads or vegetables. You can add lemon juice to this if you so desire. The best salad dressing is virgin olive oil in lemon juice.

Other Items

You may have two rice cakes daily.

Eat real butter and totally avoid all margarine.

You may have plain unsweetened yogurt but no yogurt with fruit or sugar in it.

You may have one cup of oatmeal (the old fashioned kind) per day.

One small to medium fruit per day is permitted, but no melons or grapes.

You may have any unsweetened, decaffeinated drink. Any coffee you drink should be decaffeinated and your tea should be weak. If you must drink diet drinks they should be caffeine free and sugar free and you may have no more than two each day, maximum. You may have either two packages of Nutri-Sweet® or Equal® or Aspartame® as sweetners, but no more each day, whether they are in packages or in your diet drinks. You may, however, have Sweet and Low® or saccharine in any amounts you desire. Aspartame or Nutra-Sweet metabolizes in the human body into one-half aldehydes (also a product of candidiasis). Aldehydes are responsible for diet drink "hangover."[65]

You may use salt, pepper, garlic or onions if you desire.

For those patients who tend to lose weight easily, and especially those who should not lose any weight, they should eat three or four large tablespoons of homemade mayonnaise, 120 calories, each day, made with two fresh eggs, preferably at room temperature, add two tablespoons of freshly squeezed lemon juice (no bottled lemon juice), and add one teaspoon of salt (preferably sea salt). Mix this in your blender and add slowly one and one-fourth cup of cold pressed or expeller pressed or non-hydrogenated safflower oil.

Technically, all salt comes from the sea. However, virtually all salt that is labeled "sea salt," even from health food stores, is salt that has had its valuable minerals processed out. Read the label and look at the composition. Genuine sea salt should contain nearly every micro-nutrient found in human blood, is dark in composition, and is moist, as it lacks added chemicals to improve its ability to pour. A genuine source for proper sea salt is Grain & Salt Society, Inc., PO Box DD, Magalia, CA 95954.

Of course, if you are overweight you should avoid this mayonaise.

Don't forget that the diet in the treatment against candidiasis is absolutely vital and failure to comply with this diet will result in failure of treatment of your fungus overgrowth condition.

Additional Substances Used to Control Candidiasis

Holistic minded physicians use a variety of substances in varying proportions to control or displace *Candida albicans*. Each will have favorites used singly or in combination, or they may favor commercial preparations because of known beneficial effects and standardization of beneficial characteristics. Although a physician may be holistically minded, he may also use any one of several well-known anti-fungal prescription medications.

When herbs are used, of course, it's very important that sources be appropriately harvested, pesticide and herbicide free, and also supply the active part of the plant for medicinal use, as well as be a quality product. Usually a health-care professional will recommend herbal sources that are well-known, and have demonstrated good products over the years.

Table of Natural Substances Used to Control Candidiasis

Substance	Comments
Alfalfa (*Medicago sativa*)	Found on borders of fields, in low valleys and widely cultivated
Aloe (*Aloe vera*)	Yucca Cactus; found in East and South Africa; West Indies; South Western American deserts; recommend products containing acemannan.
Anise (*Pimpenalla anisum*)	Annual plant that grows wild but is also widely cultivated.
Balm (*Melissa officinale*)	Perennial found in Mediteranean, near East, and naturalized in America.
Barberry (*Berberis vulgaris*)	Bark of root and berries of a deciduous shrub found in Northeastern states.
Basil (*Ocimum basilicum*)	Annual found growing wild in tropics and sub-tropics.
Bifido bacterium	Bacteria natural to the lower intestine; helps fight unwanted intestinal organisms; produces enzyme which completes digestion of dairy products. Klaire Laboratories, Inc. 1573 West, Seminole, San Marcos, CA 92069; (310) 289-4372;Natren Inc.(800)-992-3323.

Bitter herbs	All bitter herbs are antifugnal because they contain alkaloids that inhibit or kill fungus.
Borage oil (*Borage officinalis*)	Annual found growing wild in Mediteranean, and cultivated elsewhere; 240 mg gamma linolenic acid; 378 mg cis-linoleic acid; 10 USP Units vitamin E as d-alpha tocopherol; Bio-Tech, PO Box 1991, Fayetteville, AR 72702; (800) 345-1199.
Capyrilic acid	A naturally occurring, medium chain saturated fatty acid from coconut oil.
Cat's Claw (*Uncaria tomentosa*)	Woody vine from South America, called Una de Gato.
Colloidial Silver	Considered safe for short term uses; sold over the counter in some health food stores.
Cinnamon (*Cinnamomum zeylanicum*)	Dried inner bark of branches of small evergreen laurel tree.
Cloves (*Caryophyllus aromaticus*) or *Syzygium armoaticum*)	Evergreen native to Spice Islands, Phillipines, and grown in Sumatra, Jamica, West Indies, Brazil and other tropics.
Ergotransferrin	Sensitizes candida to nystatin; sold by Cardiovascular Research, 1061-B Shary circle, Concord, CA 94518; (415) 827-2636.
Essiac®	Special blend of cut burdock root, powdered sheep sorrel, powdered turkey rhubarb root, and powdered slippery elm bark; Flora, Inc., PO Box 950, Lynden, WA 98264; (206) 345-2110.
Fatty acids	Most organic fatty acids are fungicidal, such as oleic acid (butter; virgin olive oil); caprylic acid.
Fennel (*Foeniculum culgare*)	Perennial or biennial that grows in Mediterranean area and Asia Minor but commonly cultivated in Europe and America. Fugastatin® contains propionic, sorbic, caprylic, and tannic acids; from Molecular Biologics, Inc. 4740, E. Second St., #23, Benecia, CA 94510.
Garlic (*Alum sativum*)	Perennial widely cultivated in gardens, and used for cooking; contains allicin, a sulfur compound, as its active ingredient; Kyloic garlic extract is available from Wakunga of America Co., Ltd., 23501 Madero, Mission Viejo, CA 92691.
German chamomilla; also called "camomile" (*Matricaria chamomilla*)	Perennial found in dry fields and around cultivated ground
Ginseng (*Panex schin-seng*; *Panex quinquefolius*)	Perennial grows in damp Manchurian woodlands; cultivated in Korea; grows wild rich, cool woodlands of North America.
Ginger (*Zingiber officinale*)	Asian tropical perennial; also cultivated elsewhere, especially in Jamaica.
Goldenseal (*Hydrastis canadensis*)	Perennial found in rich, shady woods and damp meadows from Connecticut to Min-

Grapefruit (*Citrus paradisi*);

Homeopathic

Lactobacillus acidophilus

Lanthanum (chelated or colloidial)

Licorice (*Glycyrrhiza glabra*)

Mycocidin®

Molybdenum chelate

Nystatin   `

ParaMicrociden®

Pycnogenol

Oregon grape root (*Berberis aquifolium*)

Oregano Oil; also Wild Majoram (*Origanum vulgare*)

Pau d'Arco (La Pacho or taheebo)

Rosemary (*Rosemarinus officinalis*)

SAM -GLA®

Tannic acid

nesota; also cultivated.

Grapefruit and other citrus fruit seeds and other citrus.

Varied according to need; *Borax* 30c and *Candida nosode* 30c.

Bacteria that can displace unwanted intestinal organisms. Some species produce desirable vitamins. Bacteria natural to the lower intestine; helps fight unwanted intestinal organisms; produces enzyme which completes digestion of dairy products. Klaire Laboratories, Inc. 1573 West, Seminole, San Marcos, CA 92069; (310) 289-4372; Natren, Inc.(800)-992-3323.

Candida albicans may steal this element from tissues, thereby creating chronic fatigue-like disease.[249]

Perennial plant growing wild in Southern and central Europe and parts of Asia, cultivated elsewhere.

Contains ricinoleic and undecylenic acid; Thorne Laboratories, Inc., 610 Andover, Seattle, WA; (800) 228-1966; undecylenic acid is six times more effective as an antifungal agent than caprylic acid

Converts acetylhyde produced by fungus into acetic acid used in energy cycle.

Marketed as Nilstat®, Mycostatin®, and as a powder

Grapefruit seed extract; 150 mg 3 X daily; Allergy Research Group, PO Box 489, 400 Preda St., San leandro, CA 94577-0489; (800) 345-1199

From grape seed and pine bark; inhibits fungal enzyme, must be used in high dosage.

Related to barberry (*Berberis vulgaris*).

Perennial found in Mediterranean and Asia, and cultivated in America.

From a South American tree.

Evergreen shrub from Mediterranean; widely cultivated for aromatic leaves and kitchen seasoning.

Evening Primrose oil supplying 440 mg omega-6 fatty acids containing 40 mg gamma linolenic acid and 315 mg cis-linoleic acid; marine lipid concentrate supplying omega-3 fatty acids containing 150 mg eicosapenoic acid and 100 mg docosahexaenoic acid, and 10 USP units Vitamin E as d-alpha tocopherol; Bio-Tech, PO Box 1991, Fayetteville, AR 72702; (800) 345-1199.

Tanalbit®, zinc-salicylo-tannate, from Scien-

	tific Consulting service, 466 Whitney St., San Leandro, CA 94577; (510) 632-2370; liberates tannins in lower GI tract.
Tea Tree Oil	Usually used externally, for nails and vaginal douche; effective against staphyloccus infection accompanying candidiasis.
Thyme (*Thymus vulgaris*)	Cultivated in American and European gardens; small shrubby plant.
Vinegar	Recommended by fungal specialist Prof. Dr. Hans Rieth, M.D., University of Hamburg; vinegar contributes a substance (CH_3) very important for liver functions; interferes with adherence of candida; take either straight or diluted at bedtime, together with high fiber diet for three consecutive days; don't use distilled vinegar as these are made with petroleum products instead of food grade substances. One of us (Gus J. Prosch, Jr., M.D.) believes that vinegar in any form should not be used, as it contains yeast, itself.
Wormwood (*Artemesia annua*)	Silky perennial found along roadsides from Newfoundland, to Hudson Bay to Montana; native of Europe; bitter herb that is also antiparasitic.
Yellow Gentian (*Gentiana lutea*)	Perennial found in mountain meadows and pastures in Europe and Asia; related species, Blue or American Gentian (*Gentiana catesbaei*), Fringed Gentia (*Gentiana crintiana*), or Stiff Gentian (Gallweed) (*Gentiana quinquefolia*), growing in a different environment, have similar properties, and can be used for the same purposes; Bio-cidin® is a strong spectrum mixture of gentian and other traditional Chinese herbs manufactured by BioBotanicals, and available only through pharmacies. BioTonic, also by BioBotanicals, is available through health food stores
Yogurt (*Lactobaccilus bulgaris*) -	For directions on 24-hour yogurt treatment recommended by nutritionist and microbiologist Elaine Gottschall, author of *Breaking the Vicious Cycle: Intestinal Health Through Diet*; write to Kirkton Press, RR1, Kirkton, Ontario, Canada N0K 1KO; (519) 229-6795.

Toxic Drugs Used (or Can be Used) to Control Candidiasis

Name	Comments
5-nitro-imidazoles	Any one of clotrimazole, metronidazole, nimorazole, ornidazole, tinidazole; used in treating rheumatoid diseases; can wipe out infectious organisms, but also can wipe out

	good intestinal microorganisms, and therefore should be used with replacement *Lactobacillus acidopholus;* can have adverse side effects. Metronidazole, especially, can aggravate candidiasis. Clotrimazole is routinely used as an anti-fungal. t *Lactobacillus acidopholus* required to metabolize metronidazole, perhaps others.
Colchicine	Relieves gouty arthritis; research shows that gout, mycoplasm, and the yeast *Candida utilis,* and other yeasts, often go together.
Fluconazole	Antifungal; very expensive but quite effective; possible adverse reactions.
Griseofulvin	Antibiotic derived from a species of *Penicillium*; not justified for use in minor or trivial infections; anti-fungal; possible adverse reactions.
Itraconazole	Inhibits fungal synthesis of a constituent of cell membranes; possible adverse reactions.
Ketoconazole	May damage liver; must have sufficient hydrochloric acid in stomach.
Miconazole®	Canadian pharmacies; used in combination with fluconazole.
Salicylic acid	Aspirin.
Silver sulfadiazine	Antifungal and antibacterial; possible adverse reactions.
Sodium sulfadiazine	Antifungal and antibacterial; possible adverse reactions.
Sodium sulfapyridine	Antifungal and antibacterial; possible adverse reactions.
Sodium sulfathiazole	Antifungal and antibacterial; possible adverse reactions.
Sulfadiazine	Antifungal and antibacterial; possible adverse reactions.
Sulfanilamide	Antifungal and antibacterial; possible adverse reactions.
Sulfathiazole	Antifungal and antibacterial; possible adverse reactions.
Sulphasalazine	Antifungal and antibacterial; possible adverse reactions; splits in the gut into a sulfa drug and a salicylic acid.

Candida Purge

William (Bill) G. Neely, D.C.[67] of Johnson City, TN, and Nurse S. Colet Lahoz, M.S., R.N. of East West Clinic, White Bear Lake, Minnesota, successfully use a candida purge that contains a mixture of items to be taken orally that will kill overgrowth while also helping to scrape fungal candida from the intestinal tract. We believe that this mixture produces the fastest observable relief from the fungal form when used properly. The mixture contains Caprol (caprylic + oleic acids), psyllium (*Plantago ovata*), whose seeds and husks have a large capacity to absorb moisture, bentonite, an absorbant type of earth or clay, and *Lactobacillus acidophilus*. (Also see *Conquering Yeast Infections*, S. Colet Lahoz,R.N., M.S., L.Ac.; *Candidiasis: Scourge of Arthritis*, Anthony di Fabio; *Friendly Bacteria* -- Lactobacillus acidophilus & Bifido bacterium, Anthony di Fabio.)

The caprylic acid is fungicidal for *Candida albicans*. It is harmless to friendly intestinal flora, and effective against the invasive fungal or mycelial form as well as the yeast form because it is absorbed by the intestinal mucosal cells. Caprylic acid is metabolized by the liver and does not get into the general blood circulation. It must exert its fungicidal effect in the intestinal tract or not at all. According to studies, just ten minutes after oral intake of straight caprylic acid, more than 90% can be traced on its way to the liver. Consequently, Caprol should be taken with psyllium powder which will form a gel in the intestinal tract and release over a period of time the caprylic acid trapped within.

Oleic acid -- a major component of virgin olive oil: 56-83% and also found in butter -- hinders conversion of *Candida albicans* yeast to the more harmful mycelial fungal form.

Psyllium gradually scrapes away *Candida albicans'* breeding ground (fecal encrustations) from the colon wall, absorbs toxins within the colon and carries them out, reduces toxic overload ("die-off reaction" or Herxheimer effect) from poisons released by dying candida during treatment start-up, and forms the gel which binds Caprol into a timed-release formulation. This powdered product gives slippery adhesive bulk to help loosen and dig out old, congested, solidified fecal matter that often coats the colon walls, thereby providing a breeding ground for *Candida albicans* and other undesirable microorganisms. Because psyllium is not absorbed itself, toxic wastes are carried out in the feces. (Also see *Tissue Cleansing Through Bowel Management*, Berard Jensen, D.C., Ph.D.; *Guess What Came to Dinner*, Louise Gittleman.)

Lactobacillus acidophilus arrests intestinal *Candida albicans* overgrowth, primarily by using up intestinal attachment sites, and is also effective in the same manner against many pathogenic bacteria, thereby strengthening the immune system by lessening its workload.

Bentonite directly adsorbs *Candida albicans* and toxins and flushes them out reducing toxic overload ("die-off reaction") from poisons released by dying candida during treatment start-up. According to Frederic Damrau, M.D.[68] "Bentonite is a native, colloidal, hydrated aluminum silicate. . . . It has been established . . . that hydrated aluminum silicate adsorbs toxins, bacteria and viruses. This property helps explain its therapeutic usefulness in acute diarrhea of diverse cause. By virtue of its physical action bentonite serves as an adsorbent aid in detoxification of the intestinal canal."

Patients with severe candidiasis (up to 50% of the cases) may experience certain uncomfortable effects within the first week after initiation of the Candida Purge program at the intensive level of therapy, such symptoms as flu symptoms -- called "Herxheimer[48] reaction" -- (stuffiness, headache, general aches, diarrhea), skin rashes, and vaginal irritation/discharge may result from the release of toxins from a rapidly dying *Candida albicans* population. The exact symptom picture will depend upon the individual case and is often dramatic -- anything from "lead feet" to mental aberrations. The exact symptoms are neither important nor do they lend themselves to explanation, and they'll all disappear in a few days, as also happens when the Herxheimer effect is experienced in the successful treatment of other diseases.[48] (See this chapter, "The Herxheimer Effect.")

The Goodbye Candida Program® is available from Nu Biologics,® 2470 Wisconsin Street, Downers Grove, IL 60515-4019;[69] a similar product, Acu-trol®, is available % Monica O'Kane, #2 Willow Rd., North Oaks, MN 55110, (612) 484-2811.[81]

The Arthritis Trust of America, 5106 Old Harding Road, Franklin, TN 37064 can provide a catalog listing of vendors approved by health professionals. Send tax-exempt donation, self-addressed, stamped, legal-sized envelope with request.

Parasites: Candidiasis is often accompanied by parasites. Microscopic organisms, usually one or more species of protozoa, are transplanted into our intestinal tracts via air, water and food. About 50 percent of arthritic patients also have intestinal parasites, and these have got to be handled, especially if the patient has stomach cramps and bloating. Recent medical research suggests that three out of every five Americans will be infected with parasites sometime in their lives.

Diarrhea, cramps, and gastroenteritis -- sources of arthritic diarrhea and bloating -- are normal signs of parasitic infestations as well as candidiasis. These parasites contribute to a large number of different diseases. Some of the rheumatoid diseases affected are Crohn's disease, ulcerative colitis, generalized joint pain, and rheumatoid arthritis.

It's often easier and less costly to treat for parasites than it is to test for them, as often the tests' accuracies are unknown, and there are so many different tests, almost as many as there are different species of parasites, which is large, indeed.

Although special treatments may be recommended, such as colonics, which cleans out encrusted fecal matter and the inner lining of the lower intestinal tract where many parasites live, some of the treatments against parasites are similar to those against candidiasis, and therefore parasites can be treated at the same time as is the candidiasis.

Summary

We all live in a sea of microorganisms, among which are many that are organisms-of-opportunity, such as yeast/fungi and parasites. None of us will ever be completely free of such organisms. So long as we sustain a healthy immune system we'll also maintain a healthy balance between beneficial organisms and harmful organisms.

Once we've been exposed to any factors that weaken our immune system, we've automatically opened the doorway -- sent an invitation -- for organisms-of-opportunity, such as *Candida albicans* and various parasites.

Candida albicans has seven known modes of survival, changing its form and function depending upon its surrounding environment. The most inimical to us is the fungal form, where rootlets are set deep within cellular tissue lining the intestinal tract -- indeed, some scientists say candida even invades the cells themselves.

The yeast/fungus can move into any tissue, and, while there, imitate a large number of diseases, including rheumatoid arthritis and related rheumatoid diseases.

Pores opened through the intestinal mucosa by candida will also permit molecular-sized protein food particles to enter our blood stream where the protein molecules are recognized as a foreign invader. We build antibodies against these foreign invaders, thus creating an increasing number of food allergies.

There are prescription drugs, natural herbals and concentrates, and a specifically known and recommended diet, all of which have their place in getting candidiasis under control. Simultaneously, treatment against parasites should be considered.

An extremely wide variety of parasites, microorganisms, and worms inhabit the inner lining of the intestinal tract, and there sap our strength and immune system. The American public is no longer isolated from this worldwide infestation. Although parasites, including *Candida albicans*, can be decreased in numbers and effects, it is usually through the elimination of pesticides and herbicides via total body detoxification that produces the greatest improvements. Eliminating herbicides and pesticides comes about substantially only when heavy metals -- in particular dental and other mercury -- has been decreased substantially, according to Lee Cowden, M.D. Root canal and tooth extracted foci of infections as well as those remaining from improperly sterilized adnoidectomies and tonsilectomies also play hob with our ability to return to wellness.

Although some of these recommended practices can be performed by the individual, it is the wise and thankful patient who works with their health-care practitioner to insure that the disease is actually under control, and that a new generation of resistant organisms has not been developed.

Diet for Food Allergies

Often simply solving a food allergy problem will also solve various forms of arthritis, including rheumatoid arthritis. For example, a sensitivity to the solanines -- tomatoes, potatoes, tobacco, eggplant, red peppers -- will produce arthritis symptoms, and discontinuing their use will relieve those symptoms. This effect is also true with many other foods to which we've become allergic, called allergenic substances.

Allergies, and chemical sensitivities, as does candidiasis, may affect every organ and system in the body producing a multitude of symptoms that often remains unresolved by use of traditional medicines.

Foods that we regularly consume remain in our intestinal tract for longer periods, and therefore the risk of developing food allergies to them are greater than for seldom eaten foods. The basis to this higher risk, however, is often referred to as a "leaky gut syndrome," a condition caused by either a thining of the protective mucosal layer in our intestinal tract, or caused by organisms-of-opportunity, such as parasites including *Candida albicans*, the latter sending down hyphae, or rootlets into the mucosa and opening up small doorways that permit undigested food to pass directly into the blood stream to be recognized as a foreign invader by our immune system. Once a particular food, such as the molecules from corn, are recognized as a foreign invader, we have developed a biochemically conditioned reflex action to that substance -- corn -- which manifests as an allergy.

If we have an allergy to external molds and pollens at the same time that we consume foods to which we've become allergic, the condition worsens.

Physicians who treat allergies and environmental chemical sensitivities, a condition similar to allergies, view allergies as biochemically the same as a drug addiction: (1) withdrawal symptoms on removing the allergenic substance from our diet involving headaches, running nose, diarrhea, etc.; (2) craving for the allergenic substance, as, for example, a craving for chocolates; (3) restoration to a feeling of normality on supplying the allergenic substance.

There are numerous tests and treatments for determining allergenic foods, not all of the same quality or consistency. One of the most commonly used methods is both diagnostic and curative, which is known as the "elimination diet."

There are also a large number of variations on the nature of an elimination diet. Once a food is suspected as being a problem, the patient refrains from eating it totally for ten to fourteen days. On a trial consumption, physical reactions are observed, thus determining whether this food is truly an allergenic item.

Another method is the "pure water" diet, consuming nothing but pure water for five days, after which but one food at a time is introduced into the diet. Physical reactions swiftly determine which foods are offensive. How does one know? Because, if allergenic, after refraining from eating the food for a time and then resuming its consumption, you'll suffer from symptoms such as headaches, diarrhea, joint pain, etc.

When blood tests are made to determine specific allergenic foods, refraining from consuming those foods for four months will often break the allergic response.

Methods for solving the allergy problems will be discussed in the treatment sections that follow.

Other Rheumatoid Arthritis Treatments that Have Worked

Accupuncture

Acupuncture, a development of thousands of years of Oriental practices, relies on knowledge of controlling the gateways to the bioelectrical energy flow along meridian pathways that parallel one another, head to toe. Acupuncture can effectively treat hundreds of conditions, including rheumatoid arthritis and osteoarthritis. (See Chapter I, "Acupuncture.")

In addition to rebalancing our energy pathways, thus revitalizing our cells, tissues, organs, and systems, numerous scientific studies have demonstrated that the use of acupuncture stimulates the immune system to better fight microorganisms, many of which may be causes for rheumatoid diseases. Other studies have shown that acupuncture increases pain resistance, probably by increasing our output of endorphins, natural brain chemicals that act as pain desensitizers.

William Michael Cargile, D.C., Chairman of Research of the American Association of Acupuncture, describes the use of acupuncture on a fifty-six-year-old woman with a twenty-year-long medically diagnosed case of rheumatoid arthritis. Bedridden, placed on damaging toxic methotrexate -- a drug used ineffectively in the treatment of cancer -- and now ineffectively against rheumatoid arthritis -- near death, she finally agreed to accept three acupuncture treatments a week. These treatments were reduced to twice a week after the first month, and finally once a week after the third month.

Dr. Cargile reports the patient's condition as dramatically improved with a marked decrease in inflammation, a much improved range of motion, and a decrease in pain, sufficiently so, the patient was able to return to work.

Since there is no difference between the methods of acupuncture used for osteoarthritis or for rheumatoid arthritis, refer to Chapter I, "Acupuncture," Osteoarthritis, for identification of appropriate acupuncture points.

Allergies, Biodetoxification, and Chemical Sensitivities[16,75]

Lee Cowden, M.D., Dallas, Texas strongly believes in the importance of overall detoxification. Within his experience he's found that intestinal parasites won't completely leave the body until pesticides and herbicides are eliminated, and those won't go until mercury is cleaned out of the body.[261]

As most food allergies stem from the development of a leaky gut, called the "leaky gut syndrome," and as the leaky gut syndrome often stems from an invasion of fungal *Candida albicans*, one should clear up fungal candidiasis if it exists. Restoring good digestion (nutrition, enzymes, hydrochloric acid) is an obvious characteristic of achieving health for any condition. Detoxification, including the elimination of intestinal parasites, is equally important, but, in its many differing aspects, often overlooked.[173] Within these standards-of-care-procedures, there are many solutions to food allergies and chemical sensitivities related to rheumatoid disease, including rheumatoid arthritis.

Food Allergies and Chemical Sensitivities

Adequate treatment for rheumatoid arthritis must include treatment against food allergies. Just as candidiasis can mimic many diseases, so can allergies mimic rheumatoid diseases, including rheumatoid arthritis. Indeed, one of the primary causes for rheumatoid arthritis has been found through clinical trials to be chemical sensitivities and food allergies.

Since Theron Randolph, M.D. and four physicians organized the Society for Clinical Ecology in 1965 there has been a quiet revolution on how we view and test for food and other chemical sensitivities. Dr. Randolph inherited some of his knowledge, and a great deal was his own major contribution to modern medicine.

The interesting -- and distressing -- part about allergies is that foods which were perfectly safe for much of our lives suddenly become intolerable -- for no obvious reasons.

Early in the medical history of treating allergies, professional allergists had great success in testing for and finding common allergens, such as those that are airborne like the pollens of various plants. When similar tests were developed for foods, or the increasing number of environmental chemicals, there was, at best, inconsistent results. People, and their physicians, will unknowingly, and wrongly, take the skin-patch test as proof that they are or are not allergic to a particular food. Food patch tests are extremely unreliable when making the determination for a food allergic reaction.[208]

One of us (Gus J. Prosch, Jr., M.D.) feels that the tests and the methods traditionally taught to treat allergies today are ninety percent worthless, either the RAST blood test (radioallergosorbent test) which measures the immunoglobulins (IgE), or the skin test. Immunoglobulins are proteins capable of acting as antibodies.

Literally thousands of patients come to the clinic who have been taking allergy shots. When asked if the shots have helped, the typical response in ninety to ninety five percent of the patients is that -- they'll kind of scratch their heads and say -- "Well, I think they've helped." They've spent a great deal of money over years. They certainly want to believe that they've been helped. They don't want to believe that they've been a fool; but the key is, if those shots had really helped, their reaction would have been "Gosh! I couldn't have gotten by without them." This statement is seldom heard.

The Case of Tim

Leo Galland, M.D.,[118] of New York, an internist and leading practitioner of complementary medicine, and a well-known medical lecturer on nutrition, immunity, parasites and laboratory testing, wrote about Tim, a 4-year-old boy diagnosed with juvenile rheumatoid arthritis. He had been sick since age one, with joint pain, fever, general unwellness and a variety of symptoms traveling around his body. On two occasions, he was hospitalized for several weeks with intensive testing.

By the time Dr. Galland saw Tim, his parents had spent $100,000 for evaluations and vain attempts to treat Tim's illness.

Dr. Galland's approach was to review what others had already considered, and what else might be relevant without great expense and with a minimum of invasive procedures. First, Dr. Galland determined what was happening in Tim's intestinal tract. Tim didn't have diarrhea or failure to thrive so they wondered if there was anything further in the intestinal tract to pursue.

A comprehensive stool test did not show much in the way of parasites or other organisms-of-opportunity; however, an intestinal permeability test showed really abnormal results. Tim had a very leaky gut and malabsorption.

"In a child that age who does not have a severe parasitic infection, the most likely cause of this permeability is a food intolerance. But not an ordinary allergy -- something about the nature of gluten intolerance or cow's milk sensitive protein enteropathy (disease of the intestines). Gluten sensitivity in children is an important cause of chronic illness and unwellness, sometimes leading to hospitalization."

Dr. Galland suggested to Tim's parents that they try a gluten elimination diet. Within two weeks, Tim had no symptoms and has remained well since that time.

According to Dr. Galland,[119] leaky gut syndromes usually result from exposure to substances that damage the integrity of the intestinal mucosa, among which are the common causes of infectious agents (viral, bacterial, protozoal), ethanol, non-steroidal anti-inflammatory drugs (NSAIDS), surgery or shock, elevated levels of reactive oxygen metabolites (biliary, food-borne or produced by inflammatory cells), and cytotoxic drugs.

Allergy/Addiction to Foods and Chemicals

Surprisingly, allergies are also addictions, or at least there is sufficient commonality between the phenomena of food and some other allergies and addictions so as to suspect an actual biological link.

According to Warren Levin, M.D.[16] of New York City, New York, a new concept to the medical profession, but one of great importance to the healing arts, is food allergy/addiction. "You will notice that I do not speak of allergy or addiction nor of allergy and addiction, but rather of a single entity -- allergy/addiction. These two different aspects are as inseparable as heads and tails on a coin. Depending on which aspect is facing you, one or the other side may be more obvious but the obverse is always there."

Most of us are acquainted with the obvious food allergy reaction. The patient who breaks out from strawberries or swells up from shellfish or who gets asthma from peanuts is well known and recognized by the doctor or layman. However this type of acute reaction represents a very small percentage of all food allergy/addiction reactions.

The acute reaction occurs from exposure to a food which is not eaten regularly. The reaction may affect one or several organs and systems, but tends to affect the same systems in a particular patient with each repeated exposure. In other words, according to Dr. Levin, any organ in the body is capable of responding as the shock organ. If cartilage, tendons, ligaments, and joint functions respond as the shock organ, you get aches and pains -- arthritis. If the nose reacts you get hayfever. If the lungs react, asthma. If the skin is the shock organ you get eczema or hives. If the intestinal tract is the responding organ you get diarrhea or constipation or nausea and vomiting or gas or a combination.

Dr. Levin describes allergic insult to the brain as being one of the most important reactions to allergy, as the brain can show localized areas of allergic reaction similar to hives, with circulatory changes, localized swelling, and increasing pressures, all taking place in re-stricted regions. The symptoms can be severe or mild, and manifest in the form of many different physical complaints, among which can be headaches, fatigue, uncontrollable sleepiness at inappropriate times, difficulty in concentrating, memory lapses, incoordination, hallucina-tions, perceptual changes among the five senses (taste, smell, touch, sight and hearing), loss of consciousness and convulsions.

Alcoholism as a Model of Allergy/Addiction

As described by Warren Levin, M.D., the most obvious example of a serious food addiction is that of alcoholism, which is not normally considered from this viewpoint. Food addiction, allergies, and alcohol-ism exhibit the same biochemical phenomena:

• The first drink is almost always the social phenomenon. The drug affect of alcohol is experienced as pleasant and unwinding, the relax-ation effect. This may be repeated socially at irregular intervals for years, without any addiction developing.

• Then perhaps after a tough day at the office the businessman may try a martini before supper to obtain the same relaxation (still from the drug affect of alcohol). When this becomes a habit the stage is set for addiction.

• Food addiction, in a similar manner, develops slowly from frequent repeated exposures to a potentially addicting substance.

• It is at this point that the addiction phenomenon becomes manifest by its major clinical sign -- the withdrawal phenomenon. If you are addicted to something you feel better when you take it and after a period of being without it you begin to feel worse. Depending on the severity of the addiction it may be very mild and difficult to recognize, and express itself just as craving for the substance to which you're addicted. Some people just *know* that they are going to feel better if they have a cup of coffee, and other people just know they can't get started unless they have their drink of orange juice, and other people don't even recognize it -- they just think that it's perfectly logical to have bread with every meal and they don't consider a meal complete without a piece of bread. What they don't realize is that the craving is to satisfy an addiction.

• For the developing alcoholic, by now he is taking a martini regularly when he comes home from work to unwind, and very subtly and gradually he becomes addicted. Every day by supper time his addiction is beginning to have its affect, and he relieves it by taking his customary drink.

• When addiction becomes progressive the length of time that the offending substance relieves symptoms becomes less and less, and soon our harried businessman notices that somewhere around three-thirty or four o'clock he is really beginning to feel frazzled. However if he keeps a little bottle in the drawer and takes a nip about three or three-thirty he can avoid that down feeling and of course it's an easy thing to do and that's only two drinks a day, and another alcoholic is on the way.

• The addiction increases, the withdrawal period becomes sooner and now we find that in order for him to function well he's got to have a drink when he goes out with the boys at lunchtime. If he is intelligent he may skip the mid-afternoon nip from the drawer because he does not need that anymore but if he is a slave to habit he will continue to have that drink as well as the one before supper.

• It's important to notice at this time that the soon-to-be alcoholic is functioning better *with* the alcohol than he does without it, even though alcohol is a total depressant to the nervous system, interferes with reflex time and in general produces less efficient functioning. In the person with an alcohol problem the non-alcoholic state is no longer normal. It is a state of withdrawal from an addicting substance and the depression and malfunction that accompanies withdrawal is worse than the state in which the stimulation of the addicting substance is in effect.

• Eventually, we get to the point where the patient is drinking every hour or two during the day to avoid the withdrawal syndrome, and he is functioning much below par but he does function as long as he continues to take his alcohol.

• When the patient goes to bed at night, he is going to go through an eight hour period without alcohol and when he wakes up in the morning he's going to be in severe withdrawal. This of course is the classical evidence of addiction to alcohol -- the patient who wakes up in the morning hung-over, nervous, irritable, and all he has to do is take a tiny sip of his favorite alcohol and he relieves withdrawal symptoms temporarily.

• It's obvious to most people except the alcoholic that the best course of action is to go "cold turkey," to suffer through the withdrawal syndrome, to detoxify and then to avoid the offending addicting allergic substance so that optimum body function can be obtained.

• Withdrawing from addictive substances such as alcohol, tobacco, and food can all produce arthritic symptoms, and all of them can create withdrawal symptoms exactly like that described for the alcoholic.

Detoxifying or Desensitization of Foods that Cause Arthritis

Detoxification or desensitization takes about five days for food substances. Once a patient has gone through this "cold turkey" period the body no longer craves the allergy/addicting foods. The body reacts intensely to these foods on the next exposure. Dr. Levin says that this phenomena is extremely important in the diagnosis of food allergy/ addiction.

• Any food can be addicting. The more quickly a given food is absorbed from the intestinal tract, the more likely it is to produce the allergy/addiction response. This means that next in line to alcohol are substances such as carbohydrates like white sugar, white flour, and corn syrup.

• The absorption of carbohydrates is slowed down by the presence of indigestible fiber, protein and oil. The refining process eliminates these factors which retard absorption and the result is increased incidence of allergy/addiction. The combination of these refined foods with alcohol is disastrous to the susceptible patient.

• Following the refined carbohydrates in speed of absorption are the natural carbohydrates, fruits, starchy vegetables, and cereals, then the proteins: meat, fish, poultry and eggs, and finally the slowest of all -- fats and oils. It is for this reason that many severely food sensitive patients are able to tolerate foods that are fried in oil Chinese style using the classical Chinese wok technique. For anyone with multiple food allergies this method of food preparation is highly recommended.

A craving for certain foods, while almost always an addiction, can also be the human body's instinct for a needed substance that is found in that particular food. Chocolateholics are almost always addicted to chocolate, but, also according to nutritionist Nan Kathyrin Fuchs, Ph.D., "Chocolate cravings may be an indication that you have a calcium/magnesium imbalance, since cocoa powder contains more magnesium than any other food." Perhaps you simply need more magnesium, which is a simple need to answer by taking more magnesium in a form that is easily absorbed and utilized. (See *Magnesium Chloride Hexahydrate Therapy*, Raul Vergini, M.D.)

Fasting Unmasks Allergies

The technique of total fasting was developed as a diagnostic and therapeutic technique by the pioneers in clinical ecology. Although techniques of various recommended fasts may vary, the general concept is the same when viewed from the allergy/addiction point of view. When eliminating all of the offending allergic substances the body begins to function better.

"Unfortunately," Dr. Levin explains, "many patients have mutliple allergies of varying degrees to many if not most of the foods that they eat. In such a situation eliminating a single food may not produce the relief that is sought and the withdrawal symptoms are merely superimposed on the general depression and low functioning level, so that the patient feels worse and does not get relief at the end of the five day elimination."

Adrenal cortical insufficiency, Addison's disease, or other debilitating illnesses can prevent or prohibit someone from using the total fast method, however, and a physician's advice is important.

To go on a total fast for 5 days means that one does not place anything in the mouth short of pure drinking water -- and also no smoking. Usually the recommended fast period is 5 days as it takes that long for the intestinal tract to eliminate all traces of foods.

The more allergies and the more sickness, often the worse one will feel, until the addiction/allergy reaction has been surmounted. By the afternoon of the fifth day the patient should begin feeling very much better.

Dr. Levin says that, "At this point we start refeeding the patient with the idea of avoiding a demonstration of an allergic reaction or the development of an addiction." That means the following rules are to be followed:

1. Initially after the fast eat only one pure food at each feeding.

2. The first few foods eaten should be foods that are not suspected of allergy or addicting potential to the patient. That means in general foods that are not in the usual daily routine diet. In some cases one must resort to exotic foods such as venison, bear or buffalo meat, kohlrabi, endive and rutabaga as vegetables. Goat's milk products are frequently acceptable. Remember that this is only in the initial phase of eating after the fast and eventually ordinary foods should be utilized for all but the worst cases.

3. If possible the first time a food is eaten after the fast it should be a fresh organic food known to be free of pesticides, preservatives or any processing. It 's amazing how many people think that they are allergic to apples only to find that it is the chemical spray at fault. Or an allergy

to oranges turns out to be due to the artifical color and not orange itself. If there is no reaction to the organic product, the next exposure could be from the ordinary source of supply whether fresh, frozen or canned. Everything we eat should be fresh and free of processing, if possible, except as processed in our own kitchen.

4. Everything that is taken by mouth must be cleared of suspicion by individual tests. That means the first time you drink the tap water it must be all by itself. It's amazing how many patients are sensitive to the chlorine and fluorine and other pollutants in our water supply. It also means that every vitamin, mineral or food supplement as well as any medication must be independently judged by taking it and it alone and observing the effects. One of the biggest problems in the so-called neurotic patient is allergy/addiction to tranquilizers. In some cases to the medication itself, in other cases fillers in the capsule and frequently to the artificial coloring. However, you must beware of discontinuing any medication for the fast without your physician's knowledge even though any prescription can be a factor just as any food or food supplement can. Ideally nothing should be taken during the fast except distilled water.

5. Keep a diary with two columns. In column A keep an accurate exact record of everything you eat and the time that it is eaten. In column B keep a record of how you feel. Any change for the better or worse should be recorded with the time of the occurrence. In addition keep a record of your pulse rate for one minute period before you eat each feeding and every ten to fifteen minutes for an hour after each feeding. A change up or down of 12 or more beats a minute is suggestive of food allergy.

6. Continue eating single foods at each feeding until you have found a number of foods that do not produce reaction. After a few days of unusual foods start testing the most likely foods, the ones you eat regularly. Remember not to test complex foods like bread. This would be getting wheat, yeast, egg, shortening, chemical and vitamin additives all at once. Test each ingredient separately. Foods for testing can be raw or cooked without any condiments or seasonings except for genuine (non-refined) sea salt which may be used. (Most so-called "sea-salt" has been refined.) Boiling, steaming, broiling and baking are the preferred cooking methods using the same water as for the fast.

Alan Gaby, M.D., Washington, says, "I am reminded of a patient with a 7-year history of daily migraines, rheumatoid arthritis, and severe abdominal pain. He had spent $27,000 on numerous doctors and treatments, without obtaining relief. A simple elimiation and re-challenge diet determined that corn allergy was the cause of all of these problems and he was essentially cured after one visit."[260]

Blood Test for Food Allergies

When using the food challenge test, it's important to know which foods to avoid. Immuno Laboratories of Fort Lauderdale, FL has developed a sensitive blood test for food allergies, testing for two types of blood "immunoglobulins," IgE (airborne) and IgG (food sensitivities). Results of the test are reported back to the patient and doctor, having tested from your blood sample for more than 100 kinds of food allergies, also supplying you with an extensive food rotation listing.

One of us (Perry A. Chapdelaine, Sr.) for example, found that 2 items, squash mix and wheat, involved the airborne IgE fractions, whereas 23 of 104 other foods tested were IgG positive, and, of course, these were exactly the foods most often purchased and "enjoyed."[108]

Through the use of Immuno Laboratories (and other similar laboratories) testing and rotation recommendations, it's likely that the 23 IgG fractions will drop out of the system after about 3 to 4 months of their complete abstinence, but it is unlikely that the 2 IgE sensitivities will do so.

A little known food allergy phenomenon is that some foods may take as long as 3 days to create an observable allergic response. A careful diary and an astute physician can spot these. Both immediate and delayed responses (as well as candidiasis) can be determined through blood tests made by Immuno Laboratories, Inc. of Fort Lauderdale, Florida. Immuno Laboratories, Inc., 1620 W. Oakland Park Blvd., Fort Lauderdale, Florida 33311; (800) 231-9196; (305) 486-4500; Fax (305) 739-6563.

The Case of Ann Staffanson

Montana citizen Ann Staffanson,[220] 70 years-of-age, fully believing that her next move would be to the wheel chair, had been on anti-inflammatory and other debilitating drugs from a rheumatologist for years and had terrible side-effects, such as three bouts with stomach ulcers, hair loss from methotrexate, constant diarrhea, and so on.

In a blood test sent to the National Bio Tech Laboratory of Seattle, Washington, advised by a naturopath and chiropractor, Ann's food allergies were tested for IgG and IgE immuno-complexes. National Bio Tech Laboratory of Seattle, 3212 NE 125th St., Washington, (206) 363-6606; Fax (206) 363-2025.)

Ann reported that she "was sent back a very thorough, very professional listing of all the foods that I have no reaction to, and those I have low, moderate and high intolerance to. This, of course, changed all my eating habits drastically but has also changed my life.

"ALL my arthritis pain was totally gone in about 2 weeks time and I am able to move about as I did 10 years ago. The test cost me $200," very little compared to the cost for ineffective, traditional drugs.

Along with dietary constraints Ann's naturopath gives her enzymes, about 6 to 8 pills 2 times a day, but is now down to 3-4 pills, 2 times daily, also taken at bedtime so they'll work thru the night as well.

One of these is a natural thyroid supplement.

"The change in my life has been miraculous and I would like to shout it to the rooftops. My bodily functions are now totally normal and my life back to what it was before arthritis."

Ann Staffanson's original health professional, Willow Moore, N.P., D.C., has moved to Maryland, Ann now goes to Susana and Don Leathers, N.P. of Bozeman, Montana.

Other Successful Allergy Treatments
Autogenous Therapies

Urine has been used extensively for therapeutic purposes for at least 5000 years, especially in countries like Tibet and India. Indian Prime Minister Morarji Desai stunned the world when he revealed that he drank a glass of his own urine every day. He died at the age of 99.

Modern drug manufacturers long ago discovered that tens of thousands of important chemical compounds are contained in urine, and so urine is collected routinely from women, men, horses and other animals for the purpose of isolating out and condensing a particular desirable product. For example, Premarin®, estrogen, given to human females for hormone replacement therapy is actually derived from the collected urine of pregant mares.

Julian Whitaker, M.D.,[259] Editor of *Health & Healing*, writes that "Your intestines are home to billions of bacteria -- 100 to 400 different species. They outnumber the cells of your body one hundredfold." In America feces and urine are socially rejected as being "nasty" or viewed as if each were filled with deadly virus and bacteria, the source of disease. Feces does contain about 30% bacteria by weight, but urine is sterile, our blood having been processed by the kidneys to produce a fluid -- the urine -- that represents an excess of vitamins, minerals, and protective substances that are used to fight various organisms. As these are excesses in the blood stream not needed by the body for the moment, they are dumped. As urine and its dissolved products contain valuable ingredients, yeast/molds, bacteria and other microorganisms rapidly take up residence in discarded urine, thereafter making it unsterile.

What we throw away in our urine each day contains hundreds of medicines that are uniquely designed for each person, and has been called the "perfect medicine."[193]

Autogenous Vaccines: One of us (Gus J. Prosch, Jr., M.D.) has had great success with 80% of his allergy patients in eliminating allergies by use of injectable urine manufactured by the patient.

After patients wash their genitals with hydrogen peroxide (3%), they urinate in a sterile container, using a mid-stream catch. This substance is then filtered through two micropore filters -- very fine filters that will screen out any kind of undesirable object such as remotely possible germs or crystals -- leaving in the already sterile fluid, all the complex molecules -- small allergens and water -- that our body needs in order to become innoculated allergy free.

The ultra-filtered urine is tested by means of specific gravity, and if the urine is sufficiently concentrated, a hyperdermic is filled with a measured amount of the filtered fluid which is injected directly into the muscles of the buttock.

Eight treatments are given, one per week.

This is nature's way of fighting infections and allergies: When any animal gets a cut or a scratch, what do they do? They always lick it. What they're doing is getting any germs found in that cut or scratch underneath their tongue where the germs are absorbed into the blood stream. The immune system says, "Hey, there's a germ, it's not supposed to be here," and so it begins building antibodies to kill that particular germ. Those antibodies are in the blood stream, they circulate to where that cut is, and so now you've got the antibodies fighting that particular germ that's found in the infection.

All of our vaccinations are based upon this same theory. When we give a vaccination against lockjaw (tetanus), we take the dead lockjaw germ and inject it into the patient. The body recognizes a foreign invader even if the germ is dead, and it builds up antibodies to fight the live germ. By the second booster, we've built up antibodies, but by the third booster, we've built up a lot of antibodies. If we come in contact with the lockjaw germ again, our body says, "There's that germ again!," and kills it quickly.

The oldtimer physicians also knew that the same process could be used to cure all sorts of infections. When they had patients who had boils that would not heal, they'd take some of the pus from the boils, sterilize it, and inject it back into the patient, and the patient would heal themself from the knowledge the body gained.

Allergies will respond the same way. We know that all of the things that you're allergic to are in your body fluids: your blood, urine, saliva, spinal fluid -- we don't why, but when you take those fluids containing the things you're allergic to out of the body, and put them back into the body, you get the same effect as you do when you take the germs and reintroduce them in a safe form back into the body.

Autogenous Oral Vaccine: If you're not squeemish -- that is, if you can break your cultural conditioning that emotionally identifies urine as a "bad thing" -- midstream urine can be used directly without filtering it and injecting into the buttocks, that is, by drinking it. Remember, aside from rather exceptional circumstances, urine is sterile, a by-product of our blood stream, and contains virtually everything required to treat every disease, including allergies and arthritis.

Frederick H. Binford, professor of physics at Fisk University, Nashville, Tennesssee, suffered from an arthritic back ache for many years, until he began using a glass of his own urine daily.

A former prime minister of India, Morarji Desai, publicly stated that he drank a glass of his own urine a day, but you don't need such large quantities. One or two drops on the tongue will do, or, in fact, you can create a homeopathic solution, diluting a few drops in pure water until there is no taste or color.

As urine also contains many nutrients, microorganisms will quickly establish a foothold in it, and thereafter it is, indeed, contaminated. Urine should be used immediately, and not be stored for later use except under sterile conditions. Since each person manufactures enough of their own perfect medicine daily, storage should not normally be required.

The Case of Mrs. Buttrey

Mrs. Buttrey from Florida was diagnosed with rheumatoid arthritis at age 28. The swelling and pain in her joints was "unbelievable." Also, since age 8 she suffered from migraine headaches, so as a precaution she took a bottle of Excedrin® wherever she traveled. Mrs. Buttrey also suffered from a severe weight problem, weighing almost 200 pounds when rheumatoid arthritis developed.

When Mrs. Buttrey learned of urine therapy, she started taking the fluid and in 4-1/2 months she weighed but 130 pounds, her rheumatoid arthritis had disappeared as had her headaches.[193] (See *Your Own Perfect Medicine*, Martha M. Christy, Future Med. Inc., Scottsdale, AZ 85267).

Teaching the Nervous System
Not to Respond to Food or Pollen Allergies

Devi S. Nambudripad, D.C., L.Ac., R.N., Ph.D. suffered miserably from food and pollen allergies and chemical sensitivities. She lived on aspirin and a very restricted diet, but was continually suffering from various illnesses. Dr. Nambudripad's persistent search paid off with her discovery which promises to revolutionize allergy treatments, as well as the traditional medical view of the nature of allergies.

Now called the Nambudripad Allergy Elimination Technique (NAET), she combined the fields of acupuncture, chiropractic and kinesiology -- muscle testing for weakness -- in this manner.

• While holding a suspected allergen (food, pollen, or chemical element) in the hand, the patient is tested by means of kinesiology for muscle weakness. If a weakness is found, the item being held is a substance that is being interpreted by the nervous system as a threat. Unconsciously the human body will produce allergen-combating substances, such as histamine at the cellular level.

• While still holding the item, acupuncture points are opened up in such a manner that all meridians are properly flowing Qi (Chi) -- bio-electric energy.

• The patient is then advised to stay away from that known allergen for a specific time period.

• On the follow-up visit, the patient is re-tested to determine if the

treatment was effective. If not, it is repeated.
- Each successive treatment reduces the number of food, pollen and chemical sensitivity reactions, until the patient is wholly free of all effects.

Adrienne Fowlie wrote to Eleanor Chin, D.C.,[253] San Francisco, California, saying, "I want to thank you for helping me so much. I am 49 years old and was diagnosed with rheumatoid arthritis nine months ago. I was very ill and actually bed-ridden much of the time. I was in enormous pain all the time."

Dr. Chin applied NAET procedures to Adrienne, and, after several weeks, Adrienne felt an overall feeling of well-being, every part of her body rejuvenated, with a high energy level." See *An Alternative Medicine Definitive Guide to Allergies*, Future Medicine Publishing Company, Fife, Washington.)

Colon Detoxification

A living colony of microorganisms -- and often worms -- live in the gut of the average person. Rheumatologist Joel D. Taurog, University of Texas Southwest Medical Center in Dallas was not thinking of arthritis when they genetically engineered a population of rats with a particular gene (HLA-B27). The rats developed a progressive inflammation of the intestines as well as arthritis. When these same rats were raised in a sterile environment, neither arthritis nor colitis resulted. These results, along with all other evidence we've offered, surely exposes the link between microorganisms and arthritis.[262]

The skin, lymph system, kidneys, lung, and the bowel are all extremely important waste elimination systems. Accumulated toxins contribute to a huge percentage of the rheumatoid arthritics' problems. Among the variety of ways that these toxins are produced and distributed to affect tissues and joints, the most severe concentrations come through impacted feces lodged more or less permanently in the colon. The liver detoxifies as a backup system for the elimination channels.

Impacted feces contain accumulated waste materials, bacteria, fungi, viruses, parasites, and dead cellular material. Toxins from these products produces inflammation and swelling of the bowel. Absorption of these materials through the intestinal lining -- a lining that is often "leaky" -- permits molecules to flow directly into the blood stream, distributing damaging toxins throughout the body. These toxins lodge in joint tissues as well as other tissues, thereby creating the antigen/antibody tussles that appear to be gigantic allergic reactions to unknown substances. In particular, all the gradations of the collagen tissue and "auto-immune" diseases are manifested, including that of systemic rheumatoid arthritis.

Nutritionist Bernard Jensen, D.C., Ph.D.,[209] author of several books including *Tissue Cleansing Through Bowl Management* with Sylvia Bell, reports that "In 50 years I've spent helping people to overcome illness, disability and disease, it has become crystal clear that poor bowel management lies at the root of most people's health problems." Dr. Jensen also says that, "No doctor should practice any system of healing without considering the care of the five elimination channels -- skin, lymph, kidneys, lungs -- and in particular, taking care of the bowel."

The Case of Amie Buttrey

Amie Buttrey,[209] followed Dr. Jensen's colon detoxification program, later writing, "When I began the tissue cleansing program, I could hardly use my hands. My left knee was so swollen I couldn't move it. During the program, my hands became more flexible, and the swelling and soreness in the palm of my right hand improved. The swelling in my knee decreased until I could walk without pain. My back is not aching all the time now and seems stronger. My feet aren't so tender on the bottoms."

The Case of Evelyn Peterson

Evelyn Peterson[209] suffered from terrible neck pains, and was treated by traditional regimens that included non-steroidal anti-inflammatories as well as steroids (cortisone). During traditional treatment, she was wrongly told that diet had nothing whatsoever to do with arthritis. After one year on these prescription drugs, she found she was not getting any relief, and so she changed direction by starting a nutritional and detoxification program under Bernard Jensen, D.C., Ph.D.

Dr. Jensen asked Evelyn to drop all drugs, which she did with great reluctance. Her withdrawal symptoms included trembling, but she persisted.

She later reported to Dr. Jensen that "Within a week, I found myself free of pain and feeling very well without drugs. One-and-a-half months later, feeling exceptionally good, I suddenly developed a fever of 105 degrees, swollen face and eye, with a headache such as I had never experienced before. I thought my whole world would collapse.

"I was told it (the healing crisis: Herxheimer) would only last 3 days -- and it did! Then I felt good again, just as Dr. Jensen said I would. (See this chapter, "The Herxheimer Effect.")

Evelyn passed through this healing crisis producing an excessive elimination of mucus, and after nine months her neck was still free of pain without the use of any drugs.

The Bernard Jensen, D.C., Ph.D. Detoxification Program

Although all avenues (skin, lungs and bronchials, kidneys, bowels) of detoxification are extremely important -- perhaps even vital -- to achieve wellness, Dr. Jensen's long-standing success with every kind of disease has been through nutrition, skin brushing and principally cleaning out an also long-standing, neglected colon.

Dr. Jensen[209] writes, "Imagine what would be the result of a pump failure in a city's sewer system or what would happen if all the pipes got plugged up with some unmovable material so that the system failed to move waste? It wouldn't take very long before a crisis developed and a huge sanitation problem would threaten health and society.

"From open sewers in the past sprang the devasting plagues and diseases that literally destroyed whole cities and populations."

Such a broad indictment is accepted by all of us because of our public hygiene education, but what we don't realize is that Jensen's summary is precisely the description of the condition of our primary elimination system, the bowels -- especially when we suffer from a persistent degenerative disease.

Clogging up of our intestines can occur in several ways well worked out by physicians such as Dr. Jensen. One of these ways is a very gradual building up of an irritated mucus membrane and bowel wall to such an extent that feces can hardly pass through. "One autopsy revealed a colon to be 9 inches in diameter with a passage through it no larger than a pencil! The rest was caked up layer upon layer of encrusted fecal material. This accumulation can have the consistency of truck rubber tire. It's that hard and black. Another autopsy revealed a stagnant colon to weigh in at an incredible 40 pounds! Imagine carrying around all that morbid accumulated waste."

In addition to this unnatural, thickened intestinal lining, the lining itself, as well as unnatural pockets and bulges in the intestine, can harbor a vast variety of organisms-of-opportuntiy, including yeast/fungus, bacteria, protozoa, mycoplasma, virus, and parasites. These foreign invaders produce poisonous toxins, and the toxins as well as the dead protein tissues of the dying organisms cross-react with our tissues creating the so-called "auto-immune" diseases.

Roger Wyburn-Mason, M.D., Ph.D., and Thomas McPherson Brown, M.D. both tackled the problem of ridding us of undesirable organisms, thus achieving wellness, but without nutritional guidelines, and attention to a general detoxification program, wellness may not be permanent.

On the other hand, Dr. Jenson, and hundreds of other physicians, have learned that often detoxification programs by themselves can rid one of various forms of rheumatoid diseases.

Lee Cowden, M.D.,[210] Dallas, Texas, says, "The one thing I have all arthritic patients do is a bowel cleanse to get rid of the false lining, 'cause I find that always helps the arthritic condition."

One sign of this condition is the production of excessive gases, although normal, moderate gas production, itself, is of no consequence to a healthy colon.

There are numerous household substances or over-the-counter preparations that can help to manage the bowel or help to cleanse the colon, for example, Wachters' Sea-Klenz With Enzymes™, consisting of betaine HCl, malt diastaase, papain, bromelain, cellulase, plantago ovata blond, apple powder, prune powder, marine algae (blend of sea plants), lemon powder, chlorophyll, and pectin, one teaspoon to 6 ounces of water or juice.

For bowel management, Dr. Jensen recommends at least three glasses of warm liquid before breakfast every morning, reminding us that cold water stays in the stomach, but that warm water goes directly to the bowel.

For elimination, Velco 77 or 79 bulk and clay water can be used three times a day with meals over a period of 30 days. More juice can be added to your diet during that time to be taken after the bulk and clay water. At the same time, add enemas, perhaps using clay water and coffee instead of plain water.

Lindsey Duncan, C.N., founder of Home Nutrition Clinic, Santa Monica, California, and also Nature's Secret, a specialty products company, Boulder, Colorado, recommends "cleaning" all of your organs, using Super Cleanse™, Ultimate Fiber™, and A.M./P.M. Ultimate Cleanse™.

A.M./P.M. Ultimate Cleanse™ is a 2-part vegetarian detoxification formula containing 29 cleansing herbs, amino acids, antioxidants, digestive enzymes, vitamins, and minerals, and 5 kinds of fiber. Signs that the program is working are the classic Herxheimer symptoms: flu-like feeling, a cold, runny nose, transient pimples, headaches, brain-fog, or fatigue, all signs that will pass within 1-2 days, according to Duncan.

Ducan's goal is to detoxify the internal body organs, not just the bowel, addressing all five channels of elimination, as well as vital organs and tissues. At the end of the program, a person should be having 2-3 bowel movements every day. Once the internal system is cleansed, nutrient absorption is more efficient.[248]

Dr. Jensen has designed a colon cleansing enema using a specially designed board -- "colema," he calls it -- that every person can learn and use for themselves, although, in some instances, he also advises colonic help from a professional on special problems, and perhaps at the start of the self-help routine.

Colonics administered by health professionals may be important as a good jump-starter, but the individual must learn to apply good rules of bowel management to prevent the condition from recurring. (See Bernard Jensen, D.C., Ph.D., Sylvia Bell, *Tissue Cleansing Through Bowel Management.*)

The Case of Roy Hampskill

Roy developed a rheumatoid disease called psoriasis, the first symptoms being scaling of scalp and facial skin under his beard. Then three years later, he noticed that the condition became worse when finger-nails begin showing pits and creases. A year later Roy developed diabetes and began taking insulin. Six months later arthritis appeared, his first symptoms being fluid in the knee and inflammation of the elbow. He was now diagnosed as having psoriatic arthritis.

Taking 20 aspirin per day for arthritis pain relief, insulin shots for diabetes, the psoriasis grew worse, and Roy began to feel depressed and hopeless.

Dr. Bernard Jensen, using iris analysis -- a method whereby the changing appearance of the visible eye structure reveals internal changes -- determined bowel, bronchial, kidney and pancreatic weakness, a toxic thyroid condition, drug deposits in the colon and congestion in the lungs.

Dr. Jensen placed Roy on a seven-day tissue cleansing program, and found from monitoring blood sugar levels that the insulin levels could be gradually reduced and then discontinued.

Psoriatic arthritis dramatically improved. Roy could now put on his socks without pain, and walking became normal. Skin was moister, and the patient was in excellent spirits when last seen. (Also see *The Surprising Psoriasis Treatment*, Helmut Christ, M.D.)

Schizophrenia and Arthritis

Schizophrenia is a group of mental disorders involving distur-bances in thinking, mood, and behavior associated with an altered con-cept of reality. Although schizophrenia and rheumatoid arthritis are usually mutually exclusive; that is, one does not normally find both conditions in the same person, both of these illnesses can occur in the same family.[256]

Researchers have found that the two diseases result from blockage of an enzyme, preventing conversion of the amino acid tryptophane from converting to niacin (B_3). Depending upon where in the biochemi-cal conversion chain this blockage occurs, a person may develop either schizophrenia or rheumatoid arthritis, but not both.

Both of these conditions exhibit similar patterns of food and chemi-cal sensitivities, Australian doctor Chris M. Reading discovered after working with over 400 rheumatoid arthritis patients and 500 schizo-phrenic patients.

Dr. Reading recommends that those suffering from either condi-tion avoid alcohol, junk food and amine-rich foods (curry, chili, zuc-chini, capsicum), yeast and fermented foods, gluten-containing grains, cow's milk, beef, eggs, legumes-beans, solanaceae (tomato, potato, eggplant, tobacco), salicylates (plums, apricots, cherries, citrus, apples, currants, raisins, almonds), and tobacco.

After a food elimination period, as described in the preceding sec-tions, foods are gradually introduced as the patient improves.

Dr. Reading also recommends additional amino acids, essential fatty acids, manganese, zinc, magnesium and folic acid, and vitamins C, E, and B-complex.

Such treatment, he found, could reverse pain and inflammation in rheumatoid arthritics, and also allow gradual restoration of mental normality to the schizophrenic.

Botanicals
Table of Herbs Found Useful in the Treatment of Rheumatoid Arthritis

Herb	Comments
Alfalfa (*Medicago sativa*)	Perennial, low fields, widely culivated.
Barberry (*Berberis* app.)	Deciduous shrub grows in hard, gravelly soil in northeastern states, and rich soils in western states; also Oregon grape (*Berberis aquifolium*).
Black Cohosh (*Cimicifuga racemosa*)	North American perennial, hillsides, woods, higher elevations, Maine, Ontario, Wisconsin, Georgia, Missouri.
Blueberries, (*Vaccinium angustifolium, Vaccinium corymbosum*), blackberries (*Rubus villosus*), cherries (*Prunus* app.), grapes (*Vitis vinifera*), hawthorn berries (*Crataegus oxyacantha*), various flowers	Colors are sources of anthocynidins and proanthocynidins; widely cultivated and wild.
Boswellin (*Boswellia serrata*)	Large, branching tree found on dry hilly regions of India.
Cayenne Pepper (*Capsicum frutescens*)	Perennial native to tropical America; widely cultivated.
Coleus forskohlii	Strengthen immune system by stimulating macrophages and lymphocytes. Ancient Hindu and Ayurvedic traditional medicine.
Chinese remedy[257] (Rheumatoid arthritis and rheumatic fever)	Rheumatic fever considered early stages of rheumatoid disease.

	Rheumatoid Fever (*Ma-huang-chia-chu-tang*)	Rheumatoid Arthritis (*Ma-hsing-i-kan-tang*)
	Ma-huang	Ma-Huang
	Apricot seed	Apricot seed
	Licorice	Licorice
	Cinnamon	Coix
	Gypsum	
	Atractylodes (white)	

Herb	Comments
Chinese thoroughwax (*Bupleurum falactum*)	Use root; anti-inflammatory action enhanced by licorice root (*Glycyrrhiza glabra*) and ginseng (*Panex ginseng*).
Devil's Claw (*Harpagophytum procumbens*)	Found in Kalahari Desert, and African Nambian Steppes
Feverfew (*Crysanthenum parthenium*)	Widely cultivated; found wild in waste places along roadsides, wood borders; Quebec to Ohio, Maryland to Missouri, California.
Ginger (*Zingiber officinalis*)	Perennial in tropical Asia and cultivated in tropical areas, especially

Ginseng (*Panax schin-seng, Panax quinquefolius*)	Jamaica. Perennial damp woodlands Manchuria, cultivated in Korea; American ginseng perennial found in wild, rich, cool, woodlands eastern North America. Contains saponins, also called "adaptogens," which can normalize systems; i.e., restore homeostasis.
Kombucha tea (*Bacterium (xylinum/Saccharomyces)*)	From Manchurian mushroom; grows on a liquid; cultivated throughout Europe, Asia, introduced to United States, and other countries after WW II.
Meadowsweet (*Filipendula ulmaria*)	Perennial common to European damp meadows; found in eastern U.S. and Canada, as far west as Ohio.
Myrobalan (*Terminalia chebula*)	Grows in Himalayas, India; Japanese call it haritaki..
Pineapple (*Ananas comosus*)	Widely cultivated; Africa, Pacific Islands.
Prickly Ash	Native North American shrub or tree; found in Canada to Virginia and Nebraska.
Quercetin	White Oak (*Quercus alba*); Onion (*Allium cepa*), Celery (*Apium graveolens*); bee propolis, etc.; bioflavanoid.
Skullcap (*Scutellaria lateriflora*)	North American perennial found in wet places in Canada and northern and eastern U.S.
Tinospora (*Tinospora* app.)	India, China; muscle relaxant, antiinflammatory.
Tumeric Curcumin (*Curcuma longa*)	Widely cultivated Asia, India, China and tropical countries; from bulb and rhizomes.
Willow Bark (*Salix alba, Salix nigra, Salix caprea*)	Tree found in moist places in North America, North Africa, and Asia; also cultivated.
Yucca (*Yucca aborescens*)	Southwestern deserts and Mexico; use all parts of plant; also use Yucca stalk (*Yucca schidigera*) and Yucca plant extract (*Yucca filamentosa*).

Herbs can be very useful for a variety of purposes: strengthen immune system, aid in eliminative processes, vitalize energy and hormones, kill parasites, or other microorganisms that have invaded the body, dampen pain, mucoreglator, and so on. The use of herbs does not necessarily permit one to ignore all of the other important aspects of rheumatoid arthritis treatment.

In addition to allergies, Ventura, California physician and herbalist, Louis J. Marx, M.D., author of *Healing Dimensions of Herbal Medicine*, says that [240] "arthritics can be expected to have other degenerative disorders, such as arteriosclerosis," the clogging up of arteries; and he views the arthritic problem as one of bacterial infections, such as resulting from tuberculosis, various spirochetes -- slender, spiral shaped bacteria -- or "mycoplasmic bacteria," a form of bacteria that usually is without cell walls, and also from other types of microorganism infections. Further, "waste products accumulate in joints, muscles and other soft tissues because the body's eliminative systems are not properly functioning. Good bowel function is important and improved kidney action is helpful. The skin as a major eliminative organ should perspire freely. Lymphatic congestion can be a major issue in both osteoarthritis and rheumatoid arthritis. Other eliminative organs must be evaluated and treated.

Dr. Marx, in full agreement with other alternative medicine practitioners, evalutes poisons that accumulate in the body, the effect of food additives, pesticides, and many other toxic substances, as well as refined flour, sugar, processed foods, and other forms of devitalized foods, saying, "Keep in mind that food and substance intolerance can produce classic arthritis symptoms." Furthermore, "arthritics tend to have poor digestion. Therefore, much of what they eat does not become nutrition, but more toxins in the body. This is probably why symptoms improve when they eat less . . . . It is advisable to eat easy, to digest foods and eat lightly. It is important to remedy the digestive problems. Each sufferer should be evaluated for hydrochloric acid and digestive enzyme deficiencies, also other digestive problems. Thyroid and parathyroid glands should always be checked." (Also see *Wilson's Syndrome*, E. Denis Wilson, M.D.)

David Hoffman, B .Sc., M.N.I.M.H.[3] of Sebastopol, California, and past President of the American Herbalist Guild, describes antiinflammatory and alternative herbs that help to alleviate symptoms of arthritis. "Of the many possible combinations this is a safe mixture that can be taken over a long period of time: combine the tinctures of meadowsweet, willow bark, black cohosh, prickly ash, celery seed, and nettle in equal parts and take one teaspoonful of this mixture three times a day. A "tincture" is the herb steeped in a 25% mixture of alcohol and water.

"In cases of rheumatoid arthritis add wild yam and valerian to the mixture and take one teaspoonful of this mixture three times a day."[3]

Michael T. Murray, N.D., Bellevue, Washington, author of *Arthritis*, and co-author with Joseph Pizzorno, N.D. of *Encyclopedia of Natural Medicine*, recommends Yucca (cactus) and Devil's Claw (*Harpagophytum procumbens*) for its positive anti-inflammatory and analgesic effects: Devil's Claw, dried powdered root, 1 to 2 grams three times daily; 4 to 5 milliliters three times a day of tincture (1:5); or 400 milligrams three times a day of dry solid extract (3:1).[3]

In addition to beneficial effects of bromelain and ginger (*Zingiber officinalis*), Dr. Murray[211] suggests the use of Curcumin (*Curcuma longa*: tumeric) for its powerful antioxidant activity, as well as its ability to enhance the body's natural antioxidant system, the body's own anti-inflammatory mechanisms, and other beneficial effects. "Curcumin is as effective as cortisone or the potent anti-inflammatory drug phenylbutazone in models of accute inflammation. However, while phenylbutzone and cortisone are associated with significant toxicity, curcumin is without side effects," according to Dr. Murray.

Devil's Claw is a plant which is found in the Kalahari Desert and Nambian Steppes of Africa.

Yin Peida and Yang Xiuyan[189] at the Sun Yet Sen University of Medical Science were able to demonstrate objectively that a derivative of Devil's Claw (*Harpagophytum procumben*), Pagosid, had beneficial effects on both osteoarthritis and rheumatoid arthritis. In a parallel study at First Military Medical University, effectiveness was rated at 75% for those with rheumatoid arthritis.[223]

Dr. Siegmund Schmidt has written: Devil's Claw "stimulates the detoxicating and protective mechanisms of the body.... It is remarkable that after treatment has been discontinued, the healing process does not stop, nor is there any reactivation of the inflammatory process, but the healing which has already begun, continues. I have been prescribing *Harpagophytum* root for the past year for my rheumatic patients. It has provided valuable support for the usual rheumatic treatment in more than a hundred patients, and I have even been able to dispense with drugs."

Dr. Christiane Northrup recommends the use of 500 to 3,000 mg of ginger and also cayenne pepper capsules, which has a warming affect on arthritis.[166]

Often recommended herbs by Michael T. Murray, N.D. and Joseph Pizzorno, N.D. reported in *Encyclopedia of Natural Medicine* are licorice, alfalfa, feverfew, tumeric, ginger, skullcap, bupleurum, and ginseng.[3]

Dr. Murray also recommends consuming half a pound of fresh or canned cherries per day. "Cherries, hawthorn berries, blueberries, and other dark red-blue berries are rich sources of compounds that have been found to favorably affect collagen metabolism and prevent and reduce inflammation of joints."[3]

In a study conducted at the Government Medical College in Jammu, India,   nearly 70% of arthritic patients tested experienced good to excellent results against stiffness and pain, using *Boswellia serrata* -- an herbal extract of a large branching tree that grows in dry hilly areas in India.[247]

Boswellia effectively shrinks inflamed tissues, improves the blood supply and promotes the repair of local blood vessels damaged by proliferating inflammation. Such versatility is attributed to a chemical compound in the gummy extract referred to as boswellic acids, which counteract the effects of leukotrienes -- biochemical substances that cause free radical damage -- calcium displacement, autoimmune responses and the movement of inflammation-producing cells to areas of the body already inflammed.

A manchurian mushroom known as "Kombucha," produces a tea known, accordingly, as "Kombucha Tea." Famous in Asia since 221 B.C., testimonials regarding the use of this tea date back to 414 A.D. covering everything from cancer (Nobel prize winner Alexander Solzhenitzyn) and AIDS to indigestion, arthritis, constipation, hemorrhoids, chronic fatigue syndrome, weight problems and hypoglycemia.

The "tea sponge" or "tea fungus" is a jelly-like mass formed of *Bacterium xylinum* and nest-like deposits of yeast cells of the genus *Saccharomyces.*

From the historical description of its effects on animal and plant organisms, including the human, Kombucha Tea must be a combination of powerful substances that restore the body's normal balance (adaptogen) and strong anti-oxidant.

The knowledge of how to home-make Kombucha Tea was preserved by Dr. Sklenar who kept cultures of the tea alive during the post World War II years in Germany, altthough this same tea has historical precedence in the Orient and throughout Russia and related states.

According to Debbie Carson,[162] author of "Kobucha Tea" (*Trans Summer* 94, p. 14) "The fungus culture is a symbiotic colony of yeast and bacteria which resembles a rubbery gelatinous pancake in appearance. It's function as a living culture is comparable to that of the agent that creates vinegar in cider or wine. Unlike genuine ferments, these cultures do not produce spores, but multiply exclusively by fusion and budding. This process enables Kombucha's active enzymes to attach to over 200 different bacteria in the human body, thus making Kombucha a helpful therapy for people who suffer from candidiasis," which most likely includes the majority of arthritics.

The fungus is placed in a tea base where complicated biochemical processes take place. "Fermentation produces a small amount of alcohol (0.5%), carbon dioxide, B vitamins, Vitamin C and various organic acids that are essential to human metabolism." Its most important products are said to be glucuronic acid and polysaccharides.

The glucouronic acid has the property of bonding to harmful substances in the body, rendering over 200 substances harmless, and also helping to "form connective tissues, cartilage, gastric mucous membranes and the vitreous body of the eye."

The polysaccharides "strengthen the body's immunity responses to pathogenic bacteria, yeasts, viruses, and increases the body's resistance to these diseases." The culture can be ordered from Laurel Farms, 13470 Washington Boulevard, Penthouse, Venice, California 90292; (310) 289-4372.

There are many possible and interesting variations on how to make Kombucha Tea, but the newcomer is advised to follow one that is known to work before experimenting:

Growth media black tea and brown sugar are preferred, and there are many who can advise on the best recipes for home-made usage.

Elizabeth Baker,[162] author of *The Uncook Book*, and several others, reports that those who work with the tea suggest taking 5 ounces or less before breakfast, or after lunch and dinner. Eventually this may be increased to a full glass, and sometimes even a liter per day.

E.W. McDonagh, D.O., a Kansas City osteopath, "has reported success among hundreds of patients suffering from a variety of advanced muscular and skeletal conditions for whom other treatments had failed to help. . . . [the} pain was significantly reduced -- or even vanished -- in two to four weeks' time. All patients were able to eliminate other medication or reduce the dosages significantly.

"Among McDonagh's patients . . . were individuals with arthritis, muscle pain of all types, degenerative joint disease following traumatic injuries, muscle wasting and loss of function, knee, foot and ankle disease and low back pain with radiation down the leg."[180]

Paul Stamets, a mycologist in Olympia, Washington, says that he has ten Kombuchas fermenting with what he calls 'the kind of benign neglect that most people are prone to,' and several of them are currently contaminated with a brilliant yellow mold of the genus *Asperguillus*, some of whose members are carcinogenic and highly poisonous. Paul Stamets also says that there is great danger in contamination, both airborne and hand-transmitted, and the potential liabilities are too great to sell the substance.

Andrew Weil, M.D., a holistic physician, who teaches at the University of Arizona College of Medicine, warns about the long-term use of Kombucha Tea, in that it contains antibiotics, a class of drugs that can help to increase antibiotic resistant germs.[179]

Prof. L.T. Danielova, whose 40-years of research on the tea fungus, states that the quality and quantity of its antibiotic properties are absolutely harmless.

Leading mycologist Prof. Rieth says that "Home preparation of Kombucha is perfectly safe. There is absolutely no risk in drinking Kombucha."

The German Bundesgesundheitsamt (comparable to our FDA) has declared, "Kombucha is not injurious to the health."[180]

The lesson to be learned is that one must be very careful how the tea is produced and preserved.

On the brighter side, millions of people have historically (more than 2,000 years) raised and drunk their own Kombucha Tea without ill effects; indeed, most have had beneficial effects.

If rheumatoid diseases, including rheumatoid arthritis, are caused by a tissue sensitivity to the toxins or protein products of microorganisms, as many believe or have demonstrated, or an amoebae, as Roger Wyburn-Mason, M.D., Ph.D. believed when he developed the first consistently successful treatment for its cure, or a mycoplasm, according to research of Thomas McPherson Brown, M.D., a herbal approach to killing or controlling microorganisms may be well worth pursuing.

Before the introduction of antibiotics into modern medicine, herbal substances were relied upon as anti-infective agents. In some places around the world these herbal substances are still widely used; indeed, there are more people using herbal medicines than any other form of medicine, considering the Chinese and Indian populations.

Reported by *The American Journal of Natural Medicine*, is a study which compared metronidazole (Flagyl) against a herbal formulation. Metronidazole is one of the Arthrititis Trust of America's (The Rheumatoid Disease Foundation's) recommended prescription drugs. Dried and pulverized plants were extracted in ethanol together and individually, and the herbal formula was *Berberis aristata, Boerhavia diffusa, Tinospora cordifolia, Terminalia chebula* and *Zingiber officinale*.[184]

In experimental caecal amebiasis (amoebic infection of the caecal tract) in rats, this well-known Ayurvedic medicine traditional in India had a curative rate of 89% with the average degree of infection reduced to 0.4 in a group dosed with 500 mg/kg per day.

The placebo group had an average degree of infection of 3.8.

Metronidazole had a cure rate of 89% at a dose of 100 mg/kg per day -- an average degree of infection of 0.4 -- and cured the infection completely when the dose was doubled to 200 mg/kg per day.

So far as amoebic infection of the caecal tract, the herbal formula was equally effective as the metronidazole without the toxic side effects.

Also reported by the *American Journal of Natural Medicine*[242] is the beneficial use of quercetin, "often referred to as the most active bioflavonoid as it typically exerts the greatest effect when compared to other bioflavonoids in experimental studies.

"Quercetin is widely distributed in the vegetable kingdom, especially in barks and rinds. Many medicinal plants owe much of their activity to their high quercetin content (e.g., *Quercus alba, Allium cepa, Apium graveolens*, propolis, etc.)

"Quercetin has been shown to exert significant anti-allergy and an anti-inflammatory activity," which "appears to be due to direct inhibition of several steps in the initial processes of inflammation. . . . and the cascade of effects that are often a result of these processes."[242]

Donald J. Brown, N.D.,[229] in *Herbal Prescriptions for Better Health,* recommends Siberian ginseng (Eleuthero) as a "standardized, concentratred extract of the root and rhizomes, 300 to 400 milligrams daily; dry, powdered root and rhizomes, 2 to 3 grams daily in two or three divided doses. Alcohol-based extract, 8 to 10 ml in two to three divided doses. Use continuously for 4 to 6 weeks with a 1- to 2-week break before resuming." Dr. Brown adds, "This one probably comes as a bit of a surprise. However, the immune system balance and adrenal support offered by eleuthero are important factors in any autoimmune disease."[229]

Other herbal considerations offered by Dr. Brown are: Ginger rhizome powder, 2 to 3 grams daily; Devil's Claw root (*Harpagophytum procumbens*) 3 to 4 grams 3 times daily; Yucca stalk (*Yucca schidigera*), 1 to 2 grams 3 times daily.[229]

Osteopathic surgeon, Robert Bingham, M.D. advocated use of a traditional American Indian remedy, Yucca plant extract, (*Yucca filamentosa*) for his arthritic patients. Dr. Bingham wrote in *Fighting Back Against Arthritis*, that "Strong evidence supports the theory that some forms of arthritis may be caused or worsened by toxic substances occurring in the intestines and absorbed by the body. Yucca seems to inhibit these harmful intestinal bacteria and at the same time help the natural and normal forms of bacteria found in the tract. Most patients who report a reduction of joint swelling and stiffness also suffer gastrointestinal disturbances associated with arthritis. These are gradually corrected by yucca treatment.

"Recent chemical research has shown that the therapeutic agent from yucca is a food supplement containing a high concentration of a vegetable steroid and a saponin. Saponin, a safe and natural form of steroid, appears to be harmless to humans and, through its actions in the intestinal tract, is in fact therapeutic. . . . it does improve circulation and reduces abnormal fat content of blood," and lowers blood pressure.

As many diseases from migraine to arthritis can stem from allergenic response to toxic substances derived from harmful colon bacteria, "an anti-stress agent such as yucca saponin introduced into the colon might have the same beneficial effect on wastes in the body and be effective in treating arthritis by improving and protecting the intestinal ["good-guys"] flora rather than any direct action upon arthritis."[203]

In a double-blind study performed throughout a 12-month period, Dr. Bingham divided 165 patients into two approximately equal groups, one half receiving yucca tablets (300 mg extract daily) and the other half receiving a placebo. Patients included those with osteoarthritis (97) and rheumatoid arthritis (68). Less than a fourth of the placebo group reported some benefit, whereas nearly half of the yucca group made the same claim. More than 60% reported overall relief of typical arthritis symptoms such as swelling, pain and stiffness. Additional improvements in circulation, skin and hair, and relief from chronic headaches were also seen.[203]

Michael T. Murray, N.D. Natural Treatment for Arthritis

Dr. Murray[211] recommends the following for achieving wellness from rheumatoid arthritis as well as for other "autoimmune" diseases such as ankylosing spondylitis, systemic lupus erythematosus, and progessive systemic sclerosis:

* Elimination diet
* Elimination of all animal products from diet except cold-water fish. Consume rich plant foods.
* Drink 16 to 24 ounces of fresh fruit and vegetable juice each day; include 1/4" to 1/2" slice of fresh ginger in juice each day.
* Use 1 to 2 tablespoons flaxseed oil each day.
* Determine if hydrochloric acid supplementation is required.
* Use 10X pancreatic enzyme at 500 to 1,000 mg three times a day 10 to 20 minutes before meals.
* Use high potency multiple vitamin and mineral supplement providing specific levels of vitamin E (200-400 IU), selenium (50-200 mcg), zinc (30-45 gm) and manganese (5-15 mg), along with 1,000 to 3,000 mg of vitamin C daily in divided dosages.
* Use physical therapy.
* Use curcumin and bromelain at 400 to 600 mg three times daily.
* If patient has been taking corticosteroids for more than three months in the past, use a herbal formula that supports the adrenal glands.
* If there is significant secondary osteoarthritis, use 500 mg of glucosamine sulfate three times daily. (See this chapter, "Allergies, Biodetoxification, and Chemical Sensitivities," "Diet and Supplements," . Also see Michael T. Murray, N.D., *Arthritis*, Prima Publishing, PO Box 1260BK, Rocklin, California 95677.)

Chiropractic Nutritional Support

Paul A. Goldberg, M.P.H., D.C.,[205] is Professor of Clinical Nutrition, Gastroenterology, and Rheumatology at Life College in Marietta, Georgia. He operates also The Goldberg Clinic in Marietta, Georgia.

Dr. Goldberg writes, that, "Rheumatic disease cases frequently originate from disturbed gastrointestinal dysfunction. When the integrity of the gastrointestinal tract is restored giving attention to intestinal integrity, maldigestion, allergy, diet, and related immunological factors, rheumatic diseases and the stiffness, pain and swelling that accompany them disappear and good health returns."

The Case of Jenny Simpson

Jenny Simpson, 43-years-of-age, complained of fatigue, severe joint pain and swelling with generalized stiffness in many areas, including knees, ankles, wrists and low back, with frequent and moderate indigestion.

Jenny had been under medical care for 8 years and was prescribed steroids, anti-inflammatory drugs, gold and methotrexate. These had resulted in a number of side effects including liver inflammation, gastric bleeding, and fascial swelling. Jenny only got worse.

Although she'd received numerous Chiropractic adjustments, they'd given her partial, temporary relief only. As Jenny's condition was deteriorating, she was naturally anxious.

Laboratory studies revealed intestinal permeability, food allergies, abnormal sedimentation rate (the rate at which blood cells sink in a sample of blood, considered a crude measure of infection or inflammatory activity), mineral toxicities, and a "leaky gut."

Dr. Goldberg placed Jenny on a detoxification program followed by a rotation diet, with reduced carbohydrates of all kinds. A regimen was followed to reduce gut permeability, and appropriate nutrient supplementation was also given.

The first two weeks were difficult for Jenny, with an exacerbation of symptoms. During the third week she noted improvement with reduced joint pain and improved vitality. By the fifth week all joint swelling, redness and stiffness dissipated and Jenny was able to take long walks with her husband. (See this chapter, "Allergies, Detoxification, and Chemical Sensitivities.")

The sedimentation rate dropped to normal, and a follow-up of intestinal permeability showed it to be within normal limits.

Follow-up 2 years later found Jenny to be healthy and symptom free as long as she continues her diet, obtains adequate rest and observes other important hygienic factors.

In a letter to Dr. Goldberg, Jenny Simpson[205] reported that she was a new person, and that   fatigue was gone, and also joint pain 90% of the time, the remaining pain being very mild and temporary.

Her rheumatologist declared her improvement as merely coincidence, that diet, good digestion, nutrients, allergies, etc. have nothing to do with arthritis.

"He's a fool," Jenny said. I was sick with arthritis for over 8 years. I was under the rheumatologist's care for over seven of them during which time I only got sicker and more deformed. I only felt bad and worse, never any real signs of improvement while under him while being poisoned with all the damn steroids and methotrexate and gold. Now I'm consistently well for over 6 months and he says, 'It's just a coincidence.' He cannot admit that he failed where you succeeded. What pride!!!

"You know what else? I never saw any of his patients get real improvement nor any of my friends who have serious arthritis get any better under traditional medical care . . . they just go suffering and taking drugs and suffering and get worse and worse!"

The Case of Gloria Pagnotta

Gloria Pagnotta, 40-years-of-age, complained of ulcerative colitis of 18 years duration accompanied by severe arthritic pain and stiffness in hands, elbows, shoulders and knees. She also complained of chronic fatigue, ongoing bloody diarrhea, and depression, and described her condition as "desperate."

Prior care under a gastroenterologist resulted in removal of fifty percent of her colon. A rheumatologist had Gloria on steroidal drugs.

Gloria had also received care from a chiropractor for 2 years for persistent low back pain.

The patient was tested for intestinal permeability (elevated), mineral imbalances (general depletion), and food allergies (positive). Egg, wheat, and dairy products -- Gloria's major sources of allergies -- were the same foods recommended to her by her gastroenterologist and medical dietitian to "sooth the colon."

Chiropractic subluxations of the low back would not hold.

Dr. Goldberg placed Gloria on a hypoallergenic liquid diet for a period of ten days followed by a diet of cooked vegetable foods and moderate amounts of proteins excluding all allergens. Gloria was instructed on hygienic measures, and given advice for rest, sleep, fresh air, and emotional poise. She was also advised to reduce the amount of corticosteroid prescribed for colitis and arthritis.

During the first two weeks Gloria went through a stormy period of discomfort. By the 8th day her bowels began to quiet. Joint pain subsided by the 6th week accompanied by an increase in energy level. In 3 months Gloria's stools were formed without blood and joint pains had been reduced by 80%.

In her fourth month Gloria went off of her health plan and ate a variety of foods she had been warned to avoid. Within 10 days she was again passing bloody stools and experiencing severe joint/muscle pain. When she was placed back on track, she began feeling well again. "I've learned my lesson," she commented.

Paul Goldberg, D.C., M.P.H. reports that "It is common to see patients with medical diagnoses of Crohns disease and ulcerative colitis report that they also have rheumatoid arthritis, fibromyositis, etc. These patients frequently have poor digestion and allergic problems. Medical care including corticosteroids, anti-inflammatory drugs (NSAIDS), and surgery serve to aggravate and complicate the clinical picture. Resolution of the patient's digestive dysfunction frequently results in ending of the bowel problems and rheumatic complaints simultaneously."

The Case of Annie Mae Davidson

Annie Mae Davidson, 45-year-old female, and wife of a Doctor of Chiropractic, had rheumatoid arthritis for over 14 years. When she came to Dr. Goldberg the arthritis was getting worse. Her hands, shoulders, knees, and ankles were painful with much redness and swelling. A rheumatologist had placed her on prednisone and methotrexate which had produced side effects including liver inflammation from the methotrexate and dependency on corticosteroids.

Annie Mae also tried various herbal remedies, colonics, Chiropractic, homeopathics and acupuncture, none of which had provided her with lasting relief.

Laboratory tests indicated that her sedimentation rate was abnormally high, that she was anemic with elevated liver enzymes due to the methotrexate usage, and that there were mutliple food allergies. Stool cultures exhibited abnormal bacterial flora. Dietary analysis showed excessive carbohydrate intake and low B complex intake. Heavy metal indices were elevated.

Annie Mae was placed on a reduced carbohydrate diet with ample amounts of steamed non-starchy vegetables, along with free-form amino acids. After 4 weeks she was placed on a liquid diet for a period of 8 days. This was later repeated.

Food allergens were removed from her diet. Sources of heavy metals were identified and steps taken to remove them from her system. Individualized stretching and deep breathing exercises were utilized, and careful attention was given to hygienic factors such as sleep and rest.

During her first 3 weeks of detoxification, Annie Mae had exacerbated symptoms and increased fatigue. By the fifth week her sedimentation rate dropped, and she experienced a dramatic reduction in pain and stiffness.

Four years later her sedimentation rate is normal, energy level high, and she engages in swimming, walking and gardening regularly, without pain in her knees, shoulders, or ankles, and with only occasional mild stiffness in her hands.

Homeopathy

Luc De Schepper, M.D., Ph.D., Lic.Ac., D.I. Hom. writes, "Homeopathy has proven its merits for nearly two hundred years in all parts of the world and in all classes of people, rich and poor, literate and illiterate. Cancer and auto-immune disorders [such as rheumatoid arthritis] have increased dramatically over the past 20 years; most of it can be attributed to changes in lifestyles and new powerful drugs that are suppressive in nature. Homeopathy, regardless of all the new medical discoveries of recent years, still remains the most scientific method of cure known to suffering humanity. It is safe, gentle, sure, inexpensive and fairly rapid without producing additional drug pictures."[244]

As has already been stated in the chapter on osteoarthritis, homeopathic remedies used for treatment of any particular disorder depends upon the person's personality, constitution and physical condition. In general, homeopathy strengthens the immune system and decreases the pain threshold.[94]

Many success stories, with every form of disease, including rheumatoid arthritis, have been reported through the use of homeopathy.

According to Dr. Andrew Lockie, author of *The Family Guide to Homeopathy*, a study "was conducted in 1980 by Gibson and colleagues, in Glasgow. It compared homeopathic treatment of rheumatoid arthritis with orthodox treatment by the drug aspirin. The results showed that the improvement rate was higher among the former group. However, a combination of aspirin and homeopathic remedies was even more effective."[164]

According to Corazon Ilarina, M.D.,[14] of the Bio Medical Health Center, in Reno, Nevada, recommended homeopathic remedies are *Traumeel, Belladonna, Injul Farte arsemium, Album injul, Hepeel, Injul-Chal, Phosphor injul* and *Lachesis*. She reports that "*Traumeel* and *Zeel* ointments are very good for swelling and inflammation when applied topically on affected joints."[14]

Dr. Ilarina also encourages the body to rid itself of disease-producing toxins that reside in cartilage and joints by means of homeopathic remedies, describing the process as "homotoxicology."

Dr. Catherine Russell,[233] Guadalajara, Mexico, uses blood tests for the anti-streptococcus lysome produced by the body when the streptococcus germ has invaded. If the anti-streptococcus lysome measure is high, she'll administer the homeopathic remedy Streptococcus 200 X, 1time per week. She reports that "Streptococcus usually starts in the tonsils, then, after becoming chronic in the throat area, starts infiltrating in the joints. On starting the homeopathic treatment there is usually an aggravation in the joints, and the tonsils become inflamed again. The worse thing that can be done at this point is to give antibiotics which suppresses the removal of the bacteria. (See this chapter, "The Herxheimer Reaction: The Jarisch-Herxheimer Effect.")

"One must give supportive treatment to get through this throat crises. After that, the joint pain decreases, the throat crises is resolved.

"Usually 8 or 12 doses of this medicine will see the patient through the crisis. Patients definitely start getting better.

"I also use the streptococcus nosodes (homeopathic solutions whose dilutions are based on the germ) for patients with rheumatic fever."

Dr. Russell may also use The Arthritis Trust of America (The Rheumatoid Disease Foundation) treatment, starting with tinidizole (Tinidex or Fasigyn), which is easily available in Mexico over the counter. She reports that she always sees a Herxheimer reaction. (See this chapter, "The Arthritis Trust of America Treatment Protocol: Anti-Microorganism Treatment.")

Hydrotherapy

The use of water, ice, steam, and hot and cold temperatures is called "hydrotherapy," methods of maintaining and restoring health that are as old as civilization, and found in virtually every society.

Today many health practitioners prescribe baths, colonic irrigations, douches, sitz baths, jacuzzis, steam, saunas, mineral tubs, wraps, rubs, flushes, fasts, enemas, and compresses.

Applications of hot or cold water, taken internally or externally, can be effective for stress, pain, elimination of toxins, bacteria, viruses and for many other conditions.

One of the chief causes for rheumatoid arthritis, as well as other forms of arthritis, may be a tissue sensitivity to microorganisms. Whether this is the cause or not rheumatoid arthritis is also accompanied by poorly drained antigen/antibody complexes, as well as free radicals, those chemically hyperactive molecules that combine with and destroy normal functioning tissues. For these two reasons, if for no others, certain forms of hydrotherapy may be beneficial. Caution must be observed, however, that methods used do not also spread distribution and activity of microorganisms that provide the basis for rheumatoid disease.

Factors that Influence Healing

According to Agatha Thrash, M.D. and Calvin Thrash, M.D., Seale, Alabama, authors of *Home Remedies*, primary factors that influence the rate of healing are: (1) the number of white cells circulating in the blood stream; (2) the rate at which each white cell travels to its prey; (3) the "interest" white cells have in consuming particular germs; (4) the white cell's ability to kill the germs; (5) the nature of the immune system, strong or weak; (6) general health, and various other factors.

Doctors Thrash and Thrash write, "The rapidity with which the phagocytes, the 'eating cells', travel to an infection, as well as the liberation of enzymes at the site of infection are prime defense mechanisms."[201] For every $10°$ Fahrenheit temperature rise of the body, the velocity of chemical reaction, thus phagocytic activity, is approximately doubled or tripled. In rather extensive studies investigators found that white blood cell counts rose from 6,800 to 13,200, and in another study from 7,125 to 11,269, when temperature was sustained for five hours at $105°$ to $106°$ Fahrenheit.

The skin contains about 11,000 square feet of ducts of the sweat glands, and will carry away about 98% water and 2% solids, whereas urine carries away 96% water and 4% solids. The skin, therefore, is a very important organ for elimination of toxins.

Hot, Cold and Contrast Hydrotherapies

Hot Water Hydrotherapy: According to Douglas Lewis, N.D.,[3] Chairperson of Physical Medicine at the Bastyr College Natural Health Clinic, Seattle, Washington, hot water hydrotherapy stimulates the immune system and "causes white cells to migrate out of the blood vessels and into the tissue where they clean up toxins and assist the body in eliminating wastes."

Therapeutic hot water soothes, relaxes, and through reflex action of the nervous system, can affect every organ and system in the body. By increasing blood in one area through dilation of blood vessels, compensatory blood reduction occurs in another area. Drs. Thrash and Thrash believe this fact explains the pain relief given by applying heat to an arthritic joint or over a congested nerve or muscle. "As the blood vessels in the inflamed area contract, the tension in the tissues is relieved, and pain abates."

Since hot applications lower alkalinity of tissues, and the arthritic is more than likely too acidic at the start, it is always wise to end a hot application with a cold application, which will help to restore alkaliity of the blood.

Cold Water Hydrotherapy: Cold water constricts blood vessels, thus making them less permeable, and preventing inflammatory agents from passing through into tissues, such as joint cartilage. Muscles are also toned up. According to Dr. Lewis, short cold water treatments may increase fever while long cold water treatments may pull heat away from the body for fever reduction.

Cold packs have been cited as the fastest means to relieve pain and reduce inflammatory swelling, or edema.

Contrast Hot and Cold Water Hydrotherapy: Contrast hot and cold water treatment alternates between the two. "They can stimulate the adrenal and endocrine glands, reduce congestion, alleviate inflammation, and activate organ function."[3]

Agatha Thrash, M.D. and Calvin Thrash, M.D. describe contrast baths which are used for rheumatoid arthritis with "considerable relief, ... The temperatures recommended have been 50^0 to 65^0 Fahrenheit (10^0 to 18^0 C) for cold water and 99^0 to 110^0 Fahrenheit (37.8^0 to 43.3^0C) for the hot. Alternation in the temperature increases circulation to the joint.

"For advanced and crippling arthritis, the continuous or hammock bath rigged with clamps in constantly flowing water offers much relief. The water should be about 98^0 Fahrenheit, and the room somewhat warm. Continue the bath for 2 hours, five or six days a week. It is remarkable how quickly patients feel relief. Usually they are enabled to stop their medications after the second or third bath. One patient walked again after the tenth bath, which he had been unable to do for three years."[201] (See Agatha Thrash, M.D., Calvin Thrash, M.D., *Home Remedies*; Chapter I, Osteoarthritis, "Hydrotherapy," "Environmental Medicine.")

Balneotherapy and Physical Exercise: Until those suffering from rheumatoid arthritis, and other rheumatoid diseases have become well, Roger Wyburn-Mason, M.D., Ph.D.[6,7,8,9] -- the English doctor who developed the first consistently effective treatment for rheumatoid arthritis -- cautioned against use of exercise because he felt it could spread faster the organism(s) causing the disease, although some exercise is necessary for maintenance of a healthy metabolism.

One type of physical therapy in addition to massage that has proven to be beneficial   is balneotherapy, the use of mineral baths and mud packs.

In Europe, mineral baths and mud packs are a form of physical therapy often recommended for rheumatoid arthritis. Studies have shown that sulfur and mud pack therapy alone or in combination are effective in reducing inflammation and pain during an arthritic "flare-up."

Spa therapy usually consists of mud packs, sulfur packs and bathing in the Dead Sea.

A recent study was conducted in Israel along the Western shore of the Dead Sea at the Ein Gedi Spa, where there are many hot, thermal-mineral springs in large natural concentrations of mud, as well as high barometric pressures, low humidity, high temperatures, low rainfall, and absence of air pollution. Patients were divided into four groups - - Group I, daily baths in the Dead sea, Group II, sulfur baths, Group III, a combination of daily Dead Sea bathing and sulfur baths. Group 4, non-baths, served as a control group.

All patients were evaluated by a rheumatologist under standard double-blind procedures.

Statistically significant improvement was seen only in the first three "treatment" groups, lasting up to three months reduction in pain and inflammation.[157]

Dr. Herbert, New Zealand government balneologist, or specialist on spa water treatment, "recommended certain pools as beneficial for arthritis. All of these had a high boron content, but he did not know what the reasons for their curative properties were." According to Rex E. Newnham, N.D., D.O., Ph.D.[28] it's the high boron content of the water absorbed both by skin when bathing, and also when people drank some of the water while staying at the spa.

Iron Overload Therapy

There are few natural means whereby blood is lost: bleeding and menstruation being the two most common. For this reason, iron tends to accumulate especially based on our diet of fortified foods and red meat.

The condition of excessive iron is more frequent than generally known. This is one area where a knowledgable physician is required to make an accurate determination if iron overload is present. Few doctors are performing all the correct tests.

• Your doctor is most likely to give you the serum (blood) iron test. If the values, as compared against the laboratory's standards, are below a given range, a faulty conclusion may be reached of iron anemia, and your doctor may prescribe more iron, which is exactly what is not needed. A deficiency in B_6, pyridoxine, for example, can increase iron absorption. Adeena Robinson,[264] a former victim of iron overload reports in *Iron-A Double Edged Sword*, that many anemic people are overloaded with iron.

Serum iron measures only the iron present in the bloodstream, and not that iron which is in storage.

The serum ferritin test may present a more accurate picture of iron in storage in tissues. The size of serum ferritin standard required to suspect an iron overload has been steadily decreasing over the past years, but not all laboratories are keeping pace with this reduction.

If your laboratory reports that you are *iron depeleted*, this is not at all the same thing as *iron deficient* -- so don't permit your doctor to jump to the hasty conclusion that you need more iron.

To answer the question as to how much iron you are absorbing, take the transferrin saturation blood test. "In the past, the upper limit of normal was believed to be around 55%. Recently, however, investigators have shown that the risk of developing iron related illness begins to increase when transferrin saturation rises above 30%. Values below 15% may be suggestive of iron deficiency, but only when other tests are indicative of low iron. . . . . transferrin saturation levels tend to decrease during infections, inflammations, and other chronic illnesses, even when there is no other evidence of iron deficiency anemia."

If your doctor checks your homoglobin level, slighly low does not always indicate iron deficiency anemia, "and most people, even if they are iron deficient, will not show any symptoms until levels fall to around 9 g/L." When this occurs Robinson advises that the above tests also be made, as well as hematocrit and red cell count.

As blood tests, themselves, do not always tell the story, there may be other required tests to make a satisfactory determination. The caring physician will refer to various research papers presented by Adeena Robinson in her *Iron-A Double Edged Sword*.

If an iron overload condtion is determined, two general routes may usually be employed to reduce iron levels: phlebotomy, e.g. the removal of blood, such as donating blood to a worthy cause until iron levels have been reduced to a safe point; or, intravenous chelating out of excess iron through use of a chelating agent, such as deferroxamine. (See Chapter I, Osteoarthritis, "Chelation Therapy.")

Magnetic Therapy

According to Wolfgang Ludwig, D.Sc., Ph.D., Director of Biophysics in Horb, Germany, "Magnetic field therapy is a method that penetrates the whole human body and can treat every organ without chemical side effects. Magnetic field therapy has been used effectively in the treatment of: cancer, rheumatoid disease, infections and inflammations, headaches and migraines, insomnia and sleep disorders, circulatory problems, fractures, pain, and environmental stress."[3]

Richard A. Kunin, M.D., San Francisco, California writes, that "Within minutes of placing a north pole magnet over an arthritis hot spot, pain and inflammation commence to improve."[129]

"In 1974, researcher Albert Roy Davis, Ph.D., noted that positive and negative magnetic polarities have different effects upon the biological systems of animals and humans. He found that magnets could be used to arrest and kill cancer cells in animals, and could also be used in the treatment of arthitis, glaucoma, infertility, and diseases related to aging."[3]

Robert Becker, M.D., an orthopedic surgeon, discovered that weak electric currents can heal bones, and he also brought to national attention the fact that long-distance power-line grids can produce undesirable magnetic influences on people who live under or near such transmission zones.

William H. Philpott, M.D. of Oklahoma City, Oklahoma, [218] developed numerous medical treatment protocols using magnetics.[111] (See Chapter 1: Osteoarthritis, "Energy Medicine.")

For various degenerative diseases, including rheumatoid arthritis, Dr. Philpott suggests sleeping on a negative poled magnetic bed pad with magnets at the crown of the head. The magnetic bed is composed of 1-7/8" X 7/8" X 3/8" mini-block magnets which are 3,950 gauss strength, and placed 1-1/2" apart throughout the mattress bed pad. "An egg crate foam pad should be placed over the mattress pad or the mattress pad could be placed under the mattress.

"The sleeper system at the crown of the head is composed of four 5,000 gauss 4" X 6" X 1" magnets placed 3/4" apart in a wooden carrier held firmly against the headboard. The magnets may be raised or lowered depending on the height of the pillow. The magnets rest on a wooden dowel, which should be slightly below the back of the head. It's important that the head be in this 6" X 19" negative magnetic field. The top of the head should be no closer than 3" from the magnets. This provides a full magnetic field.

"A 5" X 6" X 1/8" multi-magnet flexible mat should be placed over the heart. It's well to have this both day and night. This will have the effect of magnetically treating the oxygen and water flowing through the heart."

The authors have known patients who've purchased magnetic mattresses, chairs, pillows, and so forth from vendors who apparently have no idea that area coverage and polarity is all important, or that gauss strength can make a huge difference in outcome.

One group of ladies had purchased mattresses resulting in exposure to both positive and negative polarities simultaneously, which, of course, is not the proper way to use magnets. These mattresses (or pads) should be taken apart, the magnet's polarities determined by a low-cost standard magnet furnished by Dr. Philpott, and then all of the magnets directed with the same polarities facing the same direction. The magnet's negative side (according to Philpott's standard) should then be exposed to the body, not the positive side. (Contact William H. Philpott, M.D., 17171 SE 29th Street, Choctaw, OK 73020.)

Massage Therapy

Ida P. Rolf, Ph.D.[245] was diagnosed as having rheumatoid arthritis. She did not accept the idea that her condition was incurable, and she concluded that in her case, and probably in other cases, there was a mis-evaluation of the disease condition. Through brilliant application of her own knowledge and insight she developed a new form of massage that addresses itself to "sticking fascia."

Fascia belongs to a family of related connective tissues which holds the body together and gives it shape. It surrounds all organs and, when healthy, is slightly elastic with a strong resistance to stretching. It can break or tear.

Because of Dr. Rolf's success in ridding herself of what appeared to be rheumatoid arthritis and successes with other bodily conditions -- all through her specially designed massage technique -- now there exists a Rolfing Institute to pass along her methods to students interested in applying this kind of massage. The massage technique is known, quite properly, as "Rolfing." (Information can be obtained from Rolf Institute, PO Box 1868, Boulder, CO 80306.)

Slack strands of fascia can adhere to one another forming adhesions. These adhesions shorten the fascial structure, thus also compressing, or shortening the organs and tissues which it surrounds. Shortening the muscles pulls in the skeletal framework, including tendons and ligaments, causing the body to be mis-aligned. A puckering up of external tissues based on mis-alignment of adhering fascia can be observed after surgery, as the effect of poor posture, or even from chronic emotional patterns. See Chapter 1: Osteoarthritis, "Structure.")

Often adjacent fascial structures adhere to one another and bind two structures together. Muscle groups are surrounded by fascia. As two muscle groups are intended to glide over one another, they can become yoked together, neither muscle functioning efficiently.

Fascia can even adhere to itself and change shape causing the fascial network to become distorted.

Using Rolfing massages, the practitioner can relcase these adhesions, permitting the structure to return to its natural state, straightening skeletal structure, and restoring the use of energy otherwise bound up in resistance of one muscle against another.

Dr. Rolf has taught that all muscles and ligaments that weave or support ball-and-socket joint structures, as with muscles and bones, are all proper parts of the operating joint structure. When there is trouble in one component, this is often construed to be a "joint" problem, meaning some form of "arthritis," or unrecoverable disease condition.

True arthritis, however, is deterioration of the joint characterized by chemical changes in blood and joint tissues.

"Arthritic pain is the result of joint compression. Not all cases of true arthritis are painful; where there is adequate capsular space, the individual may well be pain-free."

Your joint condition may be a pseudo-arthritis, a disorder of tendons, ligaments, or fascia. (Also see Chapter 1, Osteoarthritis, "Neural and Reconstructive Therapy.")

Rolfing, through restoration of fascial integrity, restores natural posture which, for the arthritic and pseudo-arthritic alike, means more freedom of movement and lessened pain, and also improvement of metabolism, circulation, neural transmission, joint and tissue repair, emotional stability, and, generally, an overall increase in available energy that was otherwise bound up in maintaining the poor muscular imbalances.

Zhenya Kurashova Wine,[121] a well known Russian sports massage therapist, reports on her techniques in *Massage*, cautioning that while arthritis falls under the masseur's general indications and contraindications for massage, "we cannot touch the area that is hot, or the body if it's running a temperature. We can work on the muscles surrounding the joint, but should stay at least two inches away from the joint. Massage increases inflammation if done at an inappropriate time, and will cause the condition to worsen."

If massage is desired during the inflammatory state, the masseur can do effleurage (deep or gentle stroking), light friction, and vibration on the surrounding tissue but not near the joint.

"After the inflammation has decreased you may start including the joint in your massage, spending one-third of the time on the joint, and two-thirds of the time massaging the tissue around it. Increase the time spent massaging the joint to seven-eighths of the massage by the seventh or eighth treatment."[121]

Photophoresis and Oxygen Therapies:
Hydrogen Peroxide Therapy and Ozone Therapy

Many forms of rheumatoid disease, including rheumatoid arthritis, are the result of internal tissue sensitivity to the toxins or dead protein products of invasive micro-organisms. Ozone Therapy, Hydrogen Peroxide Therapy, and Photophoresis assists the body to kill off these micro-organisms resulting in improvement and often cure of the arthritis.

Hydrogen peroxide and ozone therapies are often referred to as "Oxygen Therapies," which is somewhat of a misnomer. According to research performed by Charles H. Farr, M.D., Ph.D., one can take a breath of air and receive more additional oxygen than one can receive from hydrogen peroxide therapy or ozone therapy.[101] Although their complete biological functions are not thoroughly understood, these two therapies clearly do not supply significant additional oxygen.

Chemical reactions where electrons are transferred from one molecule to another are referred to as "oxidation/reduction reactions."

As oxygen molecules are frequently involved, the "loss of electron," reactions are called "oxidation." Donor molecules are said to be "oxidized."

Molecules that gain electrons are oxidants, like iron rust. Removing rust to form iron again is called "reduction."

Chemical reactions of the body lose electrons and gain them again in a finely tuned balance. Too much oxidation can be harmful; too much reduction can be harmful. Repeated nutritional and environmental stresses -- including toxicity from micro-organisms -- overburden oxidative functions. The proper oxidative processes, such as hydrogen peroxide or ozone therapy can give immediate assistance, permitting the body to restore its balance.

Hydrogen Peroxide Therapy

Hydrogen peroxide[104,105] is a clear, colorless liquid that easily mixes with water. Where water consists of two parts hydrogen to one part oxygen, or H_2O, hydrogen peroxide consists of two parts hydrogen to two parts oxygen, or H_2O_2. The extra oxygen atom is easily dislodged to combine with other substances. Heavy concentrations of hydrogen peroxide can be damaging to tissue, whereas dilute amounts can be very helpful when used properly.

Hydrogen peroxide has been in medical use for centuries,[101,102,103] and there are thousands of scientific studies on its successful use. The first record of its use intravenously was for a serious outbreak of influenza pneumonia, where 80 percent died. In 1920 Dr. T.H. Oliver (*The Lancet*) treated 25 critical patients with intravenous infusions and 13 fully recovered.[202]

In the 46 years that Dr. Edward Carl Rosenow worked at the Mayo clinic, he unearthed 25 major diseases of humans which could be treated with hydrogen peroxide, and published hundreds of scientific papers while at Mayo.

According to Charles H. Farr, M.D., Ph.D., one of the world's leading authorities on the properties of, and treatment with hydrogen peroxide, this treatment helps nutrients and essential materials move across the cell membrane, stimulates and regulates immune functions, regulates energy production, and, among many other purposes, has the ability to kill bacteria, virus, fungi, yeast, and a number of parasites, many of which may be related to setting up the conditions of rheumatoid arthritis.

Hydrogen peroxide is sold in all drug stores for topical sterilization of wounds. What is not well known is that hydrogen peroxide is used both internally[103] and externally for many different disease conditions. Although intravenous injection of the proper concentration is recommended, there are an increasing number of reports of successful oral usage of hydrogen peroxide in a number of diseases, including rheumatoid arthritis. Both means of delivery   strengthen the theory that infectious organisms are at least partially responsible for various rheumatoid diseases, as -- according to researcher and developer Charles Farr, M.D., Ph.D. of Oklahoma -- hydrogen peroxide kills or inhibits bacteria, yeast, protozoa, mycoplasma, protozoa, virus growth and other parasites, and also oxidizes immunocomplexes, substances formed by the combination of antigen/allergen reactions inside the body. (For information on Hydrogen Peroxide treatments, contact: International Oxidative Medicine Association, PO Box 890910, Oklahoma City, OK 73189. See Nathaniel Altman, *Oxygen Healing Therapies*; Charles H. Farr, M.D., Ph.D., *Workbook on Free Radical Chemistry and Hydrogen Peroxide Metabolism*, IBOM Foundation, PO Box 891954, Oklahoma City, OK 73189.)

Intravenous Hydrogen Peroxide Therapy

Hydrogen peroxide found in drugstores and used for topical sterilization of wounds is a 3% mixture. Six percent hydrogen peroxide is used for bleaching hair. Reagent grade hydrogen peroxide of 30% looks harmless, like water, but is very corrosive, and must be handled with extreme care. Food grade hydrogen peroxide is 35%, and is sprayed on cheese, eggs, vegetables and fruits as a general disinfectant. At 90%, hydrogen peroxide is used as a rocket fuel.

Before use in the human body, reagent grade hydrogen peroxide is finely filtered with appropriate micropore filters and diluted with sterile water to make a concentration of 0.03%. The mixture is slowly infused in the arteries for about 3 hours. Depending upon the chronic disease being treated, including that of rheumatoid arthritis, anywhere from 1 to 20 treatments may be required.

Although hydrogen peroxide intravenous injections are not normally given for allergies, one of us (Gus J. Prosch, Jr., M.D.), as well as other physicians,   have witnessed spontaneous improvement in allergies in some patients after they've received the injections.

1. To prepare the intravenous (IV) Dr. Farr begins with 30% hydrogen peroxide of USP food or cosmetic grade. **Caution: This concentration can harm tissue. Keep away from children.**

2. Dilute the 30% solution with equal amounts of sterile distilled water to make a 15% stock solution.

3. Pass the stock solution through a Millipore 0.22 μm medium flow filter for sterilization and removal of particulate matter.

4. Store in 100 ml sterile containers and keep refrigerated for future use.

5. Add 1/4 ml of the 15% stock hydrogen peroxide to sterile 5% dextrose water, producing a 0.0375% concentration. This is used for intravenous infusion. **Caution: Vitamins, minerals, peptides, enzymes, amino acids, heparin, EDTA, or other injectable materials**

should never be mixed with the hydrogen peroxide solution.

The Case of Susan Nightingale

Charles H. Farr, M.D., Ph.D.[185] has treated hundreds of patients with chronic systemic candida, or yeast infection, using intravenous hydrogen peroxide. Keep in mind that candidiasis is an infection that contributes to, and can simulate many of the rheumatoid diseases, including rheumatoid arthritis.

Susan Nightingale, age 34, had suffered from candidiasis for 5 years, having taken many antibiotics and also having practiced rotation and elimination diets without effect. She suffered from "vaginal yeast infection, intermittent diarrhea, headaches, acne, lethargy, joint pain, mental confusion, menstrual irregularities, and had been unable to work for 2 years."

Keep in mind that by the time a common vaginal yeast infection is spotted, candidiasis has already spread throughout the body -- systemically -- contrary to the belief of traditional medical practitioners. All of Susan's additional symptoms should have been clues leading to that conclusion.

Dr. Farr gave Susan intravenous infusions of hydrogen peroxide. After just 2 treatments Susan reported feeling more alert and better able to concentrate and that she was feeling much better.

By the third treatment, Susan's complexion "started to improve, all signs of her vaginitis disappeared, and her bowel function became normal.

"After 8 treatments, she was free of all the symptoms that had plagued her for 5 years."

Within 2 more months Susan went job-hunting. (See this chapter, "Arthritis By Organisms-of-Opportunity.")

Oral Hydrogen Peroxide Therapy

Dr. Farr[104] William Douglass, M.D.[266] and other physicians have shown that the intravenous usage of hydrogen peroxide has a beneficial effect on many disease states, but feel that the oral usage of hydrogen peroxide has possible damaging effects because of the potential for combining with substances such as iron in the intestinal tract, thereby creating damaging chemicals. Ascorbate (vitamin C), iron and fats in the stomach change hydrogen peroxide into superoxide free radicals which can do severe damage to the stomach lining. Studies on mice in low concentrations showed erosion of the lining, tumors and in some, cancer.

Reported benefits from the oral usage of hydrogen peroxide may be closely related to its ability to kill off unwanted organisms in the intestinal tract.

In desperation for relief -- any kind of relief -- arthritics will gradually increase their oral intake of food-grade hydrogen peroxide according to a protocol available by ECH,O Inc. (a non-profit foundation) many reporting relief of their symptoms, and sometimes their degenerative conditions.

1. Keep in mind that not all physicians approve of oral usage of hydrogen peroxide.

2. According to some advice, purchase 30-35% food grade hydrogen peroxide. **Caution: This concentration can harm tissue. Keep away from children.** (Preservatives in the hydrogen peroxide sold in drugstores as a 3% topical disenfectant are believed to be toxic, by some advisors, although at least one physician, William Campbell Douglass, M.D.[266] -- who does not approve of oral hydrogen peroxide usage -- has written that one shouldn't be concerned about the amount of preservatives contained in the drugstore over-the-counter 3% source taken for, say, 13 days; and clearly, many people take much larger dosages for months without noticeable ill effect.)

3. Dilute the food grade hydrogen peroxide to a 3% concentration, the basic solution to be diluted when used. (For 35% use 1 ounce of 35% to 11 ounces of distilled water.)

4. The 3% solution is used as:
1st day: 3 drops in a glass of distilled water, 3 times;
2nd day: 4 drops in a glass of distilled water, 3 times a day;
3rd day use 4 drops in a glass of distilled water, 3 times a day;
4th day 6 drops; 5th day 7 drops; 6th day 8 drops; 7th day 9 drops; 8th day 10 drops; 9th day 12 drops; 10th day 14 drops; 11th day 16 drops; 12th day 18 drops; 13th day 20 drops; 14th day 22 drops; 15th day 24 drops; 16th day 75 drops, each 3 times a day.

5. For more serious problems, stay at 25 drops, 3 times a day, for 1-3 weeks, then drop to 25 drops 2 times a day until the condition changes, which may take 1-6 months.

6. Taper off by reversing the above, in a manner you find comfortable.

7. You may place the hydrogen peroxide in distilled or spring water, juice or milk. Blended carrot juice, bananas, carbonated drinks or alcoholic beverages are not compatible.

For a more complete protocol on the oral use of hydrogen peroxide, write to the non-profit foundation, ECH,O Inc. founder, Walter O. Grotz, PO Box 126 Delano, Minnesota 55328, can supply an oral hydrogen peroxide treatment protocol.

The Case of Alwyne Pilsworth

Alwyne Pilsworth,[190] a potato agronomist in the United Kingdom, had researched the use and development of hydrogen peroxide on potatoes and other crops, finding great benefits to crop growth, vigour, health and yields.

Alwyne also suffered from severe arthritis pains, at last discovering the benefits obtained through the oral use of hydrogen peroxide on herself from Walter Grotz, founder of ECH,O, Inc. Walter Grotz, a retired postmaster, was a disciple of Father Wilhelm, a retired Catholic pastor from the U.S. Air Force, also another who had obtained complete relief from rheumatoid arthritis by drinking hydrogen peroxide in controlled dosages.

Alwyne used 3 to 4 small doses of 35% food grade hydrogen peroxide in pure water during the day. In 12 days he was pain free, and pain has not returned.

We again caution: 35% food-grade hydrogen peroxide is chemically very active, and must be handled with great care. Contact ECH,O, Inc., PO Gox 126 Delano, Minneosta 55328 for instructions on its handling and use.

Alwyne also found that his life-long catarrh (inflammation of mucous membranes) had disappeared; that is, his sinuses cleared. Alwyne reports that "I also felt better in body and mind, especially in the ability to concentrate."

Alwyne Pilsworth also reported that he travelled over 2000 miles by car in the United States, and met and talked with dozens of people who had experienced the wide-ranging benefits of hydrogen peroxide for themselves and for their animals and crops.

"I met Dr. Robertson, a veterinary surgeon, who has used hydrogen peroxide for over thirty years with great success.

"I met farmers who found that their animals benefited -- laying hens given hydrogen peroxide in their drinking water were suddenly clear of Salmonella infection in their oviducts and the hens produced clean eggs."

Fattening birds weighed one-half pound heavier. Pig farmers found that when they gave hydrogen peroxide in the drinking water, they had no need for antibiotics and the pigs were more efficient food converters with leaner meat. Crops with the highest yields were those that had been treated with hydrogen peroxide.

Alwyne Pilsworth has established non-profit ECH,O, UK at 13 Albert Road, Retford, Nottinghamshire DN22 6JD, Telephone 0777 71

Farmers and lay people have long known of and discovered great benefits in the oral use of hydrogen peroxide for a variety of conditions, including rheumatoid diseases.

Dr. Farr has shown that the good effects of intravenous hydrogen peroxide usage stem principally from its ability to kill off tissue-invasive organisms, disassociate immuno complexes (allergy related), stimulate oxidation enzymes, aid membrane transport, act as a hormonal messenger, regulate thermogenesis (heat production), stimulate and regulate immune functions, regulate energy production and many other important metabolic functions -- but none of these by increasing oxygen intake.

It's clear that this unpatentable form of treatment has been swept aside by many with a vested financial stake in selling patented drugs.

Ozone Treatment

Ozone therapy[106] is somewhat newer on the medical scene. The air we breathe consists primarily of two atoms of oxygen, O_2. Ozone created by lightning, electrical spark gaps, and by ultra violet radiation streaming into the atmosphere consists of three atoms of oxygen, O_3. Ozone is an unstable atom, and "wants" to give up its extra oxygen atom to another element, thus oxidizing it.

Ozone[104,105,106] is created naturally by ultra-violet radiation which adds sufficient energy to the oxygen, O_2, that we breathe to create ozone, O_3, a molecule that reacts easily with other substances. After or during a thunder storm, with lightning adding the energy to create ozone, we often smell a "fresh" odor, which is the small amount of ozone created by the lightning's action on oxygen.

Ozone was first used as an operating room disinfectant in 1856, and later to purify municipal drinking water, where it kills viruses, bacteria, and other micro-organisms, also greatly improving the taste of the water.

In 1932 ozone began to be used for medical treatments, and today there are more than 8,000 licensed German health practitioners who use ozone therapy on their patients, and 15,000 European physicians, altogether having treated one million patients with more than ten million treatments. The use of ozone for treating many diseases, including cancer, HIV, and rheumatoid arthritis has been growing rapidly, worldwide.

As ozone is very destructive to virus, bacteria, and fungi -- all suspected causative organisms for rheumatoid arthritis -- its proper use can only be beneficial for the arthritic.

Treatments usually use 0.05 parts of ozone to 99.95 parts of normal oxygen, but the actual amount may vary according to each patient. Too much can suppress the immune system, and not enough is ineffective.

There are more than a dozen ways to administer ozone, some of them listed as follows:

Methods of Treating Ozone

Method Used	Condition
Autohemotherapy (minor)	Remove 10-50 ml of blood and treat with ozone before returning it to patient via intra-muscular injection.
Autohemotherapy (major)	Remove 50-100 ml of blood and treat with ozone before returning it to patient via arteries.
Inhalation of ozone	Room ozone generators are considered dangerous by most physicians, yet small amounts of ozone are effectively used for short-term purposes. Ozonate a closed room, then 1 hour afterward one can enter, and use the room.
Intrarticular injection	Bubble ozone through water, then inject mixture directly into joints.

Intramuscular	Usually in buttocks. Treat allergies and inflammatory diseases.
Intravenous	Directed into artery or vein. For arterial disorders. Rarely used now because of dangers of accidents.
Ozonated oil	Ozone is added to oil and used to treat skin problems.
Ozonated water	Bubble ozone through water, then use water to treat wounds, burns, and slow healing infections.
Ozone bagging	Mixture of ozone and air in plastic bag surrounds area to be treated, and is absorbed by the skin.
Renal insufflation	Through rectum. For wide variety of conditions. Considered one of the safest methods.

In applying ozone therapy -- as in the application of photopheresis where a small sample of blood is removed and treated with selected ultra-violet frequencies -- a small supply of blood may be removed, treated with ozone, and then replaced in the patient. Somehow, in both instances, photopheresis and ozone therapy, the small sample of blood diffuses and spreads throughout the body, killing micro-organisms that have overburdened the immune defense system. (See this chapter, "Arthritis By Organisms-of-Opportunity.")

Photopheresis

So far photopheresis has shown promise for the treatment of various rheumatoid diseases: scleroderma, lupus erythematosus, rheumatoid arthritis, as well as autoimmune diabetes mellitus, organ transplant rejection and AIDS related complex.[86]

Photopheresis, like ozone therapy, is a treatment that exposes relatively small portions of extracted blood mixed with a light-sensitive chemical to ultra-violet radiation. The blood is then placed back in the body by means of intravenous infusion.

Carl Schleicher, Foundation for Blood Irradiation, reports that "Ultraviolet blood irradiation first evolved in the early 1930s as a means to treat persons afflicted with the poliovirus which was causing considerable anguish and fear similar to the advent"[214] of AIDS.

According to Carl Schleicher, "Much credit for the early development of this technology goes to E.K. Knott of Seattle, Washington; Louis Ripley of Danbury, Connecticut; and Dr. T. Lewis of Pittsburgh, Pennsylvania."[214]

Its object is to "immunize" the body against malignant T cells found in the immunological system. It is also quite remarkable in its ability to wipe out populations of invasive organisms. "Intravenous ultraviolet, raises the resistance of the host and is therefore able to control many disease processes. A fundamental effect of ultraviolet blood irradiation is to 'energize' the biochemical and physiological defenses of the body by the introduction of ultraviolet energy into the bloodstream that may, in part, be effective by producing small amounts of ozone from the oxygen circulating in the blood,"[214] according to Schleicher.

"The efficacy of this method is attested to by the remarkable and consistent recovery of patients with a wide variety of diseases, apparently unrelated" to cause.

This form of treatment has never been known to cause any kind of adverse side effects, or worsening of the disease condition, in short or long term follow-up.

William Campbell Douglass, M.D.,[87] of Georgia, as well as Alaskan Robert Rowen, M.D.,[192] report excellent success with many otherwise intransigent disease conditions, using photopheresis, and especially against AIDS. Photopheresis units are now operative in more than sixty care centers in the United States, according to Richard Edelson, M.D. of Birmingham, Alabama.

Qigong for Arthritis

Qigong is an ancient Chinese system that combines movement, breath regulation, and meditation, often along with other Chinese disciplines such as acupuncture and herbs, to enhance the flow of vital energy, blood circulation, and strengthen the immune function. Although it includes exercise usually of specific recommended patterns, the nature and degree of exercise can be designed to fit the patient's capabilities.

As described in the chapter on osteoarthritis, the balancing or distribution of Qi energy to body parts in need can be an important therapy for most conditions, including that of rheumatoid arthritis.[183] (See Chapter 1, Osteoarthritis,"Qigong for Arthritis.")

The Case of Emily Peterson[207]

When forty-three year-old Emily Peterson approached Roger Jahnke, O.M.D., Santa Barbara, California, about her rheumatoid arthritis, she was in an early onset of inflammatory arthritis, an acute phase.

Acupuncture and herbal treatments were useful in getting out of the acute phase and back to work.

Dr. Jahnke says that, "Because Chinese herbal medicine is tailored to the individual's energy system and symptomology, it is not appropriate to provide a formula applicable to others. However, in cases where rheumatoid arthritis is the key feature, the Oriental Medical Doctor may use Rhehmannia, Coix, Bupleurum, and Hoelen.

"In non-acute cases, where an individual wants a gentle tonic, Shou Wu formula, and Rehmannia #8 can be obtained at most health food stores."

Since Emily's family history included arthritis, she was quite intent on doing something about it before it became severe. According to Dr. Jahnke, unlike some of his clients, Emily perceived the value of early intervention -- early treatment -- so she was willing to change her diet and begin self-care.

Emily found through the process of doing Qigong on a regular basis she was able to cut her need for acupuncture by 90%. "Instead of coming two times a week as she did originally, she came 1 time every 2 months. The rest is all Qigong. . . . She's clear [of arthritis] -- this is a case where acupuncture [and Qigong] were able to return a person to normal function when used early."[207] (See Roger Jahnke, O.M.D., video tape, *Qigong: Awakening and Mastering the Medicine Within*; books *The Self Applied Health Enhancement Methods* and *The Most Profound Medicine*; audio tape, *Deeper Relaxation for Self Healing*, Health Action, 243 Pebble Beach, Santa Barbara, CA 93117; *Qigong for Arthritis*, Dr. Yang Jwing-Ming this foundation; also *The Root of Chinese Chi Kung: The Secrets of Chi Kung Training*, YMAA Publication Center, 38 Hyde Park Avenue, Jamaica Plain, Massachusetts 02130.)

References

1. *Textbook of Internal Medicine*, J.B. Lippincott Company, 1989.

2. *The Merck Manual of Diagnosis and Therapy*, 16th Edition, Merck, Sharp & Dohme Research Laboratories, Division of Merck & Co., Inc., Rahway, N.J., 1992.

3. Burton Goldberg Group, *Alternative Medicine: The Definitive Guide*, Future Medicine Publishing Co., 1994.

4. Anthony di Fabio, *Arthritis: Little Known Treatments*, The Arthritis Fund/The Rheumatoid Disease Foundation, 1995.

5. Anthony di Fabio, *The Art of Getting Well*, The Arthritis Fund/The Rheumatoid Disease Foundation,1995.

6. Anthony di Fabio, *Arthritis*, Supplement to the Art of Getting Well, The Arthritis Fund/The Rheumatoid Disease Foundation, 1992.

7. Anthony di Fabio, *Rheumatoid Diseases Cured at Last*, The Arthritis Fund/ The Rheumatoid Disease Foundation, 1985.

8. Roger Wyburn-Mason, M.D., Ph.D., *The Causation of Rheumatoid Disease and Many Human Cancers: A New Concept in Medicine*, IJI Publishing Co., Ltd., Tokyo, Japan, 1978.

9. Roger Wyburn-Mason, M.D., Ph.D., *The Causation of Rheumatoid Disease and Many Human Cancers: A New Concept in Medicine, a Precis and Addenda, Including the Nature of Multiple Sclerosis*, The Arthritis Fund/The Rheumatoid Disease Foundation,1983.

10. Ronald Davis, M.D., *A Treatment for Scleroderma & Lupus, The Art of Getting Well*, The Arthritis Fund/The Rheumatoid Disease Foundation, 1989; also published in *Townsend Letter for Doctors*, December 1989, #77.

11. Helmut Christ, M.D., *The Surprising Psoriasis Treatment, The Art of Getting Well*, The Arthritis Fund/The Rheumatoid Disease Foundation, 1989; also published in *Townsend Letter for Doctors*, June 1990, #83.

12. Jack M. Blount, M.D., Archimedes Concon, M.D., James Rowland, D.O., William Renforth, M.D., Paul Williamson, M.D., Roger Wyburn-Mason, M.D., Ph.D., *Historical Documents In Search of the Cure for Rheumatoid Disease*, The Arthritis Fund/The Rheumatoid Disease Foundation, 37064

13. Lester Winters, *Cellular Therapy*, San Diego, CA 92110.

14. Corazon Illarina, M.D., unpublished manuscript, The Holistic Book Project, Inc., Burton Goldberg Group, Future Medicine Publishing Co., 1994.

15. Theron G. Randolph, M.D., Ralph W. Moss, Ph.D., *An Alternative Approach to Allergies*, Bantam Books, 1982.

16. Warren Levin, M.D., Anthony di Fabio, *Allergies and Biodetoxification for the Arthritic*, Suplement to The Art of Getting Well, The Arthritis Fund/The Rheumatoid Disease Foundation; Warren Levin, M.D. portion published originally in *Let's Live Magazine*, used with permission of author.

17. Perry A. Chapdelaine, Sr., *In Memoriam Robert Bingham, M.D.*, The Arthritis Fund/The Rheumatoid Disease Foundation; also published with permission in *Townsend Letter for Doctors*, November 1994

18. John H. Kippel, M.D., John L. Decker, M.D., Ed., *Clinics in Rheumatic Diseases*, Vol. 9/No.3, W.B. Saunders Co., Ltd., December 1983.

19. Personal conversation, 1983.

20. Personal conversation, 1990.

21. *Physicians Desk Reference*, Medical Economics, Inc., Oradell, NJ 07649.

22. Dr. Paul K. Pybus, *Intraneural Injections for Rheumatoid Arthritis and Osteoarthritis* and *The Control of Pain in Arthritis of the Knee*, The Arthritis Fund/The Rheumatoid Disease Foundation, Copyright 1989 and 1984, respectively.

23. Lida H. Mattman, Ph.D., *Cell Wall Deficient Forms: Stealth Pathogens*, 2nd Edition, CRC Press, 1992.

24. Morton Walker, D.P.M., "The Carnivora Cure for Cancer, AIDS & Other Pathologies," *Townsend Letter for Doctors*, June 1992, p. 412; also "The Carnivora Cure for Cancer, AIDS & Other Pathologies -- Part II," Townsend Letter for Doctors, Op.Cit., May 1992, p. 329.

25. Robert Bingham, M.D., "Rheumatoid Disease: Has One Investigator Found Its Cause and Its Cure?" *Modern Medicine*, source unknown, copy provided by Robert Bingham, February 15, 1976, pp. 38-47.

26. Lectures attended by the author in the 1950s. Also, see L. Ron Hubbard, *Research and Discovery* series, *Science of Survival*, and *Dianetics: The Modern Science of Mental Health*, Bridge Publications.

27. Gus J. Prosch, Jr., M.D., *Essential Fatty Acids are Essential*, The Arthritis Fund/The Rheumatoid Disease Foundation; also permission to republish portions granted to *EXPLORE!*, Vol. 5, No. 3, p. 23, 1994.

28. Rex E. Newnham, D.O., N.D., Ph.D., *Boron and Arthritis*, The Arthritis Fund/ The Rheumatoid Disease Foundation, Op.Cit., 1994; Rex E. Newnham, N.D., D.O., Ph.D., *Away With Arthritis*, Vantage Press, Inc., 1994; Rex E. Newnham, N.D., D.O., Ph.D., *Boron and Arthritis*, The Arthritis Fund/The Rheumatoid Disease Foundation, 1994.

29. *Clinics in Rheumatic Diseases*, W.B. Saunders & Co, December 1983.

30. Maureen Salaman, *Nutrition: Cancer Answer II*, distributed by Bay to Bay Distribution, Inc.; [First book was *The Cancer Answer*, Stratford Publishing.

31. Jeffrey Bland, Ed., *Medical Applications of Clinical Nutrition*, Keats Publishing, Inc., 1983.

32. Robert F. Cathcart, M.D., Anthony di Fabio, *Vitamin C: The Great Missing Vitamin*, The Arthritis Fund/The Rheumatoid Disease Foundation; also in *The Art of Getting Well*, 1985, Ibid; also Robert F. Cathcart, "Vitamin C, Titrating to Bowel Tolerance, Anascorbemia, and Acute Induced Scurvy, *Medical Hypotheses*," 7:1359-13767, 1981.

33. William Campbell Douglass, M.D., *The Cutting Edge*, The Douglass Center.

34. Nancy Appleton, Ph.D., *Lick the Sugar Habit*, Warner Books, Inc., 1986.

35. Price/Pottenger Foundation, San Diego, CA 92115.

36. Anthony di Fabio, *Candidiasis: The Scourge of Arthritics*, The Arthritis Fund/

The Rheumatoid Disease Foundation, 1994; also in *The Art of Getting* Well, Ibid, 1985; also see John Parks Trowbridge, M.D., Morton Walker, D.P.M., *The Yeast Syndrome*, Bantam Books; William G. Crook, *The Yeast Connection*, Third Edition, Professional Books; William G. Crook, *Solving the Puzzle of Your Hard-To-Raise Child*, Ibid, 1987.

37. Warren Levin, M.D., Anthony di Fabio, *Food Allergies and Biodetoxification*, Supplement to The Art of Getting Well, The Arthritis Fund/The Rheumatoid Disease Foundation, 1994.

38. Gus J. Prosch, Jr., M.D., lecture, transcribed with permission from *The The Arthritis Fund/TheRheumatoid Disease Foundation's Second Annual Medical Convention*, Santa Monica, CA, July 16-19, 1986.

39. Robert Bingham, M.D., *Fight Back Against Arthritis*, Desert Arthritis Medical Clinic, 1993.

40. William J. Faber, D.O., Morton J. Walker, D.P.M., *Treatment of First Choice for Osteoarthritis and for Other Arthritic-like Pain: Sclerotherapy, Proliferative Therapy, Reconstructive Therapy*, Supplement to The Art of Getting Well, The Arthritis Fund/The Rheumatoid Disease Foundation, 1992; also William J. Faber, D.O., Morton J. Walker, D.P.M., *Pain, Pain Go Away*, ISHI Press International, 1995.

41. Personal communication with Lida Mattman, Ph.D., 1995.

42. Leon Chaitow, M.D., James Strohecker, *You Don't Have to Die*, Future Medicine Publishing, Inc., 1994.

43. Gerald J. Domengue, Jorgen U. Schlegel, Hannah B. Woody, "Naked Bacteria in Human Blood," *Microbia*, Tome 2, No. 2, Annee 1976.

44. John W. Mattingly, *Microscopy, Bacteriology and Gaston Naessens' Biological Theory*, Jan. 1986; also reproductions of *The Microzymas and The Blood* (1908) translated by Montague Leverson, M.D., 1990.

45. Virginia Livingston-Wheeler, Edmond G. Addeo, *The Conquest of Cancer*, Franklin Watts, 1984.

46. Antoine Bechamp, *The Blood and Its Third Anatomical Element*," (Translated from the French by Montague R. Leverson, M.D.), Boericke & Tafel, Philadelphia, 1911; made available by Mr. & Mrs. John Mattingly.

47. Barry Lynnes, *The Cancer Cure That Worked*, Bookpeople, Berkeley, CA; also Christopher Bird, "What Has Become of the Rife Microscope?" *New Age Journal*, March 1976, p. 41

48. Dr. Paul K. Pybus, *The Herxheimer Effect*, Supplement to the Art of Getting Well, The Arthritis Fund/The Rheumatoid Disease Foundation, TN, 1991.

49. Herxheimer, K. Krause: Uber eine bei Syphilitische vorkommende Quecksilerberreaktion. *Deutsch. Med. Wschr.* 28:50, 1902; Herxheimer, K. and Martin, H.: So-called Herxheimer reactions. *Arch. Derm. Syph.* 13:115, 1926; Millian, G.: Syphilis: Reaction d' Herxheimer. *Biotropisme. Paris nd.*: 37:91, 1920; Fleishman, K. and Kreibich, C.: Zum Wesen der Reaktion nach Jarish-Herxheimer. *Me. Klin.* 21:1157, 1925; Mahoney, J.F., Arnold, R.C., and Harris, A.: Penicillin treatment of early syphilis. *Amer. J. Public Health* 33:1387, 1943; Moore, J.E., Farmer, T.W. and Hoekenga, M.T.: Penicillin and the Jarisch-Herxheimer reaction in early, cardiovascular and nuerosyphilis. *rans. Ass. Amer. Phycns.* 61:176, 1948; Joulia, P., Pautrizell, R., Texier, L. and Sebra, De.: La chute des eosinophiles sanguines apre une premiere injeciton de penicilline au cours de la syphilis primo-secondaire: temoin du conflit antigene-anticorps. *ull. Soc. Franc. Derm. Syph.* 58:399, 1951; Heyman, A., Sheldon, W.H. and Evans, L.D.: Pathogenesis of the Jarisch-Herxheimer reaction. *rit. J. vener. Dis.* 28:50, 1952; Jadassohn, J.: Beitrag zur Jarisch-Herxheimer Reaktion. *Z. Haut Geschlechtskr* 19:158, 1965; Jarisch, A. Wien. *med Wschr.* 45:721, 1895; Gudjonsson, Haraldur: The Jarisch-Herxheimer Reaction, Stockholm 1972 (A summary based on the following seven publications: a. Skok, E. and Gudjonsson, H.: On the allergic origin of the jarisch-Herxheimer reaction. *Acta Dermatovfener* (Stockholm) 46:136, 1966.; b. Gudjonsson, H. and Skog, E.: The effect of

prednisolone on the Jarisch-Herxheimer reaction. *Acta Dermatovener* (Stockholm) 48:15, 1968.; c. Gudjonsson, H. and Skog, E.: Fever after inoculation of rabbits with *Treponema pallidum.* Jarisch-Herxheimer reaction? *Proc. 18. Meeting Scand. Dermatol. Ass.,* Turku 1968. ; d. Gudjonsson, H. and Skog, E.: Fever after inoculation of rabbits with *Treponema pallidum. Brit. J. vener. Dis.* 46:318, 1970.; e. Gudjonsson, H., Newman, B. and Turner, T.B.: Demonstration of a virus-like agent contaiminating amterial containing the Stockholm substrain of the Nichols pathogenic *Treponema pallidum. Brit. J. vener. Dis.* 46:435, 1970.; f. Gudjonsson, H. Newman, B. and Turner, T.B.: Screening out a virus-like agent from the testicular suspension of the Nichols pathogenic *Treponema pallidum. Brit. J. vener. Dis.* In press at time summary was written.; g. Gudjonsson, H.: Experiments to induce febrile Jarisch-Herxheimer reaction on syphilitic rabbits with penicillin and erythromycin. *Acta Dermatovener.* (Stockholm). In press at time summary was written.

50. Guy [study performed in South Africa by a Rheumatologist], reference source lost.

51. Gus J. Prosch, Jr., M.D., Personal Communication.

52. Names and addresses of compounding pharmacists or the address of Seldon Nelson, D.O. is available through The Arthritis Fund/The Rheumatoid Disease Foundation. Please include a donation and self-addressed, stamped envelope to help defray the cost of the service.

53. Anthony di Fabio et. al., *Friendly Bacteria -- Lactobacillus acidophilus & Bifido bacterium,* The Arthritis Fund/The Rheumatoid Disease Foundation, 1989.

54. Personal conversation with John Baron, D.O., 1984.

55. *Candidia Research and Information Foundation Newsletter,* No. 9-10, March 1989,94546.

56. "Candida Albicans," *Capsulations™,* No. 15, Thorne Research, Inc., October 1989.

57. Raymond Keith Brown, M.D., *Aids,Cancer and the Medical Establishment,* Trizoid Press, New York, 1993, ISBN0-9639293-0-5.

58. James P. Carter, M.D., Dr.P.H., *Racketeering in Medicine,* Hampton Roads Publishing, Inc., p. 80.

59. C. Orian Truss, M.D., *The Missing Diagnosis,* AL 35226, 1983.

60. William B. Crook, M.D., *The Yeast Connection,* Professional Books, Third Edition, 1986. Also see *Solving the Puzzle of Your Hard-To-Raise Child,* Op. Cit. 1987.

61. Morton Walker, D.P.M., John Parks Trowbridge, M.D., *The Yeast Syndrome,* Bantam Books, 1986.

62. Dennis W. Remington, M.D., Barbara W. Higa, R.D., *Back to Health,* Vitality House International, Inc., 1986.

63. Personal conversation with a Vanderbilt University pharmacologist, who chooses not to be identified, 1983.

64. Paul A. Goldberg, M.P.H., D.C., Personal letter, May 18, 1994.

65. Personal Communication from Stephan Cooter, Ph.D. May 15, 1994.

66. S.M. Peck, H. Rosenfeld, "The Effects of Hydrogen Ion Concentration, Fatty Acids and Vitamin C on the Growth of fungi," *J. Invest. Dermatol.* 1:237-265, 1938.

67. William (Bill) G. Neely, D.C., 512 E. Unaka Ave., Johnson City, TN 37601, Personal Communication, 1992. Candida Purge available from Nutri-Dyn -- Nu Biologics; Acu-Trol available from #2 Willow Rd, North Oaks, MN 55110, % Monica O' Kane.

68. Frederic Damrau, M.D.,"The Value of Bentonite for Diarrhea," *Medical Annals of the District of Columbia,* Vol. 30, No. 6, June 1961, p. 328.

69. Nu Biologics.

70. Benjamin Lau, M.D., Ph.D., *Garlic for Health,* Odyssey Publishing, Inc., Vancouver, B.C., Canada V6M 2J2, 1991. Also see:Tariq H. Abdullah, M.D., O. Kandil, Ph.D., A. Elkadi, M.D., and J. Carter, M.D., "Garlic Revisited: Therapeutic For

338   ANTHONY DI FABIO, M.A. & GUS J. PROSCH, JR., M.D

the Major Diseases of Our Times?," *Journal of the National Medical Association*, Vol. 80, No. 4, 1988; Christopher L. Marsh, Robert R. Torrey, James L. Woolley, Gary R. Barker, Benjamin H.S. Lau, "Superiority of Intravesical Immunotherapy With Corynebacterium Parvum and Allium Sativum in Control of Murine Bladder Cancer," *The Journal of Urology*, Vol. 137, February 1987, p. 359; Benjamin H.S. Lau, M.D., Ph.D., Takeshi Yamasaki, D.V.M., M.S., Daila S. Gridley, Ph.D., "Garlic Compounds Modulate Macrophage and T-lymphocyte Functions," *Mol. Biother.*, Vol. 3, June 1991; Benjamin H.S. Lau, James L. Woolley, Christopher L. Marsh, Gary R. Barker, Dick H. Koobs, Robert R. Torrey, *The Journal of Urology*, Vol. 136, September 1986; Padma P. Tadi, M.S., Robert W. Teel, Ph.D., Benjamin H.S. Lau, M.D., Ph.D., "Anticandidal and Anticarcinogenic Potentials of Garlic," *Integrated Therapies*, School of Medicine, Loma Linda University, Loma Linda, CA 92350, 1990; address correspondence to Benjmain H.S. Lau, M.D., Ph.D.; Benjamin Lau, M.D., Ph.D., Garlic Research Update, Odyssey Publishing Inc. Op. Cit, 1991.

71. Wakunaga of America Co., Ltd, Mission Viego, CA 92691; telephone 1-800-544-5800.

72. Dan Bensky, Andrew Gamble, *Chinese Herbal Medicine, Materia Medica*, Revised Edition, Eastland Press, Inc., 1993.

73. Stephen Cooter, Ph.D. "Molybdenum: Recycling Fatigue Into Energy," *Townsend Letter for Doctors*, April 1994, p. 332; an excerpt from *Beating Chronic Illness: Fatigue, Pain, Weakness, Insomnia, Foggy Thinking*, Pro Motion Publishing, San Diego, CA 92120; also see Walter H. Schmitt, Jr., D.C., *Molybdenum for* Candida albicans *Patients and Other Problems*; The Arthritis Fund/The Rheumatoid Disease Foundation; published originally in *The Digest of Chiropractic Economics*, 31:4, January-February, 1991, pp. 56-63, Livonia, Michigan 48152-3661, reprinted as it appeared with permission of the author and Chiropractic News Publishing Company, Inc., courtesy of Keith A. Tosolt, Managing Editor.

74. Paul Reilly, N.D., "Natural Therapies for Autoimmune Diseases," *Townsend Letter for Doctors*, Issue #42, p. 331, 1986.

75. Theron Randolph, M.D., Ralph Moss, Ph.D., *An Alternative Approach to Allergies*, Bantom Books, New York, ISBN: 0-553-29830-6.

76. Warren Levin, M.D., "Allergy/Addiction to Foods and Chemicals," *Let's Live Magazine*, Los Angeles, CA 90004, June 1976. Used with permission of Warren Levin, M.D.

77. Anthony di Fabio, *Chelation Therapy*, Supplement to The Art of Getting Well, The Arthritis Fund/The Rheumatoid Disease Foundation, 1993.

78. William Campbell Douglass, M.D., *The Milk of Human Kindness is not Pasteurized*, Last Laugh Publishers, Marietta, GA 30067, 1985.

79. Correspondence and literature form Immuno Laboratories, Inc., Fort Lauderdale, FL 33311.

80. Gus J. Prosch, Jr., M.D., Wyatt C. Simpson, M.D., *Chronic Systemic Candidiasis: The Fungus Among Us*, Biomed Associates, P.C., Birmingham, AL 35226.

81. S. Colet Lahoz, M.S., R.N., Director East-West Clinic, White Bear Lake, MN 55110, Personal Correspondence, 1995.

82. Perry A. Chapdelaine, Sr., personal experiences.

83. Carl J. Reich, M.D., Stephan Cooter, Ph.D., *Calcium and Vitamin D Deficiency: The Clinical Work and Theory of Carl J. Reich, M.D.*, Supplement to The Art of Getting Well, The Arthritis Fund/The Rheumatoid Disease Foundation, TN 37064, 1995.

84. F. Batmanghelidj, M.D., *Your Body's Many Cries for Water*, Global Health Solutions, Inc., 1992; also F. Batmanghelidj, M.D., *How to Deal With Back Pain & Rheumatoid Joint Pain*, Global Health Solutions, Inc., 1992; also F. Batmanghelidj, M.D., *Prevent Arthritis and Cure Back Pain*, The Arthritis Fund/The Rheumatoid

Disease Foundation, 1995.

85. William Kaufman, M.D., Ph.D., "Niacinamide: A Most Neglected Vitamin," *Journal of the International Academy of Preventive Medicine*, Vol. VIII, No. 1, Winter 1983; also William Kaufman, M.D., Ph.D., *The Common Form of Joint Dysfunction: It's Incidence and Treatment*, E.I. Hildreth & Co., Brattleboro, VT, 1949.

86. Richard Edelson, Peter Heald, Maritza Perez, Alain Rook, "Photopheresis Update," *Progress in Dermatology*,Vol. 25, No. 3, September 1991.

87. Personal Communication from William Campbell Douglass, M.D.

88. Personal visit with Tonis Pai, M.D.

89. Anthony di Fabio, *Germanium*, The Rheumatoid Disease Foundation; Sandra Goodman, Ph.D., *Germanium, The Health and Life Enhancer*, Thorsons Publishers Limited, Wellingborough, Northamptonshire; Betty Kamen, Ph.D. *Germanium: A New Approach to Immunity*, Nutrition Encounter, Inc.

90. Lester Winters, Ph.D., *Cellular Therapy*, Cellular Therapy Physician Associates of Tijuana, Tijuana, Baja California, Mexico; personal communication with Lester Winter, Ph.D.; Personal visit to William J. Saccoman, M.D. and Lester Winter, Ph.D.

91. Robert W. Bradford, D.Sc., Henry W. Allen, Michael L. Culbert, D.Sc., *The Biochemical Basis of Live Cell Therapy*," The Robert Bradford Foundation, Chula Vista, CA, May 1986.

92. Gerhard Shettler, Prof. Dr. med, "Intra-articular Cellular Therapy and Adjunctive Treatment," University of Cologne, Bunderesreupublick Deutchland.

93. Harvey Bigelsen, M.D., "The Arizona Board of Homeopathy," *Townsend Letter for Doctors*, #51, October 1987, p. 294.

94. Luc de Schepper, M.D., Ph.D., C.A., *Peak Immunity*, Santa Monica, CA 90403, 1989.

95. Ralph Wilson, Abstracter of Callinan, P., "The Mechanism of Action of Homeopathic Remedies -- Towards a Definitive Mode of Action," *Journal of Complementary Medicine*, July 1985.

96. "British Medical Journal Acknowledges the Value of Homeopathy," *The Townsend Letter for Doctors*, 98368.

97. Dr. Erik Enby, *Hidden Killers*, Peter Gosch, Michael Sheehn, Sheehan Communications, 1990.

98. Dr. Julian Whitaker, "DHEA References," *Health & Healing*," June 1992; also see "DHEA: The Closest We Can Get, Today, To A Foundation of Youth," Op.Cit., Vol.2, No. 6, June 1992; William Regelson, Roger Loria, Mohammed Kalimi, "Hormonal Intervention: `Buffer Hormones' or `State Dependency,' Neuroimmunomodulation: Intervention in Aging and Cancer," *Annales N.Y. Acad. Sci.*, Vol. 521, 1988; George Weber, Ed., "Advances in Enzyme Regulation," *Proceedings of the Twenty-Sixth Symposium on Regulation of Enzyme Activity and Synthesis in Normal and Neoplastic Tissues held at Indiana University School of Medicine, Indianapolis, Indiana*, Volume 26, Pergamon Press, September 29, 30, 1986; Jonathan V. wright, M.D., *Physiologic and `Supraphysiologic' Suppression of Allergy by Dehydroepiandrosterone*, February 26, 1990.

99. Virginia Livingston-Wheeler, M.D. Edmond G. Addeo, *The Conquest of Cancer*, Franklin Watts, 1984.

100. Julian Whitaker, M.D., *Health & Healing*, Vol. 2, No. 6, June 1992.

101. Walter O. Grotz, *Grotz: Hydrogen: Bibliography*, ECHO, MN 55328.

102. Kurt Donsbach, D.C., Ph.D., *Hydrogen Peroxide*.

103. Charles Marchand, *The Therapeutical Applications of Hydrozone and Glycozone*, Echo, Inc. republished from the 1904 18th edition 1989.

104. Charles Farr, M.D., Ph,.D., *Hydrogen Peroxide Therapy*, The Rheumatoid Disease Foundation.

105. Ed McCabe, *Oxygen Therapies*, Energy Publications, 1988.

106. Personal Communication from Helmut Christ, M.D., Germany and William

34040

ANTHONY DI FABIO, M.A. & GUS J. PROSCH, JR., M.D

Campell Douglass, III, M.D., Georgia.

107. Thomas Gervais, Courtland Reeves, Anthony di Fabio, *Lymphatic Detoxification*, Supplement to The Art of Getting Well, The Arthritis Fund/The Rheumatoid Disease Foundation, 1994.

108. College Pharmacy, Colorado Springs, CO 80903.

109. Henry Scammell, *The Arthritis Breakthrough*, M.Evans and Company, Inc., 1993; includes Thomas McPherson Brown, M.D., *The Road Back*, 1988.

110. Marion Patricia Connolly, "Price Reaffirmed," *Price-Pottenger Foundation Journal*, Vol. 12, #1, 1988.

111. William H. Philpott, M.D., *Magnetic Resonance Bio-Oxidative Therapy for Rheumatoid and Other Degenerative Diseases*, Supplement to The Art of Getting Well, The Arthritis Fund/The Rheumatoid Disease Foundation, 1994.

112. Linus Pauling, Ph.D., *How to Live Longer and Feel Better*, Avon Books, 1987.

113. Irwin Stone, *The Healing Factor*, Worldwide, New York, 1972.

114. A. Kalokerinos, *Every Second Child*, Thomas Nelson, Australia, 1974.

115. "How Vitamin C Can Prevent Heart Attack and Stroke," *The Linus Pauling Institute of Science and Medicine Newsletter*, March 1992.

116. *The Key to the Power of Vitamin C*, Ester-C Polyascorbate™, Inter-Cal Corporation, AZ 86301.

117. Nancy Chandler, Personal letter from Inter-Cal Corporation, May 3, 1989.

118. Leo Galland, M.D., "From the Doctor's Desk," Great Smokies Diagnostic Laboratories,"

119. Leo Galland, M.D., "Leaky Gut Syndromes: Breaking the Vicious Cycle," *Townsend Letter for Doctors*, August/September, 1995, p. 62.

120. Personal communication with Carl Reich, M.D.

121. Zhenya Kurashova Wine, "Russian Medical Massage: Arthritis, *Massage*, Issue Number 57, September/October 1995, p. 90-92.

122. Dr. John Mansfield, "Chemical Crippling," *What Doctors Don't Tell You*, Vol. 6, No. 7, The Wallace Press, London.

123. Martin Zucker, "Boswellia: An Ancient Herb Combats Arthritis," *The Natural Way*, June/July 1995.

124. Nan Kathyrn Fuchs, Ph.D., "Calcium Controversy," *The Natural Way*, April/May 1995, p. 12-13.

125. "Arthritis: The Price of Painkillers," *Control Your Health*, Volume 2, No. 12, The Wallace Press, London.

126. Keith W. Sehnert, M.D., Gary Jacobson, D.D.S., Kip Sullivan, J.D., "Is Mercury Toxicity an Autoimmune Disorder?" *Townsend Letter for Doctors & Patients*, October 1995, p. 134-137.

127. Personal knowledge of Connie Anderson.

128. *Essentials of Immune Response, Inflammation and the Pathogenesis of Rheumatoid Arthritis*, Smith Kline & French Laboratories, 1984.

129. Personal letter from Richard A. Kunin, M.D.

130. Harold E. Buttram, M.D., "Volatile Organic Compounds: Contributory Causes of Learning Disabilities and Behavorial Problems in Children," *Townsend Letter for Doctors*, April 1994.

131. "We Are Losing the War Against Cancer,: Re: *New England Journal of Medicine Reports, Townsend Letter for Doctors*, July 1986, p. 193.

132. "Cocaine Facts," *The Fairview Observer*, Fairview, TN, April 6, 1993, p. 5; from NIDA, U.S. Department of Health and Human Services and *800-Cocaine Survey* 2/90.

133. "Wax on Your Fruits & Vegetables," Citizen Petition, Amyherst, NH 03031.

134. James P. Carter, M.D., Dr.PH, *Racketering in Medicine: The Suppression of Alterntives*, Hampton Roads Publishing Company, Inc., 1993; Also see book review

"The Battle to Suppress the Suppressors of Medical Alternatives," *Townsend Letter for Doctors*, January 1993.

135. Susan Mix, Ph.D., "Invisible Poisons: Pesticides, *Health Freedom News*, January 1994, p. 31.

136. Jule Klotter, "Toxins in Pesticides," *Townsend Letter for Doctors*, May 1993, p. 518.

137. Maureen Kennedy Salaman, "Malathion Spells M-U-R-D-E-R," *Health Freedom News*, May 1994, p. 4; from Norma Grier, *Journal of Pesticide Reform*, Vol. 7, No. 4, Northwest Coalition for Alternatives to Pesticides.

138. "FDA v. NutriCology," *Townsend Letter for Doctors*, p. 408; from Earth Save Foundation, Santa Cruz, California 95062-2205.

139. Michael D. Lemonick, "Toxins On Tap," *Time*, November 15, 1993, p. 86.

140. Elizabeth Croteau, "Beware Parasites in Your Drinking Water, *Health Freedom News*, Monrovia, CA 91017, March 1995, p. 33.

141. Ellen Brown, J.D., "Crystal Power: Bioenergetically Treated Potatoes Reported Free of Toxic Chemicals," *Townsend Letter for Doctors*, 1993, p. 1107.

142. Dr. Michael Colgan,"The Vitamin Pushers," *Townsend Letter for Doctors*, p. 126.

143. Sam Ziff, Michael F. Ziff, D.D.S., "The Medical Profession Should Rediscover Mercury," *Townsend Letter for Doctors*, 1993, p. 1109.

144. Danila Oder, "BGH -- It Does A Body No Good," *Health Freedom News*, April, 1994, p. 30.

145. Carl L. Tellen, " Mislabeling Filthy Meat," NEWS from the QUACK-BUSTERS: National Council Against Health Fraud Newsletter (November/December 1994), *Townsend Letter for Doctors*, May 1995, p. 130.

146. Ruth Sackman, "EPA to Loosen Standards on Pesticides," *Townsend Letter for Doctors*, July 1993, p. 732.

147. "The Medical Effects of Tobacco Consumption," *Scientific American*, New York, New York, May 1995, p. 49.

148. Donald C. Thompson, M.D., D.Ph., "Tobacco's Biggest Field is Debt and Death," *Townsend Letter for Doctors*, May 1995, p. 24.

149. "Under the Microscope: The Health Care Crisis," *Health Freedom News*, November/December 1992, p. 4.

150. *What is Scientology?* Bridge Publications, 1992, p. 528.

151. Paul V. beals, M.D., "Chelation Stopped in Maryland," *Townsend Letter for Doctors*, January 1989, p. 532.

152. Ed Randegger, "Unfriendly Skies.... * Not Just for Canaries, But Everyone!" a book review of Jet Smart by Diana Fairechild, *Townsend Letter for Doctors*, 1993, p. 1140.

153. Anthony di Fabio, *Fluoridation: Governmentally Approved Poison*, Supplement to the Art of Getting Well, The Arthritis Fund/The Rheumatoid Disease Foundation, 1994.

154. Hector E. Solorzano del Rio, M.D., D.Sc., *Systemic Enzyme Therapy*, Supplement to the Art of Getting Well, The Arthritis Fund/The Rheumatoid Disease Foundation, 1994.

155. Personal letter received from W.A. Shrader, Jr., M.D. October 31, 1995.

156. Marjorie Crandall, Ph.D., *Position Paper*, received November 4, 1995 from Dr. Crandall; also see Marjorie Crandall, Ph.D. "Generalized Symptoms in Women with Chronic Yeast Vaginitis: Treatment with Nystatin, Diet and Immunotherapy Versus Nystatin Alone," *Journal of Advancement in Medicine*, 4: 21, 1991 available through C. Orian Truss, M.D., , Critical Illness Research Foundation; and Marjorie Crandall, Ph.D. letter in *New England Journal of Medicine* 324: 1593, 1991.

157. "Balneotherapy for Rheumatoid Arthritis," Clinical Research Bulletins, *American Journal of Natural Medicine*, July/August 1995, Volume 2, Number 6, p. 26-

27.

158. Dr. Tsu-Tsair Chi, N.M.D., Ph.D., *Mineral Infrared Therapy*, Chi's Enterprise, Inc., Anaheim, CA 92807, 1993.

159. Julian Whitaker, M.D., *Dr. Whitaker's Guide to Natural Healing*, Prima Publishing, 1995.

160. Christopher J. Hegarty, "Eating the 'Wright' Way, *Health Consciousness*, October 1991, p. 64; reporting on Patrick Wright, Ph.D. *Grains & Greens.*

161. Pinina Langevitz, Ilan Bank, Deborah Zemer, Mazl Book, Mordechai Pras, "Treatment of Resistant Rheumatoid Arthritis with Minocycline: An Open Study," *The Journal of Rheumatology*, 19:10, 1992, p. 1502.

161. Harold E. Paulus, M.D., "Minocycline Treatment of Rheumatoid Arthritis," *Annals of Internal Medicine*, Volume 122, Number 2, January 15, 1995, p. 147.

162. Debbie Carson, "Kombucha Tea," (reporting on Gunther W. Frank, *Kobucha*) in *Trans*, Nashville, TN, Summer 1995, p. 14; Elizabeth Baker, author of *The Uncook Book*, Indianola, WA. Kombucha,

163. Internet: #44384 S2/Holistic Medicine, 23-July-94 13:16:61; Sb: #44377-Rheumatoid Arthritis; Fm: Steve Harris, M.D. 71450, 1773 To: Larry Johansen, MS 71260, 3377.

164. Dr. Andrew Lockie, *The Family Guide to Homeopathy*, Fireside, Rockefeller Center, New York, New York 10020, 1989.

165. Personal communication from Rex E. Newnham, D.O., N.D., Ph.D., November 6, 1995.

166. Dr. Christiane Northrup, "Relief from Rheumatoid Arthritis in Body, Mind and Spirit," *Health Wisdom for Women*, Vol. 2, No. 11, November 1995.

167. "Fish Oil Relieves Rheumatoid Arthritis:" *Nutrition & Healing*, c/o Publishers Mgt. Corp., November 1994, p. 8.

168. Ricki Lewis, Ph.D., "Arthritis: Modern Treatments for That Old Pain in the Joints," *Consumer* 06/01/1991.

169. Personal communication from Gilbert Manso, M.D., November 10, 1995.

170. Jane Heimlich, *What Your Doctor Won't Tell You*, Harper Perennial, HarperCollins Publishers, 1990.

171. Elmer M. Cranton, M.D., James P. Frackleton, M.D., Free Radical Pathology in Age-Associated Diseases: Treatment With EDTA Chelation, Nutriton, and Antioxidants, *Journal of Holistic Medicine*, Vol. 6, No. 1, Human Sciences Press, Spring/Summer 1984.

172. Personal communication from Efrain Olszewer, M.D. received November 17, 1995.

173. Personal communication with Jack M. Blount, M.D., Robert Bingham, M.D., Archimedes A. Concon, M.D., Gus J. Prosch, Jr., M.D., Dr. Paul K. Pybus, William Renforth, M.D., Roger Wyburn-Mason, M.D., Ph.D.

174. Anthony di Fabio, *The Master Regulator*, The Arthritis Fund/The Rheumatoid Disease Foundation, 1989; also Broda O. Barnes, M.D., Lawrence Galton, *Hypothyroidism: The Unsuspected Illness*, Harper & Row, New York, 1976.

175. E. Denis Wilson, M.D., *Wilson's Syndrome*, Cornerstone Publishing Company, Orlando, Florida 32812, 1991.

176. Personal correspondence from James Carlson, D.O.

177. Personal interview with Shirley Holmstead, November 21, 1995.

178. References supplied by W.A. Shrader, Jr., M.D.: McEwen, L.M., Ganderton, M.A., Wilson, C.W. and Black, J.H. Hyaluronidase in the treatment of allergy, *Brit Med J* 1967: ii:507-8; McEwen, L.M., Starr, M.S. Enzyme potentiated hyposensitization I, the effect of pre-treatment with β-glucuronidase, hyaluronidase and antigen on anaphylactic sensitivity of guinea pigs, rats and mice. *Int. Arch Allerg* 1972: 42:152-8; McEwen, L.M. Enzyme potentiated hyposensitization II, Effect of glucose, glucosamine, N-acetylamino-sugars and gelatin on the ability of β-glucuronidase to block

the anamnestic response to antigen in mice. *Ann Allerg* 1973: 31:79-83; McEwen, L.M. Nicholson, M., Kitchen, I. and White, S. Enzyme potentiated hyposensitization III, Control by sugars and diols of the immunological effect of β-glucuronidase in mice and patients with hay fever. *Ann Allerg* 1973: 31: 543-9; McEwen, L.M., Nicholson, M., Kitchen, I., O'Gorman, J., White, S. Enzyme potentiated hyposensitization IV, Effect of protamine on the immunolgical behavior of β-glucuronidase in mice and patients with hay fever. *Ann Allerg* 1975: 34:290-5; McEwen, L.M. Enzyme potentiated hyposensitization V, Five case reports of patients with acute food allergy. *Ann Allerg* 1975: 35:98-103; McEwen, L.M. A double-blind controlled trial of enzyme potentiated hyposensitization for the treatment of ulcerative colitis. *Clin Ecol*: 5:47-51; Fell, P. and Brostoff, J. A single dose desenisitization for summer hay fever. *Eur J Clin Pharm* 1990: 38:77-9; Eaton, K.K. Preliminary studies with enzyme potentiated desensitization in canine atopic dermatitis. *Env Med* 1991: 8:140-1; Longo, G., Poli, F. and Bertoli, G. Efficacia clinica di un novo trattemento iposensibilizzante, EPD (enzyme potentiated desensitization) nella terapia della pollinosi. *Reforma Med* 1992: 107: 171-6; Eggar, J., Stolla, A., McEwen, L.M. Controlled trial of hyposensitization in children with food-induced hyperkinetic syndrome. *Lancet* 1992: 339 (May 9): 1150-3; Shrader, Jr., W.A., McEwen, L.M. Enzyme potentiated sensensitization: A sixteen month trial of therapy with 134 patients. *Environmental Medicine* 1993: 9/No. 3&4: 128-38.

179. Stuart Timmons, "The Fungus Among Us," *New Age Journal*, November/ December, Langley, VA, p. 81.

180. Anna Bond, letter to Peggy Taylor, Editor, *New Age Journal*, dated December 7, 1994.

181. Gus J. Prosch, Jr., M.D., Biomed Associates, P.C., Birmingham, Alabama, 35226, *Recommended Protocol for Treatment of the Rheumatoid Diseases*, patient and physician handout.

182. A.V. Costantini, M.D., *The Fungal/Mycotoxin Connections: Autoimmune Diseases, Malignanacies, Atherosclerosis, Hyperlipidemias, and Gout*, Keynote Speaker, American Academy of Environmental Medicine, Reno, Nevada, 1993.

183. Jwing-Ming Yang, *Arthritis -- The Chinese Way of Healing and Prevention*, YMAA Publication Center, Yang's Martial Arts Association (YMAA), Jamaica Plain, Massachusetts 02130, 1991.

184. "Traditional Herbal Formula vs. Flagyl in Amebiasis," *The American Journal of Natural Medicine*, Vol. 2, No. 9, IMPAKT Communications, Inc., November 1995, p.16.

185. "Candida," *Alternative Medicine Digest*, Issue 8, Future Medicine Publishing, Inc., Fife, WA 98424, 1995.

186. "Why a Single Hormone May Dictate the Future of Agiing," *Alternative Medicine Digest*, Issue 8, Future Medicine Publishing, Inc., Fife, WA 98424, 1995.

187. Julian Whitaker, M.D., *Health & Healing*, Phillips Publishing, Inc., Volume 5, Number 8, August 1995.

188. Hildegard Pickles, *Devil's Claw*.

189. Wun Peida, Yang Xiuyan, "Preliminary Clinical Observation On Treatment of 40 Cases of Arthritis with Pagosid," Branch of Rheumatology and Clinical Immunology, Department of Internal Medicine, First Affiliated Hospital, Sun Yet Sen University of Medical Science.

190. Alwyne Pilsworth, *Hydrogen Perxoide; Report by Alwyne Pilsworth*.

191. Hal A. Huggins, D.D.S., M.S., *It's All In Your Head*, Avery Press.

192. Conference lecture by Robert Rowen, M.D. attended by author.

193. Martha M. Christy, "The Newest Alternative to Antiobitoic Therapy," *Health Freedom News*, National Health Federation, November/December 1995; also *Your Own Perfect Medicine*, Future Med, Inc.1994.

194. Sherry A. Rogers, *Wellness Against All Odds*, Prestige Publishing, Box 3068

3500 Brewerton Rd., Syracuse, NY 13220.

195. Lita Lee, Ph.D., "Hypthyroidism, A. Modern Epidemic," reprint from *Earthletter*, Spring 1994, #397, Eugene, Oregon.

196. Lita Lee, Ph.D., "The 24-Hour Urinalysis According to Loomis," reprinted from *Earthletter*, Volume 2, Summer 1994, #397 Eugene, Oregon.

197. Anthony J. Cichoke, D.C., "Chiropractic & Nutrition," *Townsend Letter for Doctors & Patients*,   January 1996, p. 32.

198. Henry Kriegel, "Memorandum," Kriegel & Associates, Belgrade, MT 59714, November 7, 1995.

199. Flyer received from Rivers of Life, Mariposa, CA 95338-1913.

200. Tilley, Barbara, C., Ph.D., et. al., "Minocycline in Rheumatoid Arthritis: A 48-Week, Double-Blind, Placebo-Controlled Trial," *Annals of Internal Medicine*, January 15, 1995; 122(2):81-89.

201. Agatha Thrash, M.D., Calvin Thrash, M.D., *Home Remedies*, Thrash Publications,   Seale, Alabama 36875.

202. Charles H. Farr, M.D., Ph.D., *Workbook on Free Radical Chemistry and Hydrogen Peroxide Metabolism*, IBOM Foundation, Oklahoma City, OK 73189.

203. Robert Bingham, M.D., *Fight Back Against Arthritis*, The Arthritis Fund/ The Rheumatoid Disease Foundation, 1985.

204. Dava Sobel, Arthur C. Klein, "Bee Venom," *Arthritis: What Works*, St. Martin's Press, New York, NY, 1989; Also see *Alternative Medicine Digest*, Future Medicine Publishing, Inc., Fife, WA 98424.

205. Personal correspondence from Paul A. Goldberg, M.P.H., D.C.

206. Jay Hodin, " *Townsend Letter for Doctors*,   April 1993, p. 333; also Perry A. Chapdelaine, Sr., *Identical Religious and Medical Patterns of Suppression in the Late Twentieth Century*, Unpublished Manuscript, Franklin, TN.

207. Interview with Roger Jahnke, O.M.D.

208. James Braly, M.D., *Dr. Braly's Food Allergy & Nutrition Revolution*, Keat's Publishing, Inc., 1992.

209. Bernard Jensen, D.C., Ph.D., Sylvia Bell, *Tissue Cleansing Through Bowel Management*, Bernard Jensen, D.C., Ph.D., 1981.

210. Interview with Lee Cowden, M.D.

211. Michael T. Murray, N.D., "The Natural Approach to Rheumatoid Arthritis," *The American Journal of Natural Medicine*, Vol. 3, No. 1, IMPAKT Communications,   Green Bay, WI 54307-2496, January/February 1996, p. 8; Michael Murray, N.D., *Arthritis*, Prima Publishing, Rocklin, CA; Michael Murray, N.D. and Joseph Pizzorno, N.D., Bastyr College, Seattle, WA, *A Textbook of Natural Medicine*; *Encylopedia of Natural Medicine*.

212. Sir Gustav J.V. Nossal, "Life, Death and the Immune System," *Scientific American*, New York, NY, September 1993, p. 53.

213. Elizabeth Naugle, "Dear CDIF Friends," Candida & Dysbiosis Information Foundation publication, PO Drawer JF, College Station, TX, Vol. 2, #2, January 1996; Nolting, Siegfried, Bernd Guzek & Reinhard Hauss. *Mykosen des Verdauungstraktes*, Max Sieman KG, Hamburg, 1994; Markus, Harold & Hans Finck. *Candida, der entfesselte Hefepilz*, Ratgeber Ehrenwirth, 1995.

214. Carl Schleicher, "Application of Ultraviolet Blood Irradiation for Treatment of HIV and Other Bloodborne Viruses," *Townsend Letter for Doctors & Patients*, Port Townsend, Washington,   October 1995, p. 66.

215. Personal communication with Ronald M. Davis, M.D.

216. Personal communication with E. Denis Wilson, M.D.

217. William H. Philpott, M.D., *Amyloidosis*; *Health Strategies Self-Help Diagnostic and Therapeutic Strategies for Abudndant Health Life Styling*, Choctaw, OK 73020.

218. William H. Philpott, M.D., *Magnetic Brain Atherosclerosis, Brain Senility*

and *Alzheimer's Prophylaxis*, Choctaw, OK 73020.
219. Nancy Appleton, Ph.D., *Wellness and Body Chemistry*, Rudra Press, Portland Oregon.
220. "Interview With Dr. Nicholas Gonzalez," *Townsend Letter for Doctor & Patients*, February/March 1996, p. 136.
221. George Meinig, D.D.S., *Root Canal Cover-Up*, Bio Publishing, Ojai, California, 1994.
222. Personal letter and interview from Ann Staffanson.
223. "Arthritis," *Alternative Medicine Digest*, Issue 10, Future Medicine Publishing, Inc., Fife, Washington 98424, January 1996, p. 24.
224. *America Online*: Ofanim, 10/6/94.
225. Herbert E. Struss, "Immune Milk Treatment of Rheumatoid Arthritis -- Review," *Journal of Immune Milk*, Volume I, Number 2, December 1964, p. 23.
226. Marjorie Hurt Jones, R.N. interview with W.A. Shrader, Jr., M.D., "Enzyme Potentiated Desensitization (EPD)," *Mastering Food Allergies*, Vol. VIII, No. 3, July-August, 1993.
227. Kenneth Seaton, *Breaking the Devil's Circle*, U.S. Library of Congress, Reg. No. TX 2,826,455, Nov. 17, 1989.
228. Personal correspondence with James Braly, M.D.
229. Donald J. Brown, N.D., *Herbal Prescriptions for Better Health*, Prima Publishing, Prima Communications, Inc.
230. Peter Smrz, M.D., "Complementary Treatment of Post- and Parainfectious Rheumatoid Disorders," *Biological Therapy*, Vol. XIV, No. 1, 1996, p. 156.
231. Personal communication from George Meinig, D.D.S.
232. Karl-Heinz Ricken, M.D., "Chronic Polyarthritis and Other Immunological Diseases -- A Field for Antihomotoxic Therapy?, *Biologische Medizin*, Vol. III, 1995, P. 142-149.
233. Personal interview with Dr. Catherine Russell.
234. Information and studies provided by Lance Griffin, DNA Pacifica, 730 Summersong Lane, Encinitas, CA. Studies were conducted at several different sites following a model prepared by the San Diego Clinic, Chula Vista, CA 91912.
235. "A-Z Inventory of Popular Antifungal & Probiotic Remedies," Candida & Dysbiosis Information Foundation, PO Drawer JF, College Station, TX.
236. R. Myllykangas-Luosujarvi, "Diverticulosis -- A Primary Cause of Life-threatening Complications in Rheumatoid Arthritis," *Clinical and Experimental Rheumatology* 13: 1995, p. 79.
237. Susana Alcazar leyva, "Ribonuclease and Thiamine Pyrophosphate in The Treatment of Rheumatoid Arthritis," Bioquimia, VIII/42, p. 95, 1986; *Hypatia*, Investigaciones Filosoficas y Cientificas, S.A. de C.V. Abasolo Mexico, D.F.; Prof. Heberto Alcazar Montenegro; Dra. Susana Alcazar Leyva; Dra. rosa Maria Rivera Lopez; Dra. Maria Teresa Benitez Rodriguez, "Therapeutic Perspectives of Nucleases in Cancer," *Investigacion Medica Internacional* (1995) 22,8.
238. Phyllis Evelyn Pease, Ph.D., "L-Forms, Episomes and Auto-Immune Disease," E & S Livingstone Ltd., Edinburgh and London, 1965.
239. H. Hugh Fudenberg, Giancarlo Pizza, "Transfer Factor 1993: New Frontiers," *Progress in Drug Research*, Vol. 42, Birkhauser Verlag Basel (Switzerland), 1994.
240. Louis J. Marx, M.D., *Healing Dimensions of Herbal Medicine*, Neo-Paradigm Publishers, Ventura, CA.
241.Melissa Su, M.D., Richard S. Panush, M.D., "Antirheumatic Effects of Fasting," *IM*: Rheumatology, Vol. 12, No. 2, February 1991, p. 57.
242. Nutritional Research Bulletins, "Absorption of Quercetin," *American Journal of Natural Medicine*, Vol. 3, No. 2, March 1996, p. 15.
243. Jerome S. Mittelman, D.D.S. and Pat Connolly quotations from George

346 ANTHONY DI FABIO, M.A. & GUS J. PROSCH, JR., M.D

Meinig D.D.S. *Root Canal Cover-Up* literature.

244. Luc De Schepper, M.D., Ph.D., Lic.Ac., D.I.Hom., Homeopathy for Arthritics: Western Medicine or Homeopathy -- Which One is Real Science?" The Arthritis Fund/The Rheumatoid Disease Foundation.

245. Ida P. Rolf, Ph.D., Rolfing *The Integration of Human Structures*, Harper & Row Publishers, 1977.

246. Perry A. Chapdelaine, Sr., *How to Spot and Handle Suppression in Medicine: Identical Medical and Religious Patterns of Suppression in the Late Twentieth Century*, unpublished manuscript, Franklin, TN.

247. "Boswella," from Craig T. Kisciras.

248. "Natural Pharmacy," *Alternative Medicine Digest*, Issue 10.

249. Joel D. Wallach, D.V.M., N.D., Ma Lan, M.D., *Rare Earths: Forbidden Cures*, Double Happiness Publishing Co., Bonita, CA 91908.

250. Stratton, K., Howe, C., Battaglia S., eds., "Fetal Alcohol Syndrome Diagnosis, Epidemiology, Prevention, and Treatment," *Institute of Medicine*, Washington, D.C., National Academy Press, 1996.

251. Smuel Razin, "Mycoplasmas: The Smallest Pathogenic Procaryotes," *Ir. J. Med Sci* 17: 510-515, 1981.

252. D. Taylor-Robinson, "Mycoplasmal Arthritis in Man," *Ir. J. Med. Sci.*, 17, No. 7, July12981.

253. Personal letter from Adrienne Fowlie to Eleanor Chin, D.C.

254. Gregory S. Ellis, Ph.D., C.N.S., Allen M. Kratz, PharmD, "Homeovitic Clearing and Detox," *Alternative Health Practitioner*, Vol. 1, No. 3, Fall/Winter 1995.

255. Akil, M., Amos, R.S., Stewart, P., "Infertility May Sometimes Be associated with NSAID Consumption," *Br. J. Rheumatol* 34:76-8, 1996.

256. From *Townsend Letter for Doctors & Patients*, May 1996; reported from Dr. Chris Reading, "Relatives; Schizophrenia & Rheumatoid Arthritis; Including Nutritional Interventions," *Well Mind Association Newsletter*, March 1995.

257. Pi-kwang Tsung, Ph.D., Hong-yen Hsu, Ph.D., *Arthritis and Chinese Herbal Medicine*, Keats Publishing, Inc.

258. William Campbell Douglass, M.D., Courtesy of *Second Opinion* newsletter.

259. Julian Whitaker, M.D., *Health & Healing*, Vol. 5, No. 10, October 1995.

260. "Gaby's Literature Review," Alan Gaby, M.D., *Townsend Letter for Doctors & Patients*, November 1996, p. 30.

261. Personal interview with Lee Cowden, M.D.

262. Kathleen Facklemann, "Gastrointestinal Blues," *Science News*, Vol. 150, November 9, 1996, p. 302.

263. Harold E. Buttram, M.D., Richard Piccola, M.H.A., *Our Toxic World: Who is Looking After Our Kids?* Foresight/America Foundation for Preconception Care, Quakertown, PA.

264. Adeena Robinson, Iron: *A Double Edged Sword*, Informasearch, 1995.

265. Ross Anderson, N.D., D.C., "Parasites," *Health Freedom News*, March/April 1997, p. 28.

266. William Campbell Douglass, M.D., *Second Opinion*, March 1997, p. 8.

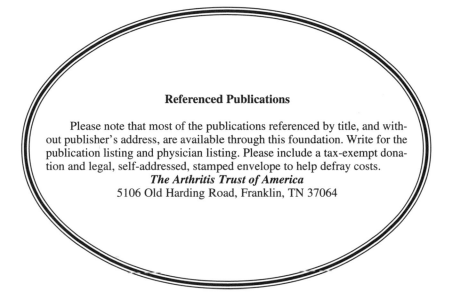

Referenced Publications

Please note that most of the publications referenced by title, and without publisher's address, are available through this foundation. Write for the publication listing and physician listing. Please include a tax-exempt donation and legal, self-addressed, stamped envelope to help defray costs.
The Arthritis Trust of America
5106 Old Harding Road, Franklin, TN 37064